Crime, Mental Health and th System in Afr

C000257384

"For a long time, African historiography has been viewed and interpreted from Eurocentric perspectives. This book is a timely contribution towards infusing Afrocentric perspectives in African scholarship by indigenous scholars. The authors' interdisciplinary topical approach, covering a gamut of topics ranging from African criminology, through mental health and psychology, to criminal justice systems, has lent a decolonizing voice toward African literary pursuit and thereby laid a solid foundation for further research by other scholars. I highly recommend it to readers, academic institutions and researchers on Africa."
—Emmanuel Onyeozili, PhD, *Professor of Criminology and Criminal Justice, Department of Criminal Justice, University of Maryland Eastern Shore, USA*

"This edited volume by an array of experts from West and Southern Africa has given a refreshing voice to psycho-criminological narratives in the continent. In a region of the world in which there is insufficient documentation of the patterns, determinants and outcomes of criminal behaviour, this book offers a culturally competent and contemporary flavour to an ancient discourse. Its focus on new areas of concern such as online dating scams, kidnapping and the mental health of officials in the criminal justice system compellingly captures the potential reader and gives good value for time. It is warmly recommended for its breadth of coverage, the authority of its claims and the multi-disciplinary outlook of its authors."
—Adegboyega Ogunwale, MBBS, FWACP, Consultant Psychiatrist, *Forensic Unit, Neuropsychiatric Hospital, Aro, Ogun State, Nigeria*

"This collection represents a significant step in the study of mental health, crime and criminal justice in sub-Saharan Africa. The breadth of topics covered is impressive, with each contribution based on methodologically-sound empirical analyses. It deserves to become a key reference for students, researchers and policy makers interested in suicide, drug use, violence, the work of prison officers, criminal investigations, and police-community interactions."
—Justice Tankebe, PhD, Lecturer, *Institute of Criminology, University of Cambridge, UK*

"Mental health and criminal justice issues are growing problems facing the world today. Questions about whether mental health affects crime or whether involvement in the criminal justice system affects an individual's health have become part of national policy discussion. This nicely written book brings together eminent scholars and experts with extensive experience in their various fields to address these and other questions related to crime, mental health, and criminal justice in Africa. The editors did well to coordinate the efforts of the contributors into a valuable pierce. I highly recommend it for all who are interested in the nexus between crime, mental health, and criminal justice systems."

—Francis D. Boateng, PhD, *Assistant Professor, Department of Criminal Justice and Legal Studies, University of Mississippi, USA*

Heng Choon (Oliver) Chan
Samuel Adjorlolo
Editors

Crime, Mental Health and the Criminal Justice System in Africa

A Psycho-Criminological Perspective

palgrave
macmillan

Editors
Heng Choon (Oliver) Chan
Teaching Laboratory for Forensics and
Criminology, Department of Social and
Behavioural Sciences
City University of Hong Kong
Hong Kong, Special Administrative Region
of China

Samuel Adjorlolo
Department of Mental Health Nursing
School of Nursing and Midwifery
University of Ghana
Accra, Ghana

ISBN 978-3-030-71026-2   ISBN 978-3-030-71024-8   (eBook)
https://doi.org/10.1007/978-3-030-71024-8

This Palgrave Macmillan imprint is published by the registered company Springer Nature Switzerland AG.
The registered company address is: Gewerbestrasse 11, 6330 Cham, Switzerland

To the Chan Family:
With deep appreciation for your unconditional love, endless support, and encouragement.
In loving memory of my mother.
Heng Choon (Oliver) Chan, Ph.D.

I dedicate this book to my lovely children: Sheena K. Adjorlolo, Samuel Adjorlolo Junior, and Gwendolyn E. Adjorlolo.
Samuel Adjorlolo, Ph.D.

Foreword: Towards the Decolonisation of the Epistemic Violence of Psychology and Criminology

This book is a reminder to criminologists and psychologists, if they need reminding, that correlation is not causation. Just because some offenders have been diagnosed as having mental illness, it does not follow that all those who are mentally ill are offenders nor does it mean that people who are sane are never guilty of crimes. The increasing knowledge-power axes of psychology-criminology call for the need to decolonise both disciplines and expose their key roles in the colonisation and criminalisation of Africans, other indigenous peoples, and the global working class around the world by European conquerors and their allies.

Prior to the enslavement and later the colonisation of Africans by Europeans, there were neither asylums nor prisons anywhere in Africa. None of the monuments built by ancient Africans thousands of years earlier was designed for the control of others by people in authority. All that changed with the emergence of the capitalist mode of production which operates by alienating the fruits of labour from the workers who provide labour power, according to Marx. The worst forms of such alien-ation were enslavement and colonisation by which the powerful claimed to own the workers and the fruits of their labour with violence deployed as the means for subjugation, exploitation and alienation.

The picture painted by Marx about the double alienation of the colo-niser and the colonised through the turning of human beings and natural resources into nothing but the means for private accumulation of profits by capitalist exploiters was supported by Frantz Fanon in *The Wretched of the Earth*. According to Fanon, both the coloniser who tortures the colonised and the tortured victims of colonial oppression tend to become mentally ill. The torturer went home to torture his wife and children, while the tortured went home after release to grab a knife and run amok down the street screaming that he was going to kill someone before being mowed down by the coloniser's machine gun. As a psychiatrist-activist who was opposed to colonial violence, Fanon was offering a description or explanation of violence and not a prescription or recommendation, contrary to popular misreadings of his work. The colonisers used psychology and criminology as technologies to demonise the decolonisation militants but Fanon reminds us that the activists were sane and their activism completely understandable as resistance against violent oppression.

The difficulty for Africa is that decolonisation remains an unfinished project given that neocolonialism came to replace colonialism as the last stage of imperialism, according to Kwame Nkrumah. This book is a reminder that decades after the regaining of flag independence and the end of apartheid, violent crimes abound in Africa and the rest of the world. The authors try to explain that it is misleading to assume that mental illness is responsible for the epidemic of violence across the world. Instead, the authors call for the criminalisation of suicide by the law that was imposed by colonisers to be decolonised and treated as a symptom of mental illness towards penal abolitionism. The violent crimes in Africa do not suggest that Africans are crazy either, they indicate that the capitalist system imposed on Africa by colonisers remains a dog-eats-dog system of plunder and domination through ruthless exploitation for primitive accumulation, white supremacy and patriarchal domination.

Michel Foucault wrote *Madness and Civilization* to argue that even Europeans did not discover madness until the age of the Enlightenment in the eighteenth century. Prior to that discovery of the repressive fetishes of modernity, mental illness was handled in the community by families that cared for those who were depressed or unwell. But with the rise of the concentration of production in capitalist factories, there also arose the industrialisation of healthcare, criminal justice and psychiatry in the prison-industrial complex. The aim was to increase the power of the dominant groups who claimed to be knowledgeable about how to control other people instead of being the result of humanitarian will to care. Unfortunately, Foucault remained silent about colonialism and the decolonisation movement in Africa. As a result, Edward Said, in *Culture and Imperialism*, dismissed Foucault and Jurgen Habermas and recommended Fanon as the theorist best able to offer a theory of decolonisation for the benefit of Africa. With *Medical Power in Prisons*, Joe Sims forced the UK government to integrate the prison healthcare system with the National Health Service because medical power in prison was not designed to heal the sick but to keep them alive to be punished.

Foucault was probably misled by the emphasis of Sigmund Freud on sexual desires as the main cause of violence and mental illness. According to Freud, incest taboos are more strictly enforced by 'neurotic' Africans and other indigenous peoples than by 'normal' Europeans. Foucault went on to analyse the history of sexuality and concluded that although Freud was wrong on the prohibition hypothesis given the preponderance of sexual images in literature and the arts, Freud had a point in the suggestion that a micro-physics of power operates to enable individuals to exercise control over their own bodies and minds while allowing the state to individualise the social control of deviance. If Foucault had tested his theory against the evidence of colonialism and imperialism the way that Fanon did, he would have realised that it is a macro-physics and not a micro-physics of power that was in operation, guided by the profit motive, sexism and white supremacy, and not driven primarily by sexual desires as such.

Unlike Freud, Emile Durkheim argued that suicide was a normal social fact sui generis in the sense that it could be explained by reference to social factors and not by atomisation through psychological or biological explanations. According to Durkheim, suicide tends to increase as a result of anomie in modern societies where what is expected is often not consistent with what is experienced in rapidly changing capitalist societies. To him, the goal of social control is not to eliminate deviance completely but to keep the energy of the collective conscience at a moderate level to avoid a permissive society where anything goes or a strict society that allows no innovation to take place. Durkheim erred by assuming that the dominant ideas represented the collective conscience of society, whereas the racist-sexist-imperialist apartheid rulers in Africa did not represent the collective conscience of the African-working-class-female majority.

Most Africans will disagree with Durkheim about the normality of deviance and insist that deviance is neither normal nor necessary for the survival of society. For instance, Chinua Achebe suggested in *Things Fall Apart* that among precolonial Igbo in present-day Nigeria, suicide was regarded as an abomination and the corpse was treated as a carcass instead of being given a befitting burial. If deviance was normal, then there would be no counselling for people who were depressed the way that the uncle of Okonkwo, Uchendu, counselled him not to be depressed just because he was forced to go into exile among his mother's kindred after he committed manslaughter of a child (no capital punishment or imprisonment). Okonkwo recovered enough to rebuild his wealth in exile through farming but he was probably still mentally ill for he returned and promptly killed an African messenger from the European colonisers, but when his kinsmen did not join him in going mad at the same time, he went off and hanged himself like a dog, falsely thinking that he was the only man left in Umuofia. In *There Was A Country*, Achebe also narrated his experience in elementary school when the village mad man walked into his class under a breadfruit tree and took the chalk from the teacher, who was discussing the geography of Britain, and instead started teaching the more relevant history of their village of Ogidi. The teacher and the students quietly allowed him to have his say and leave instead of calling the police to arrest him and detain him in an asylum as would have been the case in Europe. Buchi Emecheta suggested in *Kehinde* that women who heard voices were known as visionary people capable of foreseeing the future instead of being banged up in psychiatric wards the way the UK government did to predominantly black inmates diagnosed with mental illness. Following the publication of Emecheta's novel, the UK government closed the mental hospitals presumably to save money and released the women back into the community but none of them went on to kill anyone or to commit suicide or serious self-harm.

This book encourages Africans to continue seeking ways to reduce the increasing rates of incarceration, detention, medicalisation, suicide, violent crimes, sexual offences, corruption and armed violence across Africa instead of regarding them as normal or regarding them as signs of mental illness to be cured with pills manufactured by European pharmaceutical capitalist firms or with incarceration. The contribution of the book to knowledge is that by listening to African scholars in criminology and psychology, the world could develop new ways to reduce the violence that plagues the entire world while psychiatric practices and criminal justice institutions remain some of the most violent institutions rather than being the panacea for alienation or mental illness.

As Thomas Merton observed, the vast majority of those who are mentally ill do not commit any violent crimes and most of the violent criminals who commit genocide are actually sane or normal. The policy implication of the book is that Africans should consider the decolonisation of both the criminal justice system and the psychiatric powers, imposed by European colonisers, through the renewal of the African philosophy of non-violence, called Ubuntu by Desmond Tutu, or Mbari by Chinua Achebe, to enable us to treat deviance in the community the way that our ancestors did for thousands of years in more humane societies before contact with capitalist exploitation, oppression, humiliation and dehumanisation through imperialist knowledge-power axes of violence.

Blacksburg, VA, USA   Biko Agozino
Biko Agozino is a Professor of Sociology
and Africana Studies at Virginia Tech.

Contents

Contents xv

Notes on Editors and Contributors

Notes on Editors

Heng Choon (Oliver) Chan is Associate Professor of Criminology at City University of Hong Kong (CityU), Hong Kong, SAR. He received his PhD in Criminology from the University of South Florida, USA. Over the years, Dr. Chan has been awarded a number of awards to recognize his outstanding research performance and contributions to professional education, namely "Outstanding Criminology Ambassador Award" (2012, Department of Criminology, University of South Florida [USF]), "Early Career Award" (2014, Hong Kong Research Grants Council of University Grant Committee), "The President's Award" (2017, The President's Office, CityU), "CLASS New Researcher Award" (2017, College of Liberal Arts and Social Sciences [CLASS], CityU), "The Outstanding Supervisor Award" (2018, Office of the Provost, CityU), "CLASS Teaching Innovation Award—Team Award" (2019, CLASS, CityU), and more recently "Distinguished Alumni Award" (2021, Department of Criminology, USF).

Dr. Chan's research focuses on sexual homicide, offender profiling, sex offending, homicide, stalking behavior, and Asian criminology. As of January 2021, he has published over 90 peer-reviewed journal articles and book chapters and presented at numerous international, regional, and local academic conferences. Dr. Chan has since published four academic books, with two as the sole-authored monographs on sexual homicide (Palgrave Macmillan, April 2015; and Springer Nature, June 2019) and another two as a co-editor of edited collections on the psycho-criminological approach to Asian criminal justice (i.e., police, correctional, and legal psychology; Routledge, March 2017) and the international perspective of stalking behavior (John Wiley & Sons, April 2020). His book on the stalking behavior was awarded the CHOICE Outstanding Academic Title 2020 by the Association of College and Research Libraries of American Library Association, USA.

Dr. Chan is the senior editor of *Cogent Social Sciences* (criminology and criminal justice section), associate editor of *Frontiers in Psychology* (forensic and legal psychology specialty section), *International Journal of Offender Therapy and Comparative Criminology*, and *Heliyon Psychology* (expertise on forensic psychology and criminology). He also sits on the editorial advisory board of *Journal of Criminal Justice*, editorial board of *Sexual Abuse: A Journal of Research and Treatment*, and several more. Besides, he is an ad-hoc reviewer for over 80 peer-reviewed journals and academic publishers in the disciplines of criminology, psychology, psychiatry, forensic sciences, sociology, law, and other behavioral and social sciences. Dr. Chan has also been regularly interviewed by electronic media and quoted in print media on criminological issues; and consulted on the offending behavior of violent offenders by television program scriptwriters and movie producers.

Samuel Adjorlolo is a senior lecturer and head of Department of Mental Health Nursing, School of Nursing and Midwifery, University of Ghana. Dr. Adjorlolo holds a Ph.D. in Applied Social Sciences from the City University of Hong Kong where he received several honors and awards, including the prestigious Chow Yei Ching School of Graduate Studies Scholarship. Prior to this, he graduated from the University of Ghana where he received bachelor's and master's degrees in Nursing and Psychology and Clinical Psychology, respectively. He also received a

Master of Science degree in telemedicine and e-health from the UiT-Arctic University of Norway under the Norwegian Quota Scholarship Scheme. Dr. Adjorlolo's research focuses on mental health, including forensic mental health, child and adolescent mental health, and maternal mental health. He has published his scholarly works in peer-reviewed journals and as book chapters numbering over 30.

Dr. Adjorlolo is also a recipient of Early Career Research grant under the Queen Elizabeth Scholars-Advanced Program, a partnership program between University of Ghana (Ghana) and University of Alberta (Canada). He is a fellow of the Research Integrity program organized jointly by the University of Ghana (Ghana) and NYU Grossman School of Medicine (USA), with funding from Fogarty and National Institute of Health (NIH). He is the editor of *Cogent Social Sciences*, guest editor of *Frontiers in Psychology* (forensic and legal psychology specialty section) and *International Journal of Environmental Research and Public Health*, editorial board member of *Forensic Science International: Mind and Law*, and an ad-hoc reviewer for over 15 peer-reviewed journals and academic publishers. Dr. Adjorlolo is a board member of Anderson Care International (USA) and Executive Director of the Research and Grant Institute (REGIG), a non-governmental organization dedicated to research generation, dissemination, and utilization in Ghana. He has been regularly interviewed by major media houses in Ghana, including TV3 and GBC on mental health issues.

Notes on Contributors

Richard A. Aborisade is a reader in criminology and victimology at the Department of Sociology, Faculty of Social Sciences, Olabisi Onabanjo University, Ago-Iwoye, Ogun State. He received his doctorate from the University of Ibadan, Nigeria. He also holds an MBA in Information Technology from Coventry University, United Kingdom. He has published in both local and international journals in the areas of security management, criminal justice, criminology, victimology, and penology. His most recent works include *The Essentials of Sociology* (co-edited) and *Crime and Delinquency: A Sociological Introduction*, both published by Ibadan University Press.

Akosua A. Adu-Poku has an MPhil in Sociology at the Department of Sociology, University of Ghana, Legon. Her research interest spans across social justice, corruption, and gender and violence. She is currently conducting a doctoral research that focuses on the consequences of imprisonment for prisoners, families and children in Ghana.

Oluwagbenga Michael Akinlabi is a senior lecturer in criminology and criminal justice at Northumbria University in Newcastle, United Kingdom. He holds a PhD in Criminology and Criminal Justice from Griffith University in Australia. He was previously educated in his home country Nigeria, as well as at Cambridge University in the United Kingdom. Michael's research interests include procedural justice and police legitimacy, policing the global south, police use of force, corruption and accountability, policing youths and BAME, crime and psychopathology, and stress in police. Specifically, his current research has been exploring how perceptions of justice and fairness, corruption, and feelings of trust can go a long way to influence compliance and/or cynicism towards the law.

Thomas Akoensi holds an MPhil and PhD in Criminology from the University of Cambridge, United Kingdom, and BA in Psychology from the University of Ghana, Legon. He is currently a senior lecturer in criminology and criminal justice at the University of Kent, United Kingdom. His interests lie in penology more broadly, offender rehabilitation, prison officer culture and legitimacy in criminal justice contexts. His current project involves informal social control in informal urban settlements in Accra, Ghana (with funding from the British Academy); a longitudinal study of prison officer culture in Ghana; criminal record and employment opportunities in Ghana; the impact of COVID-19 on the work of prison officers and a study of desistance among prisoners in Ghana (with funding from the Faculty of Social Sciences, University of Kent).

Johnny Andoh-Arthur is a lecturer at the Department of Psychology, University of Ghana. His research and academic interests focus on mental and sexual/reproductive health (among men and young persons), suicide, and suicide prevention. He publishes and reviews papers in these areas for some top journals in the field. He currently serves on the editorial board for *BMC Public Health*, *Journal of Crisis Intervention and Suicide Prevention*, and *Death Studies*. He is a research fellow with the Center for Suicide and Violence Research (CSVR), Ghana.

Maria-Goretti Ane is a legal practitioner and a member of the Drug Policy Network Ghana. Maria-Goretti is an advocate for drug policy reform in Africa. As an author of a number of articles on drug use and harm reduction, she also has special interests in human rights, and drug policy reforms.

Sylvester Anthony Appiah-Honny is a trained paralegal certified by the United State Department in Ghana, and also holds a BA in Psychology from the University of Ghana. As a top management member of the POS Foundation, he provides supervision and manages activities of the organisation in the design and implementation of projects and activities, namely the Justice for All Programme, Non-Custodial Sentencing/Community Service Bill and assists in the coordination of the In-Prison Paralegal Programme, and the UN Universal Periodic Review. Sylvester is committed and passionate about the promotion of the rights of the minority in Ghana's criminal justice sector.

Mary Eyram Ashinyo is a physician specialist in public health with a background in health policy planning/management, drug policies, and quality management. She has six years working experience with the West African Drug Policy Network, now Drug Policy Network Ghana, and volunteered in Ghana's Prisons providing health care services.

Nontyatyambo Pearl Dastile is an associate professor and chair of department at the University of South Africa. She specialises in de-coloniality, gender and crime, assessment of offenders, African-centred approaches. She has taught in numerous universities throughout South Africa.

Timothy Pritchard Debrah is a registered psychiatric nurse by profession, currently working on secondment with the University of Cape Coast, as a clinical preceptor with the Department of Mental Health. He is the current focal point for Drug Policy Network Ghana. His focus is to see the youth empowered to push for drug policy reforms.

Moses Onyemaech Ede is a lecturer in the Department of Educational Foundations (Guidance and Counselling Unit), University of Nigeria. Dr Ede has published a record number of papers in peer-reviewed journals and similar outlets in the areas of human development, stress management, cognitive behavioural therapy, depression, occupational health, autism, anxiety, gambling, procrastination, rational emotive family therapy, and others. Dr Ede belongs to a number of professional organisations in the field such as Counselling Association of Nigeria (CASSON) and Nigerian Council of Educational Psychologists (NCEP).

Chiedu Eseadi is a lecturer in the Department of Educational Foundations, University of Nigeria. He serves as an editorial board member for some international peer-reviewed impact factor journals including *BMC Public Health* and *Medicine (Baltimore)*. He has published more than sixty peer-reviewed articles in both national and international journals. His research cuts across a wide array of counselling specialty including but not limited to prison counselling, mental health counselling, career counselling, stress, and burnout.

Johan van Graan served 16 years in the South African Police Service. He resigned from the police with a collection of commendations in the covert investigation of high-profile national and international crime investigations. He is currently a professor in the School of Criminal Justice at the University of South Africa. His research interests in the fields of crime reduction and prevention, community—and intelligence-led policing is being realised through dedicating his career to the study, research, and teaching in these dynamic fields. He actively contributes to his profession through professional memberships, publishing of journal articles, authoring of books and book chapters, and presenting of papers at national and international forums. Johan is currently an editorial board member of the accredited journal *Child Abuse Research: A South African Journal*, a national council member and criminology representative of the South African Professional Society on the Abuse of Children, and a member of the Criminological Society of Africa.

Samuel Cudjoe Hanu is an addiction specialist and currently works as the head of research with the Mental Health Authority, Accra, Ghana. He was a former Hubert H. Humphrey Fellow at Virginia Commonwealth University, United States; founder of –Harm Reduction Alliance, Ghana; a member of Drug Policy Network Ghana; and a fellow at WACON and GCNM. He is an advocate for decriminalisation of substance use.

Charlotte Omane Kwakye-Nuako is a trained clinical psychologist and a lawyer. She holds a PhD in Psychology from the University of Ghana, and was called to the Ghanaian Bar in 2013. She currently teaches psychology and law-related courses at the Department of Forensic Science, University of Cape Coast after a 16-year position with Methodist University College Ghana. In terms of legal practice, she joined ADU-KUSI, PRUC (formerly Law Bureau) after her pupilage at the Attorney General's Department and has been practising on adjunct basis with the firm. She boasts of being the best student in Family Law and Practice for the 2013 cohort of lawyers. Also, in 2017 she was a Fox Fellow at Yale University for a year. Additionally, she was a researcher in the Forgiveness in West Africa Project. She has published widely, and her long-term goal is to develop herself as a distinguished lawyer and legal psychologist.

Gérard Labuschagne was the commander of the South African Police Service's (SAPS) specialised Investigative Psychology Section and held the rank of Brigadier for 14 years. This section provides offender profiling services primarily focusing on serial crimes. He has been involved in over 110 serial murder investigations in South Africa and neighbouring countries. He has provided training to local and foreign law enforcement in serial investigation, and is published widely in academic literature on serial murder. He is a clinical psychologist, and Advocate of the High Court in South Africa, a SAPS-trained hostage negotiator, and a Los Angeles Sheriff's Department–trained homicide and death investigator. He is an honorary associate professor in the Department of Forensic Medicine and Pathology at the University of the Witwatersrand. He is a certified threat manager with the US Association of Threat Assessment Professionals and founder president of the African Association of Threat Assessment Professionals.

Chiamaobi Samuel Ogbonna is a graduate student at Department of Arts Education (Educational Technology unit), University of Nigeria,

Nsukka. Apart from his research interest spanning educational psychological interventions, instructional designing, educational digital technologies and educational media evaluation, he has a growing interest in online safety education.

Ifeoma E. Okoye is an assistant professor in the Department of Criminal Justice, Virginia State University (VSU), United States. She has interdisciplinary degrees in administration of justice/criminal justice, law, business administration and social sciences. She holds a PhD in Administration of Justice from Texas Southern University, United States. Her teaching and research interests revolve around quantitative analysis, idiographic and nomothetic research, innovative research methodologies, homeland security, terrorism and counterterrorism, legal aspects of criminal justice, criminological theories, and security studies. She has written and made several presentations on terrorism and contemporary approaches to countering terrorism. Among her published works, she authored *The Theoretical and Conceptual Understanding of Terrorism*; *Trends in Terrorism Incidents in Nigeria and the United States: Analysis of Data from 1980—2013*; and co-authored, *The Use and Abuse of Police Power in America: Historical Milestones and Current Controversies*; *Restorative Justice: Psychosocial Needs of Offenders, and Implications for Safety and Security*; and *The War on Terrorism in Africa: Human Rights Issues, Implications and Recommendations*.

Alaba M. Oludare is a licensed attorney in New York, and she holds a PhD in Administration of Justice from Texas Southern University. She also holds a master's degree in Tax Law from the University of Alabama, Tuscaloosa, as well as professional law degrees from Lagos State University and Nigerian Law School. Dr Oludare has worked with underserved population of first-generation college students and communities to improve the quality of life through research, service. and teaching. Her research interests include legal aspects of crime, crime prevention and administration of social control programmes and policies, domestic violence, cybercrimes, and terrorism including kidnapping and law enforcement.

Mkpoikanke Sunday Otu is a lecturer, counsellor, and researcher in the Department of Educational Foundations, and Institute of Education,

University of Nigeria, Nsukka. Mr Otu has published over 60 peer-reviewed research articles in many reputable Nigerian and international journals, including those with impact factor. He has contributed to academic textbooks. He serves as resource personnel and facilitator in training, seminars, workshops, symposiums, and conferences. He is a member of many professional associations, including Counselling Association of Nigeria (CASSON) and the American Psychology Association (APA).

Jonathan Osei Owusu is the founder and executive director of the POS Foundation, a human rights civil society organisation which has its core activities centred on human rights advocacy and has access to justice, policy reforms, youth development, and research. With over 15 years of experience in the field of advocacy, Jonathan is currently the facilitator of the renowned Justice For All Program, focal person for the UN Universal Periodic Review (UPR) NGOs platform in Ghana, Human Rights Defenders Network–Ghana, and the vice-chairman of the Ghana Human Rights NGOs Forum.

Feikoab Parimah is a psychologist and the director for Basic Research, Advocacy, and Initiative Networks. He has served as the lead researcher for West Africa Drug Policy Network, Ghana, and POS foundation on some key projects on drug policy reform and non-custodial sentencing in Ghana. As a writing and statistical coach in the Division for Postgraduate Studies, University of the Western Cape, Feikoab assists both PhD and master's students with their writing and statistical difficulties. Being a budding scholar, his research interests cover the broad areas of criminology, forensic psychology, and addiction.

Emmanuel Nii-Boye Quarshie is with the University of Leeds, United Kingdom, as a visiting research fellow in the School of Psychology. He is also a research fellow at the Centre for Suicide and Violence Research (CSVR), Ghana, and a visiting scholar in the Department of Psychology, University of Ghana, Accra, where he collaborates with faculty in the School of Social Sciences to research suicidal behaviour and suicide prevention. His research foci are self-harm and suicide prevention, child and adolescent mental health, and sexual and interpersonal violence prevention in resource-poor contexts.

Magdaleen Swanepoel holds the following qualifications: LLB (UP), LLM (Cum Laude) (UP); and LLD (Unisa). She started her law career in 2005 when she joined the University of Pretoria to complete her LLM and work as an associate. In 2007, she was appointed at Unisa as a senior lecturer. She completed her doctoral degree and was promoted to associate professor. She teaches undergraduate students as well as postgraduate students. In 2013, she was appointed as the legal representative to the Mental Health Review Board of Gauteng. She assisted in many enquiries where she had to assure that the patient's rights were protected. Prof. Swanepoel is still working at Unisa.

Lucy K. Tsado holds a bachelor's degree in Accounting. She holds a master's degree in Management Information Systems and a PhD in Administration of Justice from Texas Southern University in Houston, Texas. She is currently an assistant professor in the Department of Sociology, Social Work and Criminal Justice at Lamar University, Beaumont, Texas. She teaches corrections, class, race, gender, and crime, cybersecurity and digital forensics to undergraduates, criminal justice policy, criminal justice planning and evaluation, and cybercrime. Her research interests include re-entry programs with evidence-based practices leading to lower recidivism rates. Her other research interests focus on the cybersecurity skills gap and the pipeline deficiency that has developed as a result. Consequently, she is interested in educational and professional development opportunities that are available to students as a result of the cybersecurity skills gap.

List of Tables

1

Introduction: Exploring Crime, Mental Health, and Criminal Justice in Africa from a Psycho-Criminological Perspective

Heng Choon (Oliver) Chan and Samuel Adjorlolo

Introduction

A large majority of African countries were previously colonised by Britain, namely Gambia, Ghana, Nigeria, Southern Cameroon, and Sierra Leone in British West Africa; Kenya, Uganda, and Tanzania in British East Africa; and Malawi, Lesotho, Botswana, South Africa, Swaziland, Zambia, and Zimbabwe in British South Africa. As former British

H. C. O. Chan (✉)
Teaching Laboratory for Forensics and Criminology, Department of Social and Behavioural Sciences, City University of Hong Kong, Hong Kong, Special Administrative Region of China
e-mail: oliverchan.ss@cityu.edu.hk

S. Adjorlolo
Department of Mental Health Nursing, School of Nursing and Midwifery, University of Ghana, Accra, Ghana
e-mail: sadjorlolo@ug.edu.gh

© The Author(s), under exclusive license to Springer Nature Switzerland AG 2021
H. C. O. Chan, S. Adjorlolo (eds.), *Crime, Mental Health and the Criminal Justice System in Africa*, https://doi.org/10.1007/978-3-030-71024-8_1

1

colonies, many of these African countries are melting pots of native cultures with a substantial Western influence. As in many former British colonies, the criminal justice system in African countries is patterned after the British common law system, where the rule of law and due process is heavily emphasised. Nonetheless, revisions and amendments have been made to some legislation in the statutes of these countries since they became independent from Britain. Critical to the judicial system, especially in the sentencing process, are reports of defendants' mental states at the time of their offence. The evaluation report, which involves a mental state examination alongside collateral sources of information (e.g., risk assessment), is important for the court in making the final disposition (Adjorlolo & Chan, 2019; Adjorlolo, Chan, & Agboli, 2016).

Traditionally, criminological scholarship has been Western-centric. Some critics have contended that criminology has been dominated by white men, particularly from the United States and the United Kingdom, who have authored the most widely published and cited criminological studies (Cohn, Farrington, & Iratzoqui, 2017; Moosavi, 2019). In recent decades, movements to 'decolonise' criminology from its Western-centricity have been initiated by advocates for a 'new criminological imagination from the periphery' (Fraser, Lee, & Tang, 2017, p. 134). This movement has resulted in the development of Asian criminology (Liu, 2009) and Southern criminology (Carrington, Sozzo, & Hogg, 2016). The decolonisation and democratisation of criminology have also been observed in the African context, with the development of African criminology (Agozino, 2010). Oriola (2006) asserted that African criminology or, more precisely, post-colonial criminology, is not exclusively for Africans but rather for the entire world insofar as it aims to shy away from the punitively oriented European criminology. Simply put, these new approaches aim to de-prioritise Western concerns and place more stress on non-Western knowledge and experiences that are more relevant to specific cultures or regions. Although the African criminology movement shows promise, there is still a lack of scholarship emerging from this geographical region. Hence, the primary purpose of this edited volume is to advance knowledge by presenting up-to-date findings from research conducted among different populations within this geographical region.

The Approach Adopted in this Book

Over the years, many approaches have been proposed to study and explain crime and criminal behaviour. Many of these were put forward long before criminology emerged as a distinct academic discipline. Criminology, in the past, was often conducted within the discipline of sociology. This is similar to psychology, which also grew out of other disciplines, such as philosophy, physiology, and medicine (Hollin, 2013). As a result, most traditional (and mainstream) criminological theories are sociological in orientation. However, it is noteworthy that 'psychology and criminology emerged as distinct disciplines at a very similar historic moment—the latter half of the nineteenth century' (Hayward, 2005, p. 110).

Psychology, in a broad sense, is the scientific study of behaviour and mental processes, whereas criminology is generally regarded as the scientific study of crime and criminals. As the convergence of psychology and criminology, psycho-criminology is thus concerned with the use of psychological knowledge and skills to explain and describe (with the aim of modifying) deviant and criminal behaviour (Chan & Ho, 2017; Chan & Sheridan, 2020; Hollin, 2012). According to Bartol (2002), this sub-discipline aims to study individual offending behaviour, with attention to how the behaviour is acquired, evoked, maintained, and modified, by examining personality and social influences. In addition to taking societal influences into account, psychological criminology applies psychological theories and concepts to better explain crime, criminals, and their criminal behaviour. Psychological criminology basically addresses the question: 'What is it about the individuals and their experiences that cause them to commit crime and/or to become criminal?' (Wortley, 2011, p. 1).

This psycho-criminological approach to understanding crime and criminality is especially relevant to the focus of this edited volume. In this book, we explore different aspects and dynamics of crime, criminals and their mental health status, and the criminal justice system in the African region through a psycho-criminological lens. A highlight of this edited collection is the range of contributions to the comprehensive study of a variety of deviant and criminal behaviour and of different branches of the criminal justice system, with emphases on the Ghanaian, South African, and Nigerian contexts.

The Structure of the Book

This edited collection is written by researchers and experienced field practitioners from the African countries of Ghana, South Africa, and Nigeria. Adopting a combined theory-and practice-oriented approach, this collection attempts to introduce readers to contemporary research on deviant and criminal behaviour, mental health issues, and the criminal justice system in African countries. Written by experienced researchers and field practitioners, this book is arguably among the first to discuss different topics on African criminology and mental health studies using a psycho-criminological approach.

There are a total of 17 chapters, including this introduction and a concluding chapter. The nine chapters in the first section focus on deviance, crime, and mental health in Africa. Following this introduction, in Chap. 2, Aborisade performs a meticulous review of the existing literature on suicide, suicidal ideation, and suicidal behaviour among African youths using a multifactorial and multidisciplinary approach. Among other issues, theories of suicide proposed in different disciplines, namely sociology, psychology, mental health, and criminology, are explained. The chapter concludes with a suggested approach to addressing the problem of African youth suicide by decriminalising suicidal behaviour, along with suggestions on policies for preventive frameworks and control. In Chap. 3, van Graan first provides a brief historical background and insight into violence and crime in South Africa and follows this with a review of the nature and extent of violent crime in South Africa. A number of risk factors for crime victimisation and violence in South Africa are described. The strength of this chapter is its presentation of South Africans' perceptions and experiences of crime and violence through the narratives of the victims behind the statistics of violent crime victimisation. Chapter 4, written by Eseadi and colleagues, presents a review of contemporary online dating and romance scam issues in Africa. The authors explore the relevant concepts and platforms of online dating and romance scams, commonly observed mental health issues experienced by the victims, and tricks frequently adopted by the perpetrators of online dating and romance scams. The chapter concludes with suggestions on strategies for tackling online dating and romance scams and recommendations for future research and policy development or refinement.

In Chap. 5, Oludare and colleagues examine the crime of kidnapping in Nigeria and other countries by presenting a general understanding of kidnapping in present-day Nigeria, drawing on the rational choice and strain theoretical frameworks. The psychological aspects of this crime are explored, along with the strategies adopted by the Nigerian authorities for tackling this type of offense. Labuschagne, in Chap. 6, writes on serial murder and its investigation in South Africa. The author first reviews the existing research on South African serial murders, with an emphasis on a series of pioneer reviews of over 170 cases of serial murder identified by the South African Police Service (SAPS) since the mid-1990s. The chapter concludes with case studies to illustrate the strategies used by the SAPS in investigating these cases. Chapter 7, written by Swanepoel, primarily focuses on the constitutional position and domestic legislation in the context of the Mental Health Care Law in South Africa. This chapter introduces this act in detail, with an emphasis on how it provides mental health care users with adequate care, treatment, and rehabilitation services through a non-discriminatory approach.

Andoh-Arthur and Quarshie, in Chap. 8, introduce readers to the sociohistorical, cultural, and political antecedents to anti-suicide laws, and the dangers in the predominant binary discourse on the efforts to decriminalise attempted suicide. Specific emphasis is given to the discussion of suicide and suicide attempts within the notion of 'social suffering' in the Ghanaian context, in an attempt to foster a kinship between mental health and the legal system for an effective population-based suicide prevention campaign in Ghana. Chapter 9 by Kwakye-Nuako reports on a study of the role adopted by police prosecutors in their interactions with victims (under 16 years) of child sexual abuse and their caregivers in Ghana. The author interviewed 14 participants (i.e., six defence lawyers, seven police prosecutors, and one legal prosecutor from the Attorney General's Department) and extracted three main themes: (1) inadequate training, (2) an intimidating or friendly demeanour, and (3) a crossfire of accusations. Practical suggestions are provided to enhance the competency of Ghanaian police prosecutors in handling such cases. Finally, in Chap. 10, Eseadi first provides an overview of the common mental health issues being experienced by prison inmates in Nigeria. The author then synthesises the research conducted on the prison inmates' mental health with the policies currently adopted by the Nigerian criminal justice system to address the prison inmates' mental health challenges and concludes with a discussion of the opportunities for and threats to mental health services in Nigeria.

The next section contains six chapters on the police, correctional, and legal systems in Africa. In Chap. 11, Parimah and colleagues use interviews with 38 people who use drugs (PWUDs) to explore their experiences, particularly with the police in Ghana. Three main themes are generated in relation to their experiences and encounters with the police: (1) ecstasy use, (2) the psychosocial consequences of drug use (with the sub-themes of psychological effects, development of criminality, disruption of life, and breakdown in familial relationship), and (3) police encounters (with the sub-themes of sudden and unannounced swoops, 'ghettos', bribery, and the non-deterrence of arrest). Chapter 12, written by Akinlabi, synthesises the literature on stress and stress-related disorders associated with police work. Surveying 706 police officers in Nigeria, the author empirically examines the occurrence, prevalence, and effects of stress among police officers, and concludes with suggestions for future research and policymaking. Chapter 13 by Parimah and colleagues introduces readers to their empirical study of 253 male prisoners in Ghana, focusing on their experiences of drug use and associated sociodemographic characteristics. The findings indicate that age, childhood abuse, and previous robbery convictions were significantly associated with the prisoners' tendency to use marijuana and other drugs.

Chapter 14 is a discussion of the factors contributing to Black female incarceration in South Africa. Dastile first provides a historical overview of female offenders in Africa and follows with a general profile of Black female offenders in South Africa. The author concludes the chapter with an argument for gender-based correctional institutions. In Chap. 15,

Akoensi interviews 78 frontline prison officers in Ghana to explore their sources of job satisfaction and organisational commitment and the impact that these have on them. Seven main themes are generated related to their job satisfaction: (1) reformation, (2) benefit-finding or personal growth, (3) helping prisoners, (4) a 'good day', (5) recognition and praise for work, (6) pay and benefits, and (7) job dissatisfaction. In relation to their organisational commitment, eight main themes are found: (1) high organisational commitment, (2) continuance/calculative commitment, (3) normative commitment, (4) low organisational commitment, (5) organisational injustice, (6) pay and benefits, (7) lack of job autonomy or powerlessness, and (8) job characteristics (e.g., perceived job dangerousness, work–family conflict, and public image of the prison service). The final chapter is Chap. 16, written by Adu-Poku, which explores through in-depth interviews and observations the perceptions, attitudes, and experiences of 17 Ghanaian citizens who have come into contact with the justice system (e.g., the police and courts). The author asserts that the utilisation of the justice system in Ghana is complex and multidimensional, and that interpretations of it are context-specific. Individuals who have used formal justice mechanisms are more likely to hold negative views of the system, given the perceived shortcomings of the justice system in Ghana. At the end of the book, the concluding chapter summarises the key findings from different chapters and highlights important take-home messages to advance our limited knowledge of African criminology, mental health, and criminal justice.

Exploring Crime, Mental Health Issues, and Criminal Justice in Africa from a Psycho-Criminological Perspective

The primary aim of this book is to present a collection of original and high-quality studies conducted by researchers and practitioners in the areas of crime, mental health issues, and criminal justice in Africa. As stated by Westen and Weinberger (2004):

Collaboration between clinicians [or field practitioners] and researchers could substantially improve the quality of scientific research. …This scientific mind and the clinician [or field practitioner] mind can coexist, in a single field—indeed, in a single person—and that the dialectic between the two may be essential for a scientific [psycho-criminology]. (p. 610)

One of the common shortcomings identified with the 'international' texts on these topics is that they are mainly written by Anglo-American scholars from a Western perspective. The lack of representation of contributions from other parts of the world, in this case Africa, needs to be addressed urgently. This edited volume also recognises the wider need to foster a greater multidisciplinary and multidirectional cross-national understanding through cross-cultural research. Supported by empirical and theory-driven research findings, we envision that this edited volume could contribute significantly to the limited literature in the psycho-criminological study of African criminology, mental health, and criminal justice. Such knowledge is a prerequisite for the efficient and effective functioning of impartial criminal justice (i.e., police, correctional, and legal) and mental health systems, especially in crime prevention, criminal investigation, offender rehabilitation, and victim assistance services (Chan, Lo, & Zhong, 2016; Chan, Lo, Zhong, & Chui, 2015). The public health importance of this line of research is clear, as there is a strong potential for escalation from minor victimisation to serious offending.

References

Adjorlolo, S., & Chan, H. C. O. (2019). Risk assessment of criminal offenders in Ghana: An investigation of the discriminant validity of the HCR-20^{V3}. *International Journal of Law and Psychiatry, 66,* 101458. https://doi. org/10.1016/j.ijlp.2019.101458

Adjorlolo, S., Chan, H. C. O., & Agboli, J. M. (2016). Adjudicating mentally disordered offenders in Ghana: The criminal and mental health legislations. *International Journal of Law and Psychiatry, 45,* 1–8. https://doi.org/10.1016/j. ijlp.2016.02.001

Agozino, B. (2010). Editorial: What is criminology? A control-freak discipline! *African Journal of Criminology and Justice Studies, 4*(1), i–xx.

Bartol, C. R. (2002). *Criminal behaviour: A psychosocial approach* (6th ed.). Upper Saddle River, NJ: Prentice Hall.

Carrington, K., Sozzo, M., & Hogg, R. (2016). Southern criminology. *British Journal of Criminology, 56*(1), 1–20. https://doi.org/10.1093/bjc/azv083

Chan, H. C. O., & Ho, S. M. Y. (2017). *Psycho-criminological perspective of criminal justice in Asia: Research and practices in Hong Kong, Singapore, and beyond.* Oxfordshire, UK: Routledge.

Chan, H. C. O., & Sheridan, L. (2020). *Psycho-criminological approaches to stalking behavior: An international perspective.* West Sussex, UK: John Wiley & Sons.

Chan, H. C. O., Lo, T. W., & Zhong, L. Y. (2016). Identifying the self-anticipated reoffending risk factors of incarcerated male repeat offenders in Hong Kong. *The Prison Journal, 96*(5), 731–751. https://doi.org/10.1177/0032885516662640

Chan, H. C. O., Lo, T. W., Zhong, L. Y., & Chui, W. H. (2015). Criminal recidivism of incarcerated male nonviolent offenders in Hong Kong. *International Journal of Offender Therapy and Comparative Criminology, 59*(2), 121–142. https://doi.org/10.1177/0306624X13502965

Cohn, E. G., Farrington, D. P., & Iratzoqui, A. (2017). Changes in the most-cited scholars and works over 25 years: The evolution of the field of criminology and criminal justice. *Journal of Criminal Justice Education, 28*(1), 25–51. https://doi.org/10.1080/10511253.2016.1153686

Fraser, A., Lee, M., & Tang, D. (2017). Crime, media, culture: Asia-style. *Crime, Media, Culture: An International Journal, 13*(2), 131–134. https://doi.org/10.1177/1741659017718975

Hayward, K. (2005). Psychology and crime: Understanding the interface. In C. Hale, K. Hayward, A. Wahidin, & E. Wincup (Eds.), *Criminology* (pp. 109–137). Oxford, UK: Oxford University Press.

Hollin, C. R. (2012). Criminological psychology. In M. Maguire, R. Morgan, & R. Reiner (Eds.), *The Oxford handbook of criminology* (5th ed., pp. 81–113). New York, NY: Oxford University Press.

Hollin, C. R. (2013). *Psychology and crime: An introduction to criminological psychology* (2nd ed.). East Sussex, UK: Routledge.

Liu, J. (2009). Asian criminology—Challenges, opportunities, and directions. *Asian Journal of Criminology, 4*, 1–9. https://doi.org/10.1007/s11417-009-9066-7

Moosavi, L. (2019). A friendly critique of 'Asian criminology' and 'Southern criminology'. *British Journal of Criminology, 59*(2), 257–275. https://doi.org/10.1093/bjc/azy045

Oriola, T. B. (2006). Biko Agozino and the rise of post-colonial criminology. *African Journal of Criminology and Justice Studies, 2*(1), 104–131.

Westen, D., & Weinberger, J. (2004). When clinical description becomes statistical prediction. *American Psychologist, 59*(7), 595–613. https://doi.org/10.1037/0003-066X.59.7.595

Wortley, R. (2011). *Psychological criminology: An integrative approach*. Oxon, UK: Routledge.

Part I

Deviance, Crime and Mental Health

2

Suicide, Suicidal Ideation and Behaviour among African Youths: A Psycho-Social and Criminological Analysis

Richard A. Aborisade

Introduction

Suicide, a deadly violence against self, annually accounts for the death of an estimated one million people worldwide (World Health Organization, 2016), and globally, it is noted to account for the second highest cause of death for those between the ages of 15 and 29 years. Suicide is said to have been committed when death results from poisoning, injury, or suffocation, where it is implicitly or explicitly evident that the injury was self-inflicted and intended to be fatal (Kaslow et al., 2015; Gregory, 2020). On the other hand, suicidal ideation refers to self-reported thoughts of engaging in suicide-related behaviour (Korczak, 2015). Although, most people who have suicidal thoughts do not go ahead make suicide attempts, suicidal thoughts are nonetheless considered a risk factor for suicidal attempt (Gliatto & Rai, 1999). A WHO report (2016) has equally indicated that an estimated 10 to 20 million people attempt

R. A. Aborisade (✉)
Department of Sociology, Olabisi Onabanjo University, Ago-Iwoye, Nigeria
e-mail: aborisade.richard@oouagoiwoye.edu.ng

© The Author(s), under exclusive license to Springer Nature Switzerland AG 2021
H. C. O. Chan, S. Adjorlolo (eds.), *Crime, Mental Health and the Criminal Justice System in Africa*, https://doi.org/10.1007/978-3-030-71024-8_2

13

suicide every year. Aside from loss of lives that results from completed suicide, injuries that result from suicidal behaviour are considered a major public health problem in the world.

In spite of WHO report indicating that 79% of global suicides occur in low and middle-income countries, it is believed to be underreported in Africa. The underreporting of suicide in African countries has being identified as a key factor that undermines research and formulation of effective control and preventive programmes to addressing the apparently growing rates of suicide among youths on the continent. As a result, the knowledge and understanding about suicidal behaviour in relation to its incidence and patterns is premised on information from high-income countries, which may not capture the peculiarity of African cultural context. Much of the suicide data available on published materials are based on small studies conducted in different regions and populations within the continent. Meanwhile, information on the burden of suicide, especially among the youths on the continent, is important, in order to help inform local, regional and national policy.

In this chapter, an exposition of the incidence and patterns of African youth suicidal behaviour will be presented. Using a multifactorial and multidisciplinary approach and analysis of theories of suicide, the chapter offers perspectives in the fields of sociology, psychology, mental health and criminology as applicable to suicidal behaviour of African youths. In finding a sustainable solution to suicidal behaviour and fatality in Africa, the impact of legal instruments and other measures are evaluated.

Defining Suicide, Suicidal Ideation and Behaviour

Suicidologists and other fields related to suicide have continued to be saddled with the responsibility of defining and refining the definition of key suicide-related constructs. There have been modifications of nomenclature of some constructs of "suicide-related behaviour" (initially referred to as suicidality), which are classified as ideations (i.e., thoughts), communications and behaviours. Scholars, whose work has focused on the nomenclature of suicide-related constructs, opined that all suicide-related behaviours are *self-initiated* (Kebede & Ketsela, 1993; Neeleman, 1996).

Furthermore, there could be variations of these behaviours in respect of the presence or absence of *intent to die* and presence or absence of *physical injury* that is sustained. When there is no *intent to die*, the term *self-harm* is used.

The focus of this chapter is on suicidal ideation and behaviour that has to do with *intent to die;* as a result, the use of the term "suicidal behaviour" is preferred over and above "suicide-related behaviours." The use of suicidal behaviour in this chapter shall entail: (1) self-initiated, potentially injurious behaviour; (2) presence of intent to die; and, (3) non-fatal outcome. The use of the term *suicide* is meant to cover cases where suicide attempts lead to death. Gliatto and Rai (1999) defined suicidal ideation as thinking about, considering, or planning suicide. The acts of suicidal ideation range from fleeting thoughts, to extensive thoughts, to detailed thoughts. It has been reported that majority of people that have suicidal thoughts do not go ahead to attempt suicide even though suicidal thought has been described as being risky (Klonsky, May, & Saffer, 2016; Uddin, Burton, Maple, Khan, & Khan, 2019; Soloff, Kevin, Thomas, & Kevin, 2000). Suicidal ideation is generally connected with depression and other mood disorders; however, it appears that it is also associated with some other mental disorders, family events, and life events, all of which may increase the risk of suicidal ideation (Uddin et al., 2019). Traditionally, suicidal ideation and behaviour have been conceived as a unidimensional construct; with passive ideation, active intent and behaviour exist along a continuum (Soloff et al., 2000).

There have been a number of reports in economically advanced countries of the world identifying suicidal behaviour as the leading cause of psychiatric emergencies among children and adolescents (Klonsky et al., 2016), and one of the strongest predicators of psychiatric admission of adolescents (Korczak, 2015). Availability of reliable data that would be able to determine such trend has been scarce in Africa as suicide and suicidal behaviour remained underreported in most countries within the region. In spite of this, incidences and prevalence of suicidal behaviour in the continent based on available data and reports will be discussed in the following section.

Incidence and Prevalence of Suicide and Suicidal Behaviour in Africa

The inadequacy of systematic data collection has been reported to have impeded suicide research in Africa (Mars, Burrows, Hjelmeland, & Gunnell, 2014). Based on the report from WHO, only 10% of African countries report suicide mortality data to the organisation, and official statistics generated from these countries accounts for a mere 15% of the population of the continent. Therefore, studies on incidences and prevalence of suicide across Africa have been relied on to offer overviews on mortality and statistics on the rates and trends of suicide in the continent.

In a systematic review of published literature on suicidal behaviour across African countries, Mars et al. (2014) reported an estimated number of 34,000 suicides per year, with an overall incidence rate of 32 per 100,000 population. They equally found suicide rate in men to be three times higher than that of women. Mars et al. further reported a higher suicide fatality rate among young adults (aged 15–30 years) in the continent based on information gleaned from eleven publications from seven countries. Meanwhile, in a recent systematic analysis, Naghavi (2019) reported a significant decrease in the age-standardised suicide mortality rate in sub-Saharan Africa (ASMR 16.3 per 100,000), which accounts for the third highest regional mortality rate with approximately 11,000 suicide deaths contributing to the burden of disease.

In a study of 8573 suicide cases in South Africa, Kootbodien, Naicker, Wilson, Ramesar, and London (2020) found that 73% (6237) occurred between men and women aged 15 and 44 years with the odds of dying by suicide found to be highest among the 15–29-year age group. Meanwhile, the WHO report for 2016 identified Lesotho, Ivory Coast, Equatorial Guinea, Uganda, Cameroon, Zimbabwe, Nigeria, and Togo as African countries in the global top 20 suicide cases. Consequently, Africa, with eight countries in the top 20 of the global list of suicide portends an ominous trend of suicide rate in the region and ASMR is indicative of a growing rate of suicide among the African youths.

In respect of common methods used for suicide in Africa, reports from nine publications of research conducted in seven African countries revealed that the predominant method used for suicide attempt among the youths was poisoning, which ranged from 26% to 91% of attempts (Chibanda, Sebit, & Acuda, 2002; Ikealumba & Couper, 2006; Kedebe & Alem, 1999; Kinyanda, Hjelmeland, & Musisi, 2004; Ndosi & Waziri, 1997). While overdose of drugs was more common than pesticide poisoning in Namibia, South Africa, United Republic of Tanzania and Zimbabwe, the use of pesticide was marginally more common in Uganda. Medications that were most frequently used include antidepressants, antimalarial and psychotropic medications. Two studies reported that cutting was commonly used (Adinkrah, 2011; Ikealumba & Couper, 2006), while three studies reported frequent use of hanging (Adinkrah, 2011; Alem, Kebede, Jacobsson, & Kullgren, 1999; Kedebe & Alem, 1999).

Theoretical Considerations

Suicide is widely acknowledged as a global public health problem. In spite of this, few theories have been developed for its aetiology and effective prevention. Indeed, there had been a strong dominance of psychiatrists in suicide research and prevention, mainly as a result of the categorisation of high percentage of the suicides in the world as being due to at least a type of mental disorder based on diagnoses. However, there are growing interests in sociological evaluation of suicidal behaviour as well as completed suicide. As a result, sociological autopsy of suicide is gaining some currency in contributing to the body of suicidology literature. Considering the psycho-social approach adopted in this chapter, theories that offer both psychological and sociological explanation of suicidal ideation and behaviour among African youths will be examined.

Interpersonal Theory of Suicidal Behaviour

The theory of interpersonal suicidal behaviour is founded on the assumption that people's death resulting from suicide is a factor of their ability and desire to commit suicide (Van Orden et al., 2010). According to the theorists, there are three constructs that are central to the suicidal behaviour. Of the three constructs, two are primarily related to suicidal desire—thwarted belongingness and perceived burdensomeness—while one is related to capability—acquired capability for suicide.

Thwarted Belongingness

The concept of thwarted belongingness rests on the condition of social isolation as a strong and reliable predictor of suicidal ideation and behaviour across the lifespan. It is conceived as assessing one facet of the higher order construct of social connectedness (or social integration), which can be measured at several levels (Berkman, Glass, Brissette, & Seeman, 2000). In addition, other facets of social connectedness (e.g., loneliness and loss of a spouse) have been identified as predictors of lethal suicide behaviour. It is, therefore, postulated that variables of social connectedness are connected with suicide because of their observable indicators that fundamental human psychological needs remain unmet. These needs have been described as the "needs to belong" (Baumeister & Leary, 1995, p. 1). As the theory posits, when these needs are unmet—a state being referred to as thwarted belongingness—a desire for death develops (also referred to in the suicidology and clinical literature as passive suicidal ideation). This is similar to some other suicide theories that proposed central role for social connectedness; although, the manner of connection between social connectedness and suicide differs from one theory to another.

Several authors of suicide literature in Africa have identified social isolation as the strongest and most reliable predictor of suicidal ideation, attempts, and lethal suicidal behaviour among youths on the continent (Adewuya & Oladipo, 2019; Adinkrah, 2016; Mars et al., 2014; Omigbodun, Dogra, Esan, & Adedokun, 2008; Wanyoike, 2015). Although isolation has been noted to be very common among the elderly, there are growing literature that affirm the developing level of social isolation of youths in contemporary African society. In Africa, social isolation, also referred to as relational deprivation, is posited as a relevant dimension of poverty and a barrier to well-being and capability. The lived experiences of African youths that are living in poverty are enmeshed in isolation, humiliation, and shame. Aside from Africa, several empirical studies have established the connection between social isolation and lethal suicidal behaviour (Conwell, 1997; Dervic, Brent, & Oquendo, 2008; Joiner & Van Orden, 2008).

Perceived Burdensomeness

This concept is premised on the risk posed by family conflict, unemployment, and physical illness as factors that possess strong connection with suicide. The three aforementioned factors are acknowledged as types of negative life events. Pertinent questions that probe the association between these factors and suicide have been asked. The theorists proposed that the elevated likelihood of developing perceptions of burdensomeness on others is the common thread between family conflict, unemployment, and physical illness that can account for the connections with suicide. Similar to this proposition, Sabbath's (1969) family systems theory of adolescent suicidal behaviour also identified the importance of family in suicidal ideation. Emphasis was laid by the theory on the perceptions of adolescents that they are the expendable members of their family. According to the theory, the causal factor leading to adolescent suicidal behaviour is pathogenic parental attitudes toward the adolescent. The adolescent may then interpret these parental attitudes as indicating that he/she is not needed in the family, and in fact, that the family would be better off if he/she dies.

Research on family risk factors for youth suicidal behaviours in Africa indicates that both fatal and nonfatal suicidal behaviours have been associated with negative parent–child relationship (e.g., low closeness, high conflict), residing with single-parent household, child maltreatment, alcoholic/substance abuse, family history of affective and antisocial disorders (Amare, Woldeyhannes, Haile, & Yeneabat, 2018; Kebede & Ketsela, 1993; Shilubane et al., 2013; Dunlavy, Aquah, & Wilson, 2015). For example, high level of family conflict and negative parent–child relationship were found to be associated with suicidal ideation among adolescents in southwest Nigeria (Omigbodun et al., 2008). Similarly, in a study conducted in Zambia, Muula, Kazembe, Rudatsikira, and Siziya (2007) found that suicidal behaviour among the adolescents was associated with the family history of alcoholic/substance abuse and child maltreatment.

Research works directed at testing Sabbath's theory have found a positive correlation between perceptions of expendability and suicidal behaviours among adolescents (Rosenthal & Rosenthal, 1984; Woznica & Shapiro, 1990). However, Sabbath's theory is limited because of its failure to account for the fact that majority of youths that perceive that their family is better off with them dead do not go ahead and commit suicide. On the other hand, interpersonal theory is consistent with past conceptual work as it affirms that there is an important role played by perceptions of burdensomeness in the aetiology of suicide.

Acquired Capability for Suicide

Models of suicide generally show that incidences of suicide are caused by several factors, in such a way that suicidal ideations emanate from the fewest number of co-occurring risk factors (Joiner & Van Orden, 2008). Also, suicide attempts are caused by a greater number of factors, while completed suicide stems from the co-occurrence of the greatest number of factors. The main assumption of these models is that the risk for suicide is aggravated by the greater risk for suicidal desire and, maybe, increasing severe forms of suicidal desire. However, this assumption is challenged by Interpersonal theory that argued that the desire to die by suicide alone is not enough to result in lethal suicidal behaviour. In other words, it is not that easy to commit suicide. As posited by the theory, individuals who will be able to commit suicide must do away with some of the fears that are associated with suicide. This is premised on the belief that human beings are biologically prepared to have fear for suicide because there are involvement of stimuli and cues in suicidal behaviour which are associated with threats for survival.

The theory, however, postulated that acquiring the capability for suicide, which entails higher tolerance for physical pain and reduced fear of death, is quite possible. The exposure of African youths to suicidal acts through stories in the social media might be responsible for the recent surge in the number of lethal suicide and suicidal behaviour on the continent (Ntseku, 2019; Alabi, Alabi, Ayinde, & Abdulmalik, 2014). Media channels have exposed youths to different ways of engaging in "painless" suicide (Abdulai, 2020). For example, the use of insecticides/pesticide like Sniper for suicide acts by youths has been widely reported on social media. This inevitably exposes and encourages other youths with suicidal ideation to use similar methods or chemicals to commit suicide.

The Strain Theory of Suicide

Unlike other strain theories, the strain theory of suicide (STS) is a recently propounded theory to focus exclusively on suicide (Zhang, 2005). The formulation of the STS is to offer socio-psychological mechanisms to understand suicidal behaviour (Zhang & Lester, 2008). The postulation of the theory is that the act of suicide is usually preceded by psychological strains. The assumption of the theory is that the strain that results from psychological suffering as a result of competing pressures may lead to engagement in suicidal behaviour, perceived as a solution to ending the strain (Zhang, 2005; Zhang & Song, 2006). The STS put forward four types of sources of psychological strain that may cause suicidal ideation. Each of the four types of strain consists of at least two conflicting social facts (Zhang & Lester, 2008). If there are no contradictions between two social facts, then there will be no strain.

Differential values: Differential values have to do with two conflicting social values or beliefs competing in the daily life of an individual, leading the person to experience value strain. The two conflicting social facts are the two competing personal beliefs internalised in the value system of the individual. African youths may experience strain as the mainstream societal culture and deviance sub-group culture are considered to be important in the individual's daily life (Mars et al., 2014). Value strain in African youths may also occur based on the effects of differential values of traditional collectivism and modern individualism.

Reality versus aspiration: Reality versus aspiration occurs if there is discrepancy between the aspirations or a high goal of an individual and a non-ideal reality that the person has to live with, which may lead the individual to experience aspiration strain. In this case, the two conflicting social facts are the splendid goal or ideal that the individuals want to achieve and the reality that may prevent the individual from achieving it. Merton (1968) was the first to use this concept of strain to explain crimes in the United States. In Africa, everyone is socialised to aspire toward high achievement and success; however, access to legitimate opportunities to realising the goal is blocked off with the high incidence of unemployment, nepotism and favouritism in the society (Huschka & Mau, 2006). In this case, a lot of African youths are faced with strong strain, as the aspiration they were socialised into aiming for, are impeded or constrained by their disadvantaged social status or gender.

Relative Deprivation: There are situations where individuals that are poor realise that their situation is worse than that of other people of the same or similar background, thus, leading the person to experience deprivation strain. In this case, the two conflicting social facts are the miserable life of an individual and the perceived wealth of comparable others. A person living in absolute poverty, where there is no basis for comparison with others, does not feel necessarily bad, deprived, or miserable. However, if this person living in absolute poverty gets to find out that other people living under the same condition with him/her are getting to live a better life, he or she may feel deprived and become upset about the situation.

Most African cities are economically polarised societies, where the poor and rich live geographically close to each other. This situation may increase the likelihood of people feeling this discrepancy. There is a high level of economic and social deprivation in African communities, which raises high consciousness of discrepancies and comparativeness among African youths with some studies strongly relating it to suicidality (Adinkrah, 2011; Dunlavy et al., 2015).

Individuals suffer relatively greater strains when they experience increased perception of deprivation (Zhang & Tao, 2013). For example, in large cities in Africa like Lagos, Johannesburg, and Accra, there is a high level of social exclusion felt by economically disadvantaged people. Research has reported that youths in these urban areas that suffer relative deprivation are less tolerant of their disadvantaged conditions and more prone to deploying all means to acquiring wealth or engaging in suicidal behaviour (Khasakhala, Ndetei, & Mathai, 2013; Amare et al., 2018).

Deficient coping: There are different ways and different capacities of individuals when it comes to coping with life crisis, which may lead people to experiencing coping strain. In this case, the two conflicting social facts are life crisis and the appropriate coping capability. Experiencing strain is not compulsory for everybody that is confronted with life crises. Crisis could just be the routine pressure or stress that one faces on a daily basis; theefore, only those people that are unable to cope with such crises experience strain. Crises like these could include loss of source of income, divorce, death of a partner, and loss of status. Individuals who are unable to cope with these negative life events may experience serious strain. There have been reports of suicide or suicide attempts by adolescents who are dropped from desired programmes in universities across Africa (Wanyoike, 2015). Zhang and Tao (2013) asserted that people who are less experienced in coping with negative life events are more likely to suffer stronger strain when a crisis eventually occurs.

Deficient coping appears to be distinct from other three types of strain in a number of ways. A person may be angered and frustrated by value conflict, unrealisable goals, relative deprivation or lack of coping skills and environment; however, coping stands to play a moderating role in the relationship between anger, frustration, psyche or suicidality. The chance of an individual settling for suicide or suicidal ideation may be reduced if the person possesses good coping skills and environment. Among African youths, religion and religiosity have been identified as being formidable in preventing suicide and offering protection (comfort and strength) against suicidality (Alabi et al., 2014; Chibanda et al., 2002; Offiah & Obiorah, 2014).

Durkheim's Theory of Suicide

In spite of the sparse contribution of sociology to the discipline of suicidology, the influence of Emile Durkheim ([1897] 1951) who made use of sociological approach to study suicide remains remarkable. Studying the social context of a widely perceived individual act of suicide was of considerable interest to Durkheim. He examined the connections between suicide rates and various social factors (such as regulation and integration). There have been some remarkable debates generated from this approach. Despite the debates generated by Durkheim's theory of suicide, it remains very relevant in sociological approach in discussing suicide. Durkheim identified four types of suicide, which were categorised into two dimensions of the social structure: social integration and moral regulation. The four types are egoistic, altruistic, anomic and fatalistic suicides.

Egoistic suicide: Durkheim related egoistic suicide to a lack of social integration, which leads to incidences of suicide occasioned by coping strain. Danigelis and Pope (1979) documented that there are lower rates of incidences of suicide among married people as compared to single, widowed, or divorced people, as a result of higher social integration of married people. Lower level of social support and psychological security has been identified as increasing coping deficiency, which therefore manifests in lack of social integration. In Africa, the family institution has been recently reported to have been failing in one of its basic functions of providing social and emotional support for its members (Amare et al., 2018; Mars et al., 2014). Therefore, the increase in suicide rates among the youths has been partly associated with the dwindling fortunes of family as a social institution on the continent (Vawda, 2012; Adewuya & Oladipo, 2019).

Altruistic suicide: This is the type of suicide that is related to too much social integration. This type of suicide is related to deprivation strain. There have been some factual supports for Durkheim's theory including the actions of the Japanese kamikazes in World War II, the suicide bombers in the Middle East and the recent Boko Haram suicide bombers. As against the solidarity that is related to ordinary soldiers, it is very likely that members of close-knit terrorist groups will die of altruistic suicide when they become suicide bombers, as a result of their excessive integration into their organisation. In her study of Boko Haram suicide squad, Markovic (2019) noted that girls and young women were mostly used as suicide bombers. Over half of the bombers were women and girls, some as young as 7 years old, while there were more than 60 incidents where the bombers were below the age of 15.

Anomic suicide: This type of suicide refers to lack or inadequacy of moral regulation, which is similar to aspiration strain. There are reports of higher rates of anomic suicides in rich countries than what is obtainable in poor countries. This is because the citizens of rich countries, being less socially regulated, are likely to have higher expectations from life and, as a result, will likely have greater frustration if their expectations fail to materialise (Thio, 2004). In African countries, city dwellers are also likely to have higher rates of anomic suicide compared to those that live in the rural areas, as those in the cities get to be socialised to expect a lot from life and will be more frustrated if their expectations cannot be met due to social constraints. (Adewuya & Oladipo, 2019; Chibanda et al., 2002; Shilubane et al., 2013).

Fatalistic suicide: This has to do with suicides that occur as a result of too strict moral regulation. When control and regulation become too much, there might be frustration exhibited by some individuals. A young rural African woman who faces troubles with conflicting values may at the same time experience greater social and/or parental control than what will be experienced by her brothers. This is because the woman may have a higher level of social regulation than her brothers. This may explain why African women who are sexually assaulted sometimes resort to suicide, especially when they lose their virginity in the process. African women's sexuality is highly regulated and attached to their honour and dignity as against that of males that are less regulated.

Legal Status and Criminalisation of Suicide in Africa

A review of the legal statuses of most African countries reveal that attempted suicide, also referred to as "nonfatal suicidal behaviour," "failed suicide attempt," "nonfatal suicidal attempt," or "parasuicide," "completed suicide," and "assisted suicide," have multidimensional recognition. In some countries, the criminal and penal codes prescribe punishment for attempted suicide and accomplices in an act of attempted suicide. These countries include Nigeria, Ghana, Gambia, Kenya, Sudan,

Tanzania and Myanmar (Adinkrah, 2016). Meanwhile, in some other African countries, suicidal behaviour or attempted suicide is not criminalised and no punishment is applied on whoever attempts to take their own life. These countries include Angola, Botswana, Cameroon, Egypt, South Africa, Ethiopia and Eritrea (Adinkrah, 2016). Finally, there are African countries with no legal status attached to suicidality.

In the Nigeria Criminal Code, section 327, it is stated that any person who attempts to kill himself is guilty of a misdemeanour and is liable to imprisonment for one year. Meanwhile, in section 326, it is further stated that anybody that aids the suicide of another person by procuring another to kill himself, counselling another to kill himself and thereby inducing him to do so, or aiding another in killing himself, is guilty of felony, and is liable to imprisonment for life. Similarly, suicide and suicidal attempt is illegal in Ghana and punishable under the country's penal code. According to Act 29 section 57, subsection 2 of the Consolidation of Criminal Code (1960), "whoever attempts to commit suicide shall be guilty of a misdemeanour." It is also illegal and a crime to assist suicide in Ghana. Under Act 29, section 57, subsection 1 of the penal code, "whoever abets the commission of suicide by any person shall whether or not the suicide be actually committed, be guilty of first degree felony."

On the other hand, there are a significant number of countries within the continent where attempted and completed suicide are legal, though assisted suicide is illegal. These countries include Angola, Botswana, Cameroon, Egypt, South Africa, Ethiopia and Eritrea (Adinkrah, 2016). In South Africa, attempted or completed suicide used to be criminalised and penalised between 1886 and 1968, but the legislation criminalising the act has been relaxed. However, assisted suicide remains a crime on the country, although it is believed that the legislation on it will eventually be relaxed.

According to Adinkrah (2016), most African countries where suicide is illegal are formal British colonial territories. He affirmed that the anti-suicide statutes of most of these countries consisted of a corpus of laws imposed on the countries during the colonial periods. However, in spite of the United Kingdom, the colonial master of these countries, abrogating the laws criminalising suicide in 1961, these former colonies of the UK have maintained the legal codes. Although, the enforcement of anti-suicide laws in Ghana, Kenya and Gambia has been reported to be strict, the reverse is however the case in Nigeria as the prosecution of attempted suicide is rare in the country.

These countries have proceeded to criminalise, prosecute and penalise attempted suicide in spite of recent entreaties from suicidologists, suicide prevention advocates, mental health professionals and social analysts for suicide to be decriminalised (Adinkrah, 2016). In retaining the laws prohibiting suicide in these countries, pertinent questions have been raised on the enforcement of the laws and the impact of the laws in preventing suicide in the countries (Neeleman, 1996). For instance, the prevalence of suicide in Nigeria, one of the countries with such anti-suicide laws, is highest on the continent and sixth globally, according to the WHO 2016 Report (International Centre for Investigative Reporting, 2019). This raises the question as to whether the legal prohibition of attempted suicide results in fewer suicide deaths and suicide attempts in the country. However, questions have also been raised on whether the decriminalisation of suicide will bring about a significant decrease in the number of suicidal behaviour in the society. South Africa, one of the countries that have decriminalised suicide, still has a relatively high rate of completed suicide and suicidal behaviour. With an estimated suicide rate of 13.4 people per 100,000 South Africa's rate is approximately four times the global rate of 3.6 per 100,000 (The Citizen, 2019).

Assessing the Legal Status of Suicide in Africa

Even though in some criminological literature suicide is referred to as a "victimless crime," contemporary scholars in the field of criminology have come to identify the direct and proximate victims of suicide. Hjelmeland and Knizek (2011), O'Connor (2011) and Platt (2011) affirmed that suicide is an act that has serious negative social-psychological and mental health consequences on the society. Also, there are substantial empirical evidences that some people who are exposed to suicidal models in the media do, in fact, copy the behaviour (Stack, 2005). Suicide is also noted to have considerable effects on the health of the community.

There is a strong possibility of the families, friends, or acquaintances of people who attempt suicide to suffer shock, guilt, depression, or anger.

Controversies have continued to trail the legal prohibition of suicide in African countries. There have been a number of points raised by those who favour or are against the criminalisation of suicide on the continent. For those who support the use of legal instruments against attempted suicide, they argued that it is objectionable and inherently evil for an individual to take his/her own life (Gregory, 2020; Khasakhala et al., 2013). Hinging their belief on religious injunction, they opined that God is the provider of life and only God has the authority to take life. If this assertion holds for murder, then it can as well hold for suicide.

Also, advocates for the criminalisation of suicide submit that punishing acts of suicide will make fear of punishment attached to attempted suicide to serve as deterrence from the act (Offiah & Obiorah, 2014). It is their belief that people will abstain from suicidal behaviour if they are aware that failure to succeed in their suicidal act will lead them to be apprehended, prosecuted, convicted and penalised. Furthermore, those that oppose the decriminalisation of suicidal behaviour believe that the abrogation of the current laws against suicide will be conceived as recognition of suicide as a legitimate option for dealing with personal problems (Neeleman, 1996; Platt, 2011). Therefore, there will be increase in suicidal ideations and behaviours.

The criminalisation of suicidal behaviour is further justified by the perceived importance of apprehending and incarcerating those convicted for attempted suicide. It is believed that the period of incarceration that a person convicted for attempted suicide spends in prison will enable a rethinking of the suicide bid and may prevent additional attempts by the person or the chance of the person completing the suicide act (Mishara & Weisstubb, 2016; Neeleman, 1996). The incarceration will offer the person the opportunity to reflect on the suicidal behaviour and fashion a non-suicidal approach to addressing his personal problems after being released from prison. This will particularly hold true for those that engage in impulsive suicidal behaviour.

The main argument of those that oppose the criminalisation of suicidal behaviour is that the exhibition of the act is a manifestation of symptoms of treatable mental illness (e.g., depression, schizophrenia), despair, economic and social problems (Gliatto & Rai, 1999; Khasakhala et al., 2013). This school holds that governments across the African continent should strive to address the underlying problems that drive people into states that will make them consider suicide when they fail in their quest for decent living (Adinkrah, 2016; Offiah & Obiorah, 2014). This is considered as a sustainable way of reducing suicidal behaviour than prosecuting and penalising those that engage in nonfatal suicidal behaviour (Uddin et al., 2019). Therefore, proponents of the decriminalisation of suicide hold that suicidal persons are in need of mental health treatment modalities such as psychological counselling, psychotherapy, or economic and material assistance. These were noted to have stronger and sustainable effects than punishments that may serve to worsen the mental state of such persons. They further argued that suicide prevention programmes are aimed towards preventing incidences of suicide.

Furthermore, oppositions to criminalisation of suicidal behaviour argued that countries that criminalise suicidal behaviour often fail in obtaining factual and reliable data and rates of suicidal behaviour (Adinkrah, 2016; Mishara & Weisstubb, 2016). This, they opined, will be as a result of the fear of apprehension that will lead to underreporting of the act as it is a criminal offence. Therefore, those that engage in suicidal ideation and non-medically serious suicide attempts are not likely to report their acts to designated authorities, and may even refuse to seek help from therapists. This may make those at risk of engaging in suicidal behaviour not to be available to receive requisite psychological counselling necessary to prevent a recurrence of suicidal attempts.

Addressing Suicidal Behaviour among Youths: An African Imperative

In this chapter, a socio-psychological and criminological analysis of the growing problem of African youth involvement in suicide has been provided. From the literature explored, the psychosocial factors associated with suicide ideation and behaviour among African youths were presented and discussed. In addition, a broad overview of suicide laws in Africa and an assessment of legal statuses in African countries in controlling and preventing suicide were also done. It became evident from the assessment that the criminalisation or decriminalisation of suicide in Africa will not be sufficient to check the growth of suicide and suicidal behaviour, especially among the youths in Africa. Meanwhile, there is no evidence that indicates that decriminalisation increases suicide; on the contrary, there are reports of reduction in suicide rates in countries that decriminalise suicide. There is equally the possibility of decriminalisation engendering increase in suicide reporting as the fear of legal recrimination would have diminished.

Intervention strategies that will address the socio-psychological factors promoting suicidal ideation and behaviour among the youths should be deployed. First, there is a need for government and nongovernment agencies across the continent to develop protective factors that will guard the youths against the risk of suicide. The psychological theory of suicide has demonstrated the importance of resilience as having a buffering effect on suicide risk. Therefore, if the youths are highly resilient, association between the risk of suicide and suicidal behaviour will diminish.

As gleaned from the psychological and strain theories of suicide, there is an increase in suicidal behaviour when people suffer from relationship conflict, discord or loss. Therefore, healthy close relationships are capable of boosting the resilience of youths and acting as protective factors against the risk of suicide. In this case, healthy relationships with family members, peers, friends, partners and significant others, who are part of the closest social circle of the youths, are important, as they usually serve as supports in a time of crisis. In particular, some scholars have pointed to the dwindling level of solidarity and support of family and friends for the increase in African youth engagement in suicidal behaviour. Therefore, emphasis needs to be laid on the revival of family institution across the continent to provide social, emotional and financial support to the youths in order to buffer the impact of external stressors.

In Africa, and among African youths, religious and spiritual beliefs are important factors in conferring protection against suicide. However, some measure of care and caution should be applied. While faith itself can serve as a protective factor against suicidal behaviour, many religious and cultural beliefs and behaviours may also contribute towards stigma related to suicide, as a result of moral stances on suicide that may not encourage help-seeking behaviours. Durkheim's explanation of fatalistic suicide can also be used to understand why strict moral regulation of some religious doctrines may serve to cause rather than control suicide occurrences.

Psychologists and mental health practitioners should evolve ways of promoting lifestyle practice of positive coping strategies and well-being. Healthy lifestyle choices that have been found to be potent in promoting mental and physical well-being should be encouraged in schools and out of schools. These include regular exercises and sport, adequate sleep and diet, effective management of stress, abstinence from drugs and alcohol, and healthy relationship and social contacts. Also, practitioners and other stakeholders need to formulate measures that will help African community to desist from stigmatising mental disorder. These measures will encourage many people to seek help in order to address their mental health problems and reduce the risk of suicide.

Conclusion

Suicide may be underreported in Africa, but there is no gainsaying that it is a daunting social problem that decimates human resources, particularly those of the youths on the continent. First, it is imperative for the continent to engage in proper documentation of suicide cases so as to be conscious of possible increase and mitigate factors leading to the growth of suicide and suicidal behaviour in the continent. Also, African countries need to activate national responses to the growing rate of suicide among the youths through decriminalisation of suicide and implementation of sustainable intervention strategies to preventing suicide. Such responses should be strategic and multisectoral, which will not just involve the health sector but also other sectors like the media, education, labour, social welfare, agriculture, law, justice, business, and politics. The strategy should be tailored to the cultural and social context of each country.

In adopting a national suicide prevention strategy, it is imperative for African countries to consider the elements contained in the WHO's strategic approach in preventing suicide, which includes identification of key stakeholders in suicide prevention, undertaking situation analysis with the use of available data, assessing required resources (human and financial), achieving political commitment that is sustainable, addressing stigma related to suicide, increasing awareness about suicide, identification of risks and protective factors at individual, family, community, and societal levels, selection of effective interventions having considered the risks, protective factors and other situational analysis, improvement in suicide case registration for availability and quality of data, and conduct-monitoring, evaluation, and research for understanding the risks, protective factors and vulnerability (WHO, 2018).

References

Abdulai, T. (2020). Trends of online news media reported suicides in Ghana (1997–2019). *BMC Public Health, 20,* 35. https://doi.org/10.1186/s12889-020-8149-3

Adewuya, A., & Oladipo, E. (2019). Prevalence and associated factors for suicidal behaviours (ideation, planning, and attempt) among high school adolescents in Lagos, Nigeria. *European Child & Adolescent Psychiatry, 29*(11), 1503–1512. https://doi.org/10.1007/s00787-019-01462-x

Adinkrah, M. (2011). Epidemiologic characteristics of suicidal behaviour in comtemporary Ghana. *Crisis, 32*(1), 31–36. https://doi.org/10.1027/0227-5910/a000056

Adinkrah, M. (2016). Anti-suicide laws in Nine African Countries: Criminalization, prosecution and penalization. *African Journal of Criminology and Justice Studies, 9*(1), 279–292. Retrieved from https://www.researchgate.net/publication/303809758_Anti-Suicide_Laws_in_Nine_African_Countries_Criminalization_Prosecution_and_Penalization

Alabi, O., Alabi, A., Ayinde, O., & Abdulmalik, J. (2014). Suicide and suicidal behaviour in Nigeria: A review. *Dokita Journal, 5,* 50–62. Retrieved from https://www.researchgate.net/publication/271748010_Suicide_and_Suicidal_Behavior_in_Nigeria_A_review

Alem, A., Kebede, D., Jacobsson, L., & Kullgren, G. (1999). Suicide attempts among adults in Butajira, Ethiopia. *Acta Psychiatry Scandinavica, 100*(S397), 70–76. https://doi.org/10.1111/j.1600-0447.1999.tb10697.x

Amare, T., Woldeyhannes, S. M., Haile, K., & Yeneabat, T. (2018). Prevalence and associated factors of suicide ideation and attempt among adolescent high school students in Dangila Town, Northwest Ethiopia. *Hindawi Psychiatry Journal, 2018*, 1–9. https://doi.org/10.1155/2018/7631453

Baumeister, R., & Leary, M. (1995). The need to belong: Desire for interpersonal attachments as a fundamental human motivation. *Psychological Bulletin, 117*, 497–529. https://doi.org/10.1037/0033-2909.117.3.497

Berkman, L., Glass, T., Brissette, I., & Seeman, T. (2000). From social integration to health: Durkheim in the new millennium. *Social Science & Medicine, 51*, 843–857. https://doi.org/10.1016/s0277-9536(00)00065-4

Chibanda, D., Sebit, M., & Acuda, S. (2002). Prevalence of major depression in deliberate self-harm individuals in Harare, Zimbabwe. *East Africa Medical Journal, 79*(5), 263–266. https://doi.org/10.4314/eamj.v79i5.8866

Conwell, Y. (1997). Management of suicidal behavior in the elderly. *Psychiatric Clinics of North America, 20*, 667–683. https://doi.org/10.1016/s0193-953x(05)70336-1

Danigelis, N., & Pope, W. (1979). Durkheim's theory of suicide as applied to the family: An empirical test. *Social Forces, 57*, 1081–1106. https://doi.org/10.2307/2577260

Dervic, K., Brent, D. A., & Oquendo, M. A. (2008). Completed suicide in childhood. *Psychiatric Clinics of North America, 31*, 271–291. https://doi.org/10.1016/j.psc.2008.01.006

Dunlavy, A., Aquah, E., & Wilson, M. (2015). Suicidal ideation among school-attending adolescents in dar es salaam, Tanzania. *Tanzania Journal of Health Research, 17*(1), 147–161. https://doi.org/10.4314/thrb.v17i1.5

Durkheim, E. (1951). *Suicide*. Free Press.

Gliatto, M., & Rai, A. (1999). Evaluation and treatment of patients with suicidal ideation. *American Family Physician, 59*(6), 1500–1506. Retrieved from https://www.aafp.org/afp/1999/0315/p1500.html

Gregory, C. (2020, March 2). *Suicide and suicide prevention: Understanding the risk factors, prevention, and what we can do to help*. Psycom. Retrieved from https://www.psycom.net/depression.central.suicide.html

Hjelmeland, H., & Knizek, B. L. (2011). What kind of research do we need in suicidology today? In *International handbook of suicide prevention: Research, policy and practice* (pp. 181–198). John Wiley.

Huschka, D., & Mau, S. (2006). Social anomie and racial segregation in South Africa. *Social Indicators Research, 76*(3), 467–498. https://doi.org/10.1007/s11205-005-2903-x

Ikealumba, N., & Couper, I. (2006). Suicide and attempted suicide: The Rehoboth experience. *Rural Remote Health, 6*(535), 1. Retrieved from https://pubmed.ncbi.nlm.nih.gov/17073530/

International Centre for Investigative Reporting. (2019). *Nigeria has highest suicide rate in Africa, sixth globally.* Abuja: The ICIR. Retrieved February 15, 2020, from https://www.icirnigeria.org/nigeria-has-highest-suicide-rate-in-africa-sixth-globally/

Joiner, T., & Van Orden, K. (2008). The interpersonal psychological theory of suicidal behavior indicates specific and crucial psychotherapeutic targets. *International Journal of Cognitive Therapy, 1,* 80–89. https://doi.org/10.1521/ijct.2008.1.1.80

Kaslow, N., Sherry, A., Bethea, K., Wyckoff, S., Compton, M. T., Grall, M. B., et al. (2015). Social risk and protective factors for suicide attempts in low income African American Men and Women. *Suicide and Life-Threatening Behaviour, 35*(4), 400–411. https://doi.org/10.1521/suli.2005.35.4.400

Kebede, D., & Ketsela, T. (1993). Suicide attempts in Ethiopian adolescents in Addis Abeba high schools. *Ethiopian Medical Journal, 31*(2), 83–90. Retrieved from https://pubmed.ncbi.nlm.nih.gov/8513783/

Kedebe, D., & Alem, A. (1999). Suicide attempts and ideation among adults in Addis Ababa, Ethiopia. *Acta Psychiatry Scandinavica, 100*(S397), 35–39. https://doi.org/10.1111/j.1600-0447.1999.tb10692.x

Khasakhala, L. I., Ndetei, D. M., & Mathai, M. (2013). Suicidal behaviour among youths associated with attending outpatient psychiatric clinic in Kenya psychopathology in both parents and youths. *Annals of General Psychiatry, 12*(13), 2–8. https://doi.org/10.1186/1744-859x-12-13

Kinyanda, E., Hjelmeland, H., & Musisi, S. (2004). Deliberate self-harm as seen in Kampala, Uganda. *Social Psychiatry Epidemiology, 39*(4), 318–325. https://doi.org/10.1007/s00127-004-0748-2

Klonsky, E. D., May, A. M., & Saffer, B. (2016). Suicide, suicide attempts, and suicidal ideation. *Annual Review of Clinical Psychology, 12*(1), 307–330. https://doi.org/10.1146/annurev-clinpsy-021815-093204

Kootbodien, T., Naicker, N., Wilson, K., Ramesar, R., & London, L. (2020). Trends in Suicide Mortality in South Africa, 1997 to 2016. *International Journal of Environmental Research and Public Health, 17*(6), 1850. https://doi.org/10.3390/ijerph17061850

Korczak, D. J. (2015). Suicidal ideation and behaviour. *Paediatric Child Health, 20*(5), 257–260. Retrieved from https://www.ncbi.nlm.nih.gov/pmc/articles/PMC4472054/

Markovic, V. (2019). Suicide squad: Boko Haram's use of the female suicide bomber. *Women & Criminal Justice, 29*(4–5), 283–302. https://doi.org/1 0.1080/08974454.2019.1629153

Mars, B., Burrows, S., Hjelmeland, H., & Gunnell, D. (2014). Suicidal behaviour across the African continent: A review of the literature. *BMC Public Health, 14*, 606. https://doi.org/10.1186/1471-2458-14-606

Merton, R. (1968). *Social theory and social structure.* Free Press.

Mishara, L., & Weisstubb, D. (2016). The legal status of suicide: A global review. *International Journal of Law and Psychiatry, 44*, 54–74. https://doi. org/10.1016/j.ijlp.2015.08.032

Muula, A., Kazembe, L., Rudatsikira, E., & Siziya, S. (2007). Suicidal ideation and associated factors among in-school adolescents in Zambia. *Tanzania Health Research Bulletin, 9*(3), 202–206. https://doi.org/10.4314/thrb. v9i3.14331

Naghavi, M. (2019). Global, regional, and national burden of suicide mortality 1990 to 2016: Systematic analysis for the Global Burden of Disease Study 2016. *British Medical Journal, 364*, 194. https://doi.org/10.1136/bmj.l94

Ndosi, N., & Waziri, M. (1997). The nature of parasuicide in Dar Es Salaam, Tanzania. *Social Science Medicine, 44*(1), 55–61. https://doi.org/10.1016/ s0277-9536(96)00094-9

Neeleman, J. (1996). Suicide as a crime in the UK: Legal history, international comparisons and present implications. *Acta Psychiatrica Scandinavica, 94*(4), 252–257. https://doi.org/10.1111/j.1600-0447.1996.tb09857

Ntseku, M. (2019). *Social media pinpointed for rise in youth suicide.* Cape Argus: Independent Media. Retrieved May 3, 2020, from https://www.iol.co.za/ capeargus/news/social-media-pinpointed-for-rise-in-youth-suicide-34446427

O'Connor, R. C. (2011). Towards an integrated motivational-volitional model of suicidal behaviour. In *International handbook of suicide prevention: Research, policy and practice* (pp. 181–198). John Wiley.

Offiah, S. A., & Obiorah, C. (2014). Pattern of suicide in Nigeria: The Niger Delta experience. *Journal of Medical Investigations and Practice, 9*, 8–11. Retrieved from https://www.ajol.info/index.php/jomip/article/view/104670

Omigbodun, O., Dogra, N., Esan, O., & Adedokun, B. (2008). Prevalence and correlates of suicidal behaviour among adolescents in Southwest Nigeria. *International Journal of Social Psychiatry, 54*(1), 34–46. https://doi. org/10.1177/0020764007078360

Platt, S. (2011). Inequalities and suicidal behaviour. In *International handbook of suicide prevention: Research, policy and practice* (pp. 211–234). John Wiley.

Rosenthal, P., & Rosenthal, S. (1984). Suicidal behavior by preschool children. *American Journal of Psychiatry, 141*, 520–525. https://doi.org/10.1176/ajp.141.4.520

Sabbath, J. (1969). The suicidal adolescent: The expendable child. *Journal of the American Academy of Child Psychiatry, 8*, 272–285. https://doi.org/10.1016/s0002-7138(09)61906-3

Shilubane, H. N., Ruiter, R., Van Den Borne, B., Sewp, R., James, S., & Reddy, P. (2013). Suicide and related health risk behaviours among school learners in South Africa: Results from the 2002 and 2008 national youth risk behaviour surveys. *BMC Public Health, 13*(1), 926–935. https://doi.org/10.1186/1471-2458-13-926

Soloff, P., Kevin, G., Thomas, M., & Kevin, M. (2000). Characteristics of suicide attempts of patients with major depressive episode and borderline personality disorder: A comparative study. *American Journal of Psychiatry, 157*(4), 601–608. https://doi.org/10.1176/appi.ajp.157.4.601

Stack, S. (2005). Suicide in the media: A quantitative review of studies based on nonfictional stories. *Suicide and Life-Threatening Behaviour, 35*(2), 121–133. https://doi.org/10.1521/suli.35.2.121.62877

The Citizen. (2019). *South Africa's suicide rate four times the global rate.* The Citizen South Africa. Retrieved March 11, 2020, from https://citizen.co.za/lifestyle/fitness-and-health-your-life-your-life/2189197/south-africas-suicide-rate-four-times-the-global-rate/

Thio, A. (2004). *Deviant Behaviour* (7th ed.). Pearson Education.

Uddin, R., Burton, N., Maple, M., Khan, S., & Khan, A. (2019). Suicidal ideation, suicide planning, and suicide attempts among adolescents in 59 low-income and middle-income countries: A population-based study. *The Lancet Child & Adolescent Health, 3*(4), 223–233. https://doi.org/10.1016/S2352-4642(18)30403-6

Van Orden, K., Witte, T., Cukrowicz, K., Braithwaite, S., Selby, E., & Joiner Jr., T. (2010). The interpersonal theory of suicide. *Psychological Review, 117*(2), 575–600. https://doi.org/10.1037/a0018697

Vawda, N. (2012). Associations between family suicide and personal suicidal behaviour among youth in KwaZulu-Natal, South Africa. *South African Family Practice, 54*(3), 244–249. https://doi.org/10.1080/20786204.2012.10874222

Wanyoike, B. W. (2015). Suicide among university students in Kenya: Causes, implications and intervention. *Journal on Language, Technology and*

Entreprenuership in Africa, 6(1), 35–53. Retrieved from https://www.ajol. info/index.php/jolte/article/view/125003

World Health Organization. (2016). *Preventing suicide: A community engagement toolkit.* Geneva: WHO Press. Retrieved February 17, 2017, from http://www.who.int/mental_health/suicide-prevention/en/

World Health Organization. (2018). *National suicide prevention strategies: Progress, examples and indicators.* WHO Press.

Woznica, J., & Shapiro, J. (1990). An analysis of adolescent suicide attempts: The expendable child. *Journal of Pediatric Psychology, 15*, 789–796. https://doi.org/10.1093/jpepsy/15.6.789

Zhang, J. (2005). Conceptualizing a Strain theory of suicide. *Chinese Mental Health Journal, 19*(11), 778–782. Retrieved from https://www.researchgate.net/publication/281399869_Conceptualizing_a_strain_theory_of_suicide_review

Zhang, J., & Lester, D. (2008). Psychological tensions found in suicide notes: A test for the strain theory of suicide. *Archives of Suicide Research, 12*(1), 67–73. https://doi.org/10.1080/13811110701800962

Zhang, J., & Song, Z. (2006). A preliminary test of the Strain theory of suicide. *Chinese Journal of Behavioral Medical Science, 15*(6), 487–489.

Zhang, J., & Tao, M. (2013). Relative deprivation and psychopathology of Chinese college students. *Journal of Affective Disorders, 150*(3), 903–907. https://doi.org/10.1016/j.jad.2013.05.013

3

Perspectives on the Violent Nature of Crime Victimisation in South Africa

Johan van Graan

Introduction

According to the national statistics (South Africa, 2019a) on violent crimes, which include murder, attempted murder, rape, assault with the intent to inflict grievous bodily harm, robbery with aggravating circumstances, robbery at residential premises and motor vehicle hijacking, the daily average of crimes in 2018–2019 was 58 murders; 53 attempted murders; 114 rapes; 468 assaults with the intent to inflict grievous bodily harm; 384 robberies with aggravating circumstances; 61 households robberies; and 44 motor vehicle hijacking. Media headlines such as the ones below constantly remind South Africans of the risks and dangers associated with living in a country that has reached pandemic levels of violent crime victimisation:

J. van Graan (✉)
Department of Police Practice, University of South Africa,
Pretoria, South Africa
e-mail: vgraajg@unisa.ac.za

© The Author(s), under exclusive license to Springer Nature Switzerland AG 2021
H. C. O. Chan, S. Adjorlolo (eds.), *Crime, Mental Health and the Criminal Justice System in Africa*, https://doi.org/10.1007/978-3-030-71024-8_3

Murders 'leave South Africa cold'. (Underhill & Rawoot, 2011)

Exposure to violent crime is taking its toll on mental health, say experts. (Masweneng, 2020)

Aussie travel advisory paints bleak picture of crime and violence in SA. (Saal, 2018)

Crime: We are under siege. (Koko, 2019)

SA tormented by violence. (Gumede, 2018)

SA has become a war zone. (Mkhwanazi, 2018)

The frequency of violence and crime is a major challenge for South Africa (SA), and the annual national crime statistics signify that the state's responsibility of guaranteeing every citizen's safety is far from being realised. There is communal unease about the violent nature of crime in SA, as well as the constant snowballing numbers of crime, which places an enormous burden on the resources of the judiciary. The purpose of this chapter is to provide perspectives on the violent nature of crime victimisation in SA by providing insight into why commentators often remark on the high frequency of violent crime in SA and regularly describe SA as one of the most violent countries and as a country that has a subculture of violence and delinquency. It is therefore important to explore the violent nature of crime victimisation in SA by asking, first, why crime is so violent in the country and, second, whether it can be accepted that SA is one of the most violent countries in the world and has a subculture of violence and criminality. In order to understand SA's high levels of crime and violence, this chapter provides perspectives on the basis of the context in which crime and violence take place.

Historical Context of Crime and Violence in South Africa

In order to contextualise the violent nature of criminal victimisation in South African, it is important to provide a historical perspective on crime and violence in the country. The question of what factors contribute to the excessive levels of crime and violence in SA should also be explored. According to Gould (2014), one should look back on the country's (political) past to comprehend the scope of violence and crime in SA. Gould cites the manner in which SA has managed its fierce history; an increase in hardship and disparity; and a lack of faith in and regard for the law as principal causes of excessive violence and crime in the country. According to a study by the Centre for the Study of Violence and Reconciliation (CSVR) (2007) on the reasons for and the nature of violent crime in SA, apartheid[1] appears to be one of the primary promoters of the excessive degree of violent crime. The CSVR, in its study, examined government rules in terms of which many youths and adolescent men were subjected to degrading police provocation and a violent penitentiary structure during apartheid as a cause of violent crime in the country. Rules and regulations were also opposed by the government backing of township violence in that period. These distinctively South African problems encouraged a culture of violence. The CSVR furthermore found doubtful frames of mind concerning crime and the law, and the normalisation and prevalent acceptance of violence, to be significant factors in violent crime. Referring to additional explanations for crime and violence in SA, the CSVR, in its study, also determined that the fundamental dilemma of crime in SA is its subculture of violence and criminality. This subculture is exemplified by young men who are "invested in a criminal identity and engaged in criminal careers".

Does SA have a culture of violence? SaferSpaces (2020), an electronic information-sharing and networking portal for community safety and violence and crime prevention experts from government, civil society and the research community in SA, answers this question by explaining that

---

[1] A system of decree that defended enforced separation of diverse ethnic groups against non-white inhabitants of SA (History, 2020) from 1948 until the early 1990s.

many researchers specialising in the topic of violence in SA agree that the predicament of violence and crime in the country largely involves a culture of violence, which has to be perceived and apprehended against the background of a very violent history. However, what does a culture of violence mean? SaferSpaces explains that a culture of violence speaks of a greater trend than normal within a particular society to resort to the use of violence in daily life, which does not mean that South African society has a violent moral fibre but that it views violence as tolerable overall, perhaps since South Africans observe, commit and are the victims of violence more frequently than people in many other countries. A culture of violence means that the majority of South Africans grow up and live in a milieu in which violence has become a "norm" to some degree. SaferSpaces furthermore explains that when violence is standardised in a civilisation, some forms of violence turn out to be more universal. These forms of violence include:

- intrafamilial violence, violence between parents and violence of parents towards their children;
- the idolisation of violence;
- violence as a way of managing thoughts of subordination or creating a sense of belonging, for instance, to a gang;
- violence committed by men against girls and women as part of male identity; and
- the standardisation of political violence.

Contact crimes are, by description, crimes that typically happen because of values held by communities, families and individuals and that are related to the use of physical violence to resolve disagreements and domestic violence as a way of proclaiming power. South Africa is a country where much of the male populace traditionally connected in a violent and militarised setting. It is also frequently seen as customarily appropriate to use violence to settle disputes and to impose discipline. Additionally, strong, hostile and competitive masculinity is encouraged and "softness" is looked down upon. Because of situations such as these, numerous South Africans practise a "culture of violence" or, as a minimum, settle for violence as unavoidable under specific conditions (SaferSpaces, 2020).

The study of violence in SA demonstrates that socio-economic disparity, unfulfilled machismo and an absence of social unity link and intersect to propel violence, particularly in association with alcohol and firearms. Inequality, demonstrated by exhibitions of prosperity alongside hardship, high unemployment, gender standards that are demanding to meet in view of a shortage of resources and life possibilities, divided societies and competition for resources generate the settings that facilitate violence. Collectively, these factors intensify the possibility of murder, gender-based violence, youth violence, violence against children and combined violence (Brankovic, 2019). The 2020 Global Peace Index (Institute for Economics & Peace, 2020) confirms SA's high unemployment rate of 27%. Acts of violence in the country are mirrored in the extreme degree of violent crime, including rape and murder. However, Lamb and Warton (2016) refer to a study undertaken by Philip Davies and Kristen MacPherson in which they examined why crime is so violent in SA. Davies and MacPherson found that there are several other countries in Africa, and globally, that have similar, and even graver, socio-economic situations than SA, but these countries do not exhibit similar degrees of either crime or violence. Van Wilsem, de Graff, and Wittebrood (2003) are of the view that societies characterised by an uneven dissemination of physical resources are likely to have a high number of motivated offenders.

The Nature and Extent of Violent Crime Experienced by South African Citizens

What makes SA's crime problem particularly daunting is not only the high frequency of crime but also the violent nature of criminal victimisation. Crimes associated with violence against the person are categorised by the South African Police Service (SAPS) as contact crimes, also referred to as crimes against the person.[2] Subcategories of contact crime include

---

[2] Contact crimes refer to crimes where the victims themselves are the targets of violence or where property is targeted and the victims in the vicinity during the commission of the crimes are subjected to threats of violence or the use of violence. These crimes include murder, attempted murder, sexual offences (including rape and sexual assault), assault with the intent to cause grievous bodily harm, common assault, common robbery and aggravated robbery (including carjacking/truck

aggravated robbery and sexual offences. Sexual offences include rape and sexual assault. According to the 2016 Global Peace Index (Institute for Economics & Peace, 2016), SA ranked 10th worst in global violence reduction and 19th worst in relation to safety and security. The country ranked poorly in categories such as the number of violent crimes, forceful demonstrations, murders, undemanding access to weapons and a general perception of criminality. The 2018 Global Peace Index (Institute for Economics & Peace, 2018) listed SA as one of the utmost violent and unsafe locations globally, ranking the country 125th overall out of 163 countries. Despite SA's improvement in the 2020 Global Peace Index rankings to 123rd overall, the country faces numerous difficulties in the safety and security sphere, in particular, a very high murder rate and very high levels of violent crime (Institute for Economics & Peace, 2020). Comparisons between the crime rates of countries present certain challenges and should only be used as general measurements as opposed to precise quantifiable correlations. However, SA surpasses many other countries in respect of the nature and extent of crime.

The number of reported contact crimes experienced by South African households and individuals remains alarmingly high. Indicators of safety and security in SA remain a cause for concern, according to the 2020 Global Peace Index. South Africa competes inadequately in relation to its murder rate, which is the sixth highest globally and the second highest in sub-Saharan Africa, where it only ranks behind the murder rate of Lesotho. The standard murder ratio in sub-Saharan Africa is 9.1 per 100 000 while the murder ratio in SA is 35.9, nearly four times greater than the regional standard. The high degree of contact crime and related violence in SA is mirrored in the total number of violent crimes reported to the SAPS in 2018/2019 (South Africa, 2019a). A total of 21 022 murders, 18 980 attempted murders, 170 979 incidents of assault with the intent to do grievous bodily harm, 16 026 robberies with aggravating circumstances such as carjacking, 22 431 robberies at residential premises (home invasions), 183 cash-in-transit robberies and 52 420 sexual

---

hijacking, house robbery/home invasion, business robbery, robbery of cash in transit and bank robbery). Robbery with aggravating circumstances occurs when a person uses a gun or a weapon to commit a robbery.

offences, of which 41 583 were rapes, were reported to the police in this period. However, it is probable that the real figure of crime is higher than that reported to the police since the Victims of Crime (VOC) report that is extracted from the Governance, Public Safety and Justice (GPSJS) survey for 2018/2019 (South Africa, 2019b), which is based on a sample of 27 071 households, estimates that the number of victims of various types of crime is much higher. The VOC, for example, recorded 183 998 incidences of home invasions, 198 199 carjackings and 97 938 sexual offences.

The extreme degree of crime and violence suffered by SA residents is furthermore reflected in the Mexican Council for Public Security and Criminal Justice 2019/2020 global ranking report (Citizen Council for Public Security and Criminal Justice, 2020). This report disturbingly ranks four SA cities on its list of the 50 most violent cities on the basis of the number of murders reported per 100 000 inhabitants in cities with populations of more than 300 000 and where murder data is made available. The report ranks Cape Town as the eighth most violent city globally and the African continent's most violent city. Nelson Mandela Bay (24th), Durban (35th) and Johannesburg (41st) are the other most violent cities in the world, according to the report. The ongoing violence in Cape Town, mostly gang and drug related, prompted the SA government to deploy the military to hotspot areas in 2020. Moreover, women and children in SA live in persistent anxiety every day and not without reason. The World Health Organisation (WHO) (2018a) estimates that 12.1 in every 100 000 women are victims of femicide (the intentional murder of females (women or girls)) in SA every year, which is five times worse than the global average of 2.6 in every 100 000 women. Only three countries have a higher femicide rate than South Africa, namely, Honduras (32.7 in every 100 000 women), Jamaica (15.5 in every 100 000 women) and Lesotho (15.4 in every 100 000 women).

Risk Factors of Criminal Victimisation and the Perpetration of Violence and Crime in South Africa

Brankovic (2019) observes that numerous risk factors converge in distinctive respects, conditional on circumstances, to facilitate violence in SA. In order to prevent violence and deal with its consequences, one should comprehend how these various and overlapping factors combine to bring about violence. Brankovic further explains that while the forms and the levels of violence differ, research indicates that the four risk factors of violence mentioned below represent a series of universal and overlapping risk factors—which Brankovic labels as the drivers of violence in SA. According to Brankovic, the most noteworthy risk factors are socio-economic disparity, aggravated machismo, lack of social unity, and alcohol and firearms. These risk factors are summarised below.

Socio-economic Inequality

Brankovic (2019) regards inequality as "a super-driver of violence" and cites research conducted by Butchart and Engstrom (2002) that shows that lethal violence has a tendency to happen in places with high levels of social and economic inequality, frequently in union with other risk factors. Brankovic (2019) further explains socio-economic inequality as a driver of crime and violence in SA, citing several studies that cast light on these drivers. The studies in question propose that the desperation, embarrassment, remorse and tension related to inequality, limitations on life prospects and constrained resources give rise to violence in SA (Altbeker, 2007; Gilligan, 2000).

Socio-economic inequality is particularly aggravated in the context of high unemployment rates (Philip, Tsedu, & Zwane, 2014). According to the Quarterly Labour Force Survey (QLFS) released by Statistics South Africa, the unemployment rate was 29.1% in the third part of 2019, the highest unemployment level since Statistics South Africa began calculating unemployment by way of the QLFS in 2008 (South Africa, 2019c).

According to Ratele (2008), a situation where SA's male-controlled population do not have the means to play the part of strong breadwinners generates the circumstances for violence. According to Jewkes (2002), poverty amplifies the probability of being both an offender and a victim of gender-based violence, particularly intimate partner violence. Jewkes's finding is highlighted in the annual crime statistics of reported crimes to the SA police in 2018/2019 (South Africa, 2019a), according to which 2 771 women were murdered in SA, meaning, on average, a woman is murdered every three hours. Moreover, more than half of the South African population (55.5%), 30.4 million people, were living in poverty according to the poverty margin of R992 per individual per month in 2015 (South Africa, 2017a). Foster (in Ward, van der Merwe & Dawes 2013) explains that socio-economic exclusion influences the quality of the youth's basic education and their potential to attain tertiary schooling, restricting their life prospects and promoting violence as a manner of ensuring social status and claiming material goods, frequently by way of gang-related events. According to von Holdt (2013), violence, both interpersonal and mutual, can appear as a rightful way of bettering one's economic position in light of others' extravagant exhibitions of affluence.

Gender and Frustrated Masculinity

The second driver of crime and violence in SA, as identified by Brankovic (2019), relates to a populace where authoritative heads of families are regarded highly but inequality restricts resources, causing aggravated masculinity, which can facilitate violence in several respects. Seedat, van Niekerk, Jewkes, Suffla, and Ratele (2009) point out that in SA, men are seven times more likely to be the victims of murder than women, and men are disproportionately the offenders. The highest rate of male murder is among men aged between 15 and 45, when men are most likely to pursue macho ideals. Murders between men usually happen in a milieu of recreation where alcohol is used. In violence between men and women, men are overwhelmingly the offenders. According to Swart, Seedat, and Nel (2018), this gender-based violence typically involves the assertion of supremacy and domination, as in the case of intimate partner violence.

Swart et al. (2018) further indicate that research demonstrates that gender control is a motivation in youth violence, including individual rapes and murders, predominantly for juvenile males in gangs. Brankovic (2019) elucidates that gender roles can drive certain types of group violence. Brankovic (2019) cites research conducted by von Holdt et al. (2011), which found that in protest-related group violence, men count on demonstrations of support and admiration by women to engage in violence. Violent demonstrations are frequently extremely gendered, with men instigating violence while women approve it.

Lack of Social Cohesion

Research conducted by Matzopoulos, Bowman, Mathews, and Myers (2010) shows that a rapid turnover in neighbours, relocation from rural to metropolitan areas and growing poverty—familiar trends in SA—tend to undo community bonds and associations in neighbourhoods, diminishing social unity. Low social unity can be tied to a decreased ability to deal with the pressures of low-income living and high degrees of violence (Matzopoulos et al., 2010). Hirschfield and Bowers (1997) remark that disturbances in social systems, or a shortage of them, may isolate and intensify the likelihood of intimate partner violence among women who are already vulnerable. These factors may also encourage youth to create new social relationships that lead to violence and substance reliance. Brankovic (2019) remarks that, strangely, members of marginalised societies may single out mutual grievances that foster social unity in such a way that it supports violence. For example, research proposes that a consciousness of economic exclusion has steered diverse communities to find a mutual relationship as South Africans and to engage in xenophobic attacks on foreign nationals. The absence of social unity is a multifaceted and, at times, a counterintuitive impetus of violence. According to Mlilo and Misago (2019), 42 reported incidents of xenophobic violence occurred in 2018 alone. A total of 12 people died, 1 145 persons were displaced and 139 businesses were looted in these attacks.

Alcohol and Firearms

Brankovic (2019) emphasises that alcohol and firearms, particularly in sync, are principal forces of both lethal and non-lethal violence. This finding is confirmed by Seedat et al. (2009), who state that more than 50% of murder victims test positive for alcohol, and studies on femicide demonstrate that the majority of both victims and offenders have alcohol in their blood when the crimes are committed. According to the Global Status Report on Alcohol and Health 2018, SA has the fifth highest rate of alcohol use globally (World Health Organisation, 2018b). Firearms were the greatest cause of death among youths in SA between 2001 and 2009, and the rate of women murdered by firearms in the country has been the highest globally (Abrahams, Jewkes, & Mathews, 2010). Recent research conducted by the University of Washington's Institute for Health Metrics and Evaluation indicates the number of registered mortalities ascribed to firearms throughout the world in 2016 (The Global Burden of Disease 2016 Injury Collaborators, 2018). South Africa ranks high on this list—12th place—with Ethiopia (13th place) being the only other African country ranked in the top 20. According to this research, 3 740 mortalities were ascribed to firearms in SA, resulting in 6.9 deaths per 100 000 people. Matzopoulos, Truen, Bowman, and Corrigall (2014) found that the combination of alcohol and firearms, together with glamorised masculinity in SA's male-controlled milieu, meaningfully increases the probability of several forms of violence.

Willman, Gould, Newham, and Puerto Gomez (2018) also explain risk factors of criminal victimisation and the perpetration of violence and crime in SA, observing that SA's present violence cannot be described on the basis of one particular aspect or event. They refer to the environmental structure, the most universally applied model to understand risk factors of violence, which theorises violence as the result of a range of unified factors at the individual, interpersonal, community and societal levels. Mathews et al. (2016), the WHO (2013), Jewkes, Sikweyiya, Dunkle, and Morrell (2015) and Machisa, Jewkes, Morna, and Rama (2011) summarise these four interrelated risk factors at each level as follows.

At the *individual level*, risk factors include observation of violence in the home or community; values that tolerate interpersonal violence; poverty; age; gender; and alcohol or drug use. Willman et al. (2018) explain that, at the individual level, directly suffering or observing violence in the home is a significant risk factor for developing into a victim or an offender in future. According to the WHO (2013), gender furthermore influences vulnerability: men and boys are more prone to committing violence or to being injured or murdered while partaking in a violent event, whereas women and girls are more prone to becoming victims of violence committed by a family member or an intimate companion. Willman et al. (2018) found that poverty enhances exposure to violence and makes it more challenging for the victims and their families to manage its effects.

At the *relationship level*, risk factors comprise male-controlled or physically violent family settings and substance use by parents. Willman et al. (2018) state that at the family level, constructive and safe relations between children and their guardians are crucial to social and physical growth and the establishment of fundamental protective qualities as opposed to violence. Willman et al. (2018) identify key risk factors for being victimised, namely, substance abuse in the home, a disorderly family composition, imprisonment of a family member and a family philosophy of punitive punishment or one where disagreements are frequently settled with violence.

At the *community level*, risk factors include weak policing; access to firearms, drugs and alcohol; poverty; and tolerance of interpersonal violence. Machisa et al. (2011) and Mathews et al. (2016) found that environmental factors, such as the accessibility of weapons, drugs and alcohol, encourage proneness to violence at the community level. Mathews et al. (2016) found that access to alcohol seems to be a significant risk factor in relation to several forms of violence, referring to one assessment that indicated that children who had been subjected to adults abusing alcohol were at an increased risk of being victimised or of committing violence if they, too, used alcohol. According to the 2018/2019 crime statistics for SA (South Africa, 2019a), gang-related violence was the second most causative factor of murder in the country, with 1 120 incidents. The majority of these incidences occurred in the Western Cape, which is notorious for its gang-related violence. More murder victims were murdered with firearms (7 156 incidents) than any other instrument.

At the *societal level*, risk factors comprise insufficient laws regulating firearms; rules that uphold disparity or bias founded on race or gender; a culture of male sexual privilege; and pro-violence standards. At the societal level, SA ranks as the country with the highest inequality globally (Brankovic, 2019). According to the findings of a report by the CSVR (2007) on the reasons behind and the nature of violent crime in SA, the high level of inequality in the country promotes crime and violence. In 2008, the wealthiest 10% of families in SA earned almost 40 times more than the poorest 50%. According to transnational research, populations with high levels of disparity are likely to have high levels of violence—a sign that inequality is a significant driver of crime and violence. In addition, according to the World Inequality Database (2018), the upper 1% of South African earners are paid nearly 20% of all income in the country, while the upper 10% are paid 65% of all revenue in the country. The remaining 90% of South African earners receive merely 35% of all income in the country.

South Africans' Perceptions and Experiences of Crime and Violence

Crime and violence have dreadful consequences for family life, community unison, the effective performance and reliability of the economy and public health results. The present crime situation significantly contributes to an atmosphere of distress and anxiety among SA citizens, which constrains individuals and families' participation in daily activities. Direct experiences of being subjected to crime or anxiety over the risk of falling victim to crime result in high levels of fear. The Victims of Crime Survey 2016/2017 (South Africa, 2017b) shows that, owing to the fear of crime, most families were prevented from going to open areas (31.5%), letting children play in their neighbourhood (19.9%) and walking to town (15.0%). About 13.9% of families with children did not permit their children to walk to school owing to the fear of crime.

SaferSpaces (2020) indicates that a lack of safety in public areas and within societies severely influences the movement and quality of life of residents and their prospects to play a part in public life and progressive activities. Every year that violence persists, the number of South Africans who suffer and witness violence increases. While these figures demonstrate that the degree of violence and crime in SA is higher than what is encountered in many other countries, one cannot ascertain accurate figures of violence in SA owing to challenges such as underreporting. According to SaferSpaces (2020), the available data suggests that a considerable effort is required to reduce crime and violence and to increase peoples' sense of safety, beginning with recognising what circumstantial dynamics specific to SA could make its residents more likely to act in an unlawful or violent manner. The following verbatim narratives summarise SA citizens' feelings of safety and security:

> It is unfortunate that we have to live in a fortress, but we are forced to do so given the high crime rate in the country. I travel with two bodyguards all the time and there is substantial cost involved.
> Vivian Reddy, businessman, August 2006 (South African Crime Quotes, 2006)

> The sheer arrogance and excessive force used by gangsters in heists has had a devastating impact on ordinary people's feelings of safety and security. People feel vulnerable, not least because the underpaid police seem incapable of combating the criminals.
> Fred Bridgland, 9 August 2006 (South African Crime Quotes, 2006)

> Whatever the police or politicians may tell us, this is a violent and threatening place. Living here is dangerous.
> Peter Bruce, editor of *Business Day*, 9 August 2006 (South African Crime Quotes, 2006)

Everyone in SA is influenced by violent crime, and the result of this is an awareness of uncertainty that arises from living in fear, regardless of status, gender or ethnic group. All ethnic groups and classes in SA are impacted by crime (Silber & Geffen, 2009). The victimisation of people and the commission of crime and violence in SA are not restricted to specific groups of society. The following violent crimes received a great deal of attention in local and international media and are testimony to crime and violence across societal class categories in SA.

The "Blade Runner" Killer

Oscar Pistorius, a former professional Paralympic sprinter and international champion, was found guilty and convicted in 2015 for fatally shooting his girlfriend, model Reeva Steenkamp, at his residence on 14 February 2013. Pistorius had shot four rounds through a locked bathroom door, wounding Steenkamp three times. He received a prison sentence of 13 years and 5 months for murder. Pistorius's trial and conviction for Steenkamp's murder attracted international attention. An American entertainment channel made a movie, *Oscar Pistorius: Blade Runner Killer*, about the Pistorius case.

Cold-blooded Axe Family Murderer: The Van Breda Case

On 27 January 2015, Martin van Breda, the managing executive of the Australian division of a real estate business, his wife, Teresa, and their son, Rudi, were discovered murdered in their family residence in a luxury residential golf estate in Stellenbosch, SA. They had been murdered with an axe. Their daughter, Marli, was in a life-threatening condition, suffering from severe head wounds. The family's youngest son, Henri, only had minor cuts. On 21 May 2018, Henri was found guilty on three charges of murder, a charge of attempted murder and a charge of defeating the ends of justice. He was sentenced to three life terms' imprisonment for the massacres of his mother, father and brother, 15 years for attempted murder on his sister and an additional 12 months for obstruction of justice.

Devil in Disguise: The Karabo Mokoena Murder

Sandile Mantsoe was sent to prison for 32 years for the murder of his ex-girlfriend, Karabo Mokoena. A pedestrian discovered Mokoena's burnt body in April 2017. Mantsoe confessed that he had burnt Mokoena's body using pool acid, petrol and a tyre.

Killer Husband: The Susan Rohde Case

Jason Rohde, chief executive officer of a high-end real estate business and millionaire property mogul, was handed an 18-year sentence for killing his wife, Susan, in 2016 and five years for tampering with the crime scene to make it look like she had committed suicide. Susan's naked body was found in the bathroom of the couple's hotel room with the cord of her curling iron wrapped around her neck.

The Victims Behind South Africa's Crime Statistics

South Africa has one of the world's most advanced legal frameworks relating to the constitutional rights of and assistance offered to victims of crime. However, the relentless escalation of crime and violence in SA proves that intensifying legislation is important but not enough for improving public safety and security. South Africans have high rates of exposure to traumatic events, with specific reference to violent crime victimisation, whether by means of direct exposure as crime victims or by means of indirect exposure as witnesses of crimes or through hearing about crimes from others. Violent crime and the accompanying trauma affect communities across all social-economic spectrums since practically all communities in the country are affected or hypothetically affected by crime. All communities are vulnerable to the physical, emotional and psychological suffering brought about by crime. Crime victimisation is a frightening and often tragic part of life for South Africans. The lives of ordinary people—people who kiss their families goodbye as they walk out the front door to go to work, to drop off their children at school, to open up a restaurant or to enjoy a holiday—change instantly when they become victims of violent crime.

The nature and the magnitude of criminality and violence in SA have caught the imagination of movie directors. The following narrative from a scene from *Tsotsi*,[3] a South African film nominated for an Academy award, depicts the brutal reality of violent crime in SA (Carroll, 2006):

> Rain hammers down on a Johannesburg night as a woman pulls up outside a suburban house, steps from her car, the engine running, and rings the bell. A man breaks cover from bushes across the street. He slides into the vehicle and begins to reverse. The woman whirls around and screams—her baby is in the back seat. She lunges for the driver's door. The thief points his revolver and fires. A bullet enters the mother's stomach and she collapses onto the kerb. Her car and baby vanish into the night.

A carjacking survivor summarises his ordeal as follows:

> It was an ordinary day for me, I was on my way to work around 5 am. It was bright outside and as I reversed from the garage, I noticed a car pull up at the stop street behind me. I waited in the driveway for them to take off, but they did not. I assumed they were courteous and were letting me drive off first. As I reversed onto the road, they began driving forward as well. The next thing I saw was three men get out of the vehicle and run towards mine. My mind was blank, I did not realise what was happening. The men pointed a firearm at my window and asked me to get out of the car. They ransacked my pockets and pushed me into the back seat and asked me to put my head between my legs. A road which I travelled on for years seemed so different. All I could think of was my family and that I might never see them again. The men kept pushing the gun against my head and asking me for my bank pin number, which I gave. (Naicker, 2017)

A restaurant manager describes his experience of crime and violence in SA as follows:

---

[3] A *tsotsi* is a young criminal, especially one from an informal South African township area.

I remember it was [on a] Sunday. It was cleaning day. It was just before my 25th birthday. I was the manager at Dros [Restaurant]. People were coming into the restaurant. I was saying hello to them. The robbers were among them.

Munyaradzi 'Tom' Sundawo, robbery survivor (Hosken, 2017)

The robbers forced him to his knees before one of them shot him in the head. Three weeks later, he woke up in hospital, unable to speak or move.

Conclusion

This chapter presented and discussed perspectives on the violent nature of crime victimisation in SA by providing insight into why commentators often remark on the high frequency of violent crime in SA and regularly describe SA as one of the most violent countries and as a country that has a subculture of violence and delinquency. The exploration of perspectives on the violent nature of crime victimisation in South Africa presents a selection of key findings. These findings are based on a review of existing knowledge and evidence, which includes, in particular, official South African police crime statistics, world-leading measurements of global peacefulness, national surveys related to crime and crime victims, global safety and security indexes, global rankings on crime and violence, global statistics on mortality attributed to firearms, narratives summarising SA citizens' feelings of safety and security, and accounts of the lived experiences of survivors of violent crimes in SA.

The following key findings are highlighted: First, based on the official crime statistics on violent crimes committed in the country, it is evident that the degree of violence and crime in SA is higher than what is normally experienced internationally. SA outperforms many other countries, not only in sub-Saharan Africa but also elsewhere in the world, as far as the degree of violence and crime is concerned. The 2020 Global Peace Index (Institute for Economics & Peace, 2020) confirms that South Africa surpasses many countries in respect of criminality and associated violence—countries such as Peru, Kosovo, Ecuador, Tunisia, Lesotho, Mozambique, China, Uganda, El Salvador, Thailand, Algeria, the United

States of America and Burkina Faso. It is therefore no surprise that four South African cities are included on a list of the 50 most violent cities in the world, which are selected on the basis of the number of murders reported. Second, it was further elucidated that the nature and extent of crime and violence in the country influence citizens' well-being and have an overwhelming effect on the social structure of communities. The present degree of crime and violence considerably contributes to citizens' opinions of fear and anxiety resulting from crime and violence. Third, SA's violent history, coupled with people's mistrust in and disregard for the rule of law, contributes to the continuous excessive levels of crime and violence. Fourth, numerous risk factors, including, socio-economic inequality, gender and frustrated masculinity, lack of social cohesion, and alcohol and firearms combine in distinctive respects, conditional on circumstances, to stimulate crime and violence in SA. Given SA's high unemployment rate, socio-economic inequality and poverty increase the likelihood that an individual will either become an offender or a victim of crime and violence, particularly in association with alcohol and firearms.

Though this finding does not suggest that the general South African public has a deep-rooted violent character, it does suggest that South African citizens, to some extent, have become accustomed to the high degree of habitual crime and violence. This phenomenon could be ascribed to the fact that South Africans are witnesses, perpetrators and victims of crime and associated violence more frequently than people in many other countries. Based on the national crime statistics and international crime and violence surveys and indexes, it can be accepted that SA is one of the most violent countries in the world. A large part of South African society is characterised by violence and criminality.

In summary, crime and violence in South Africa remain significant challenges. The effective and sustainable prevention of crime and violence is not the sole responsibility of the SAPS. Crime and violence require a comprehensive, proactive, multifaceted strategy. Recommendations on a viable approach that should be adopted to mitigate crime and violence, with a view to creating an environment of assurance and peace, relate to socio-economic inequality, the rule of law, police–community cooperation and firearms. These recommendations are not all-encompassing, but they could promote increased knowledge of crime and violence. Socio-economic inequality, resulting from factors such as the high unemployment rate, should be addressed, and there should be an emphasis on persistent employment creation and implementation systems. The rule of law should be instilled in citizens and meticulously implemented by the criminal justice system. There should be a renewed focus on police–community cooperation, and practical partnerships should be established to address crime and violence. South Africa's high rate of mortalities ascribed to firearms calls for stricter regulation of laws and stringent penalties for perpetrators.

References

Abrahams, N., Jewkes, R., & Mathews, S. (2010). Guns and gender-based violence in South Africa. *South African Medical Journal, 100*(9), 586–588. Retrieved from https://journals.co.za/docserver/fulltext/m_samj/100/9/m_samj_v100_n9_a20.pdf?expires=1593264806&id=id&accname=guest&checksum=C2067B9027D348D3372E31DAC4C99306

Altbeker, A. (2007). *A Country at war with itself: South Africa's crisis of crime.* Jonathan Ball.

Brankovic, J. (2019). *What drives violence in South Africa? Research brief.* Centre for the Study of Violence and Reconciliation.

Butchart, A., & Engstrom, K. (2002). Sex- and age-specific relations between economic development, economic inequality and murder rates in people aged 0–24 years: A cross-sectional analysis. *Bulletin of the World Health Organization, 80*(10), 797–805. Retrieved from https://pubmed.ncbi.nlm.nih.gov/12471400/

Carroll, R. (2006). Carjacking: The everyday ordeal testing South Africa. Retrieved June 12, 2020, from https://www.theguardian.com/world/2006/mar/02/film.oscars2006

Centre for the Study of Violence and Reconciliation. (2007). *The violent nature of crime in South Africa. A concept paper for the Justice, Crime Prevention and Security Cluster.* Centre for the Study of Violence and Reconciliation.

Citizen Council for Public Security and Criminal Justice. (2020). *Ranking newsletter 2019 of the 50 most violent cities in the world.* Citizen Council for Public Security and Criminal Justice.

Foster, D. (2013). Gender, class, 'race' and violence. In *Youth violence: Sources and solutions in South Africa*. University of Cape Town Press.

Gilligan, J. (2000). Violence in public health and preventive medicine. *The Lancet, 355*(9217), 1802–1804. https://doi.org/10.1016/S0140-6736(00)02307-2

Gould, C. (2014). Comment: Why is crime and violence so high in South Africa? Retrieved August 9, 2016, from https://africacheck.org/2014/09/17/comment-why-is-crime-and-violence-so-high-in-south-africa-2/.

Gumede, W. (2018). *SA tormented by violence*. Pressreader. Retrieved from https://www.pressreader.com/south-africa/the-star-south-africa-late-edition/20181218/281848644703982

Hirschfield, A., & Bowers, K. J. (1997). The effect of social cohesion on levels of recorded crime in disadvantaged areas. *Urban Studies, 34*(8), 1275–1295. https://doi.org/10.1080/0042098975637

History. (2020). Apartheid. *History*. Retrieved from https://www.history.com/topics/africa/apartheid

Hosken, G. (2017). 'I survived': The people behind the crime stats tell their stories. *Timeslive*. Retrieved from https://www.timeslive.co.za/news/south-africa/2017-10-25-i-survived-the-people-behind-the-crime-stats-tell-their-stories/

Institute for Economics & Peace. (2016). *Global Peace Index 2016: Measuring peace in a complex world*. Sydney, June 2016. Retrieved from https://reliefweb.int/sites/reliefweb.int/files/resources/GPI%202016%20Report_2.pdf

Institute for Economics & Peace. (2018). *Global Peace Index 2018: Measuring peace in a complex world*. Vision of Humanity. Retrieved from http://vision-ofhumanity.org/reports

Institute for Economics & Peace. (2020). *Global Peace Index 2020. Measuring peace in a complex world*. Sydney, June 2020. Retrieved from http://visionof-humanity.org/app/uploads/2020/06/GPI_2020_web.pdf

Jewkes, R. (2002). Intimate partner violence: Causes and prevention. *The Lancet, 359*(9315), 1423–1429. https://doi.org/10.1016/S0140-6736(02)08357-5

Jewkes, R., Sikweyiya, Y., Dunkle, K., & Morrell, R. (2015). Relationship between single and multiple perpetrator rape perpetration in South Africa: A comparison of risk factors in a population-based sample. *BMC Public Health, 15*(616). https://doi.org/10.1186/s12889-015-1889-9

Koko, K. (2019). Crime: We are under siege. *Pressreader*. Retrieved from https://www.pressreader.com/south-africa/the-star-south-africa-late-edition/20190913/281509342885939

Lamb, G., & Warton, G. (2016). *Why is crime in South Africa so violent? Updated rapid evidence assessment on violent crime in South Africa.* Safety and Violence Initiative, University of Cape Town. https://doi.org/10.13140/RG.2.2.10212.88969

Machisa, M., Jewkes, R., Morna, C. L., & Rama, K. (2011). *The war at home: Gender based violence indicators project.* Gender Links and South African Medical Research Council.

Masweneng, K. (2020, January 4). Exposure to violent crime is taking its toll on mental health, say experts. *Timeslive.* Retrieved from https://www.timeslive.co.za/news/south-africa/2020-01-03-exposure-to-violent-crime-is-taking-its-toll-on-sas-mental-health-say-experts/

Mathews, S., Govender, R., Lamb, G., Boonzaier, F., Dawes, A., Ward, C., et al. (2016). *Towards a more comprehensive understanding of the direct and indirect determinants of violence against women and children in South Africa with a view to enhancing violence prevention.* Safety and Violence Initiative, University of Cape Town.

Matzopoulos, R., Bowman, B., Mathews, S., & Myers, J. (2010). Applying upstream interventions for interpersonal violence prevention: An uphill struggle in low- to middle-income contexts. *Health Policy, 97*(1), 62–70. https://doi.org/10.1016/j.healthpol.2010.03.003

Matzopoulos, R. G., Truen, S., Bowman, B., & Corrigall, J. (2014). The cost of harmful alcohol use in South Africa. *South African Medical Journal, 104*(2), 127–132. https://doi.org/10.7196/SAMJ.7644

Mkhwanazi, S. (2018, September 12). SA has become a war zone. *Pretoria News.* Retrieved from https://www.iol.co.za/pretoria-news/sa-has-become-a-war-zone-17023199

Mlilo, S., & Misago, J. P. (2019). *Xenophobic violence in South Africa: 1994–2018. An overview.* African Centre for Migration & Society, University of the Witwatersrand.

Naicker, K. (2017). Hijacking survivor speaks of his ordeal. *News24.* Retrieved from https://www.news24.com/news24/southafrica/local/hillcrest-fever/hijacking-survivor-speaks-of-his-ordeal-20170509

Philip, K., Tsedu, M., & Zwane, M. (2014). *The impacts of social and economic inequality on economic development in South Africa.* New York, NY: United National Development Programme.

Ratele, K. (2008). Masculinity and male mortality in South Africa. *African Safety Promotion: A Journal of Injury and Violence Prevention, 6*(2), 19–41. Retrieved from https://0-journals-co-za.oasis.unisa.ac.za/docserver/fulltext/

safety/6/2/safety_v6_n2_a2.pdf?expires=1593885571&id=id&accnam
e=58010&checksum=FA79FACCED82D7123251F546A4FEAADA

Saal, P. (2018, April 18). Aussie travel advisory paints bleak picture of crime and violence in SA. *Pressreader*. Retrieved from https://www.pressreader.com/south-africa/the-herald-south-africa/20180418/281616715960265

SaferSpaces. (2020). What is the situation in South Africa? *Safer Spaces*. Retrieved from https://www.saferspaces.org.za/understand/entry/what-is-the-situation-in-south-africa

Seedat, M., van Niekerk, A., Jewkes, R., Suffla, S., & Ratele, K. (2009). Health in South Africa 5: Violence and injuries in South Africa: Prioritising an agenda for prevention. *The Lancet, 374*(9694), 1011–1022. https://doi.org/10.1016/S0140-6736(09)60948-X

Silber, G., & Geffen, N. (2009). Race, class and violent crime in South Africa: Dispelling the 'Huntley thesis'. *SA Crime Quarterly, 30*, 35–43. https://doi.org/10.17159/2413-3108/2009/v0i30a897

South Africa. (2017a). *Poverty on the rise in South Africa*. Department Statistics South Africa. Retrieved from http://www.statssa.gov.za/?p=10334

South Africa. (2017b). *Victims of Crime Survey 2016/17*. Statistics South Africa.

South Africa. (2019a). *Annual Crime Statistics 2018/2019*. Statistics South Africa. Government Printer.

South Africa. (2019b). *Governance, Public Safety and Justice Survey (GPSJS) Victims of Crime Report 2018/2019*. Department Statistics South Africa.

South Africa. (2019c). *Unemployment rises slightly in third quarter of 2019*. Department Statistics South Africa.

South African Crime Quotes. (2006). Retrieved from https://www.southafrica.to/people/Quotes/crime.php

Swart, L.-A., Seedat, M., & Nel, J. (2018). The situational context of adolescent murder victimization in Johannesburg, South Africa. *Journal of Interpersonal Violence, 33*(4). Retrieved from https://link.gale.com/apps/doc/A526565638/AONE?u=usa_itw&sid=AONE&xid=b0ded79f

The Global Burden of Disease 2016 Injury Collaborators. (2018). Global mortality from firearms, 1990–2016. *JAMA, 320*(8), 792–814. https://doi.org/10.1001/jama.2018.10060

Underhill, G., & Rawoot, I. (2011, June 2). Murders 'leave South Africa cold'. *Mail & Guardian*. Retrieved from https://mg.co.za/article/2011-05-27-murders-leave-south-africa-cold/

Van Wilsem, J., de Graff, N. D., & Wittebrood, K. (2003). Cross-national differences in victimization: Disentangling the impact of composition and context. *European Sociological Review, 19*(2), 125–142. Retrieved from https://0-academic-oup-com.oasis.unisa.ac.za/esr/article/19/2/125/537105

von Holdt, K. (2013). South Africa: The transition to violent democracy. *Review of African Political Economy, 40*(138), 589–604. https://doi.org/10.108 0/03056244.2013.854040

von Holdt, K., Langa, M., Molapo, S., Mogapi, N., Ngubeni, K., Dlamini, J., et al. (2011). *The smoke that calls: Insurgent citizenship, collective violence and the struggle for a place in the new South Africa.* Centre for the Study of Violence and Reconciliation (CSVR) and the Society, Work and Development Institute (SWOP), University of Witwatersrand.

Willman, A., Gould, C., Newham, G., & Puerto Gomez, M. (2018). *An incomplete transition: Overcoming the legacy of exclusion in South Africa. Systematic country diagnostic.* World Bank. Retrieved from https://openknowledge. worldbank.org/handle/10986/29793

World Health Organisation. (2013). *Global and regional estimates of violence against women: Prevalence and health effects of intimate partner violence and non-partner sexual violence.* World Health Organisation.

World Health Organisation. (2018a). *Global health estimates 2016: Deaths by cause, age, sex, by country and by region, 2000–2016.* Geneva, Switzerland: World Health Organisation.

World Health Organisation. (2018b). *Global status report on alcohol and health 2018.* Geneva, Switzerland: World Health Organisation.

World Inequality Database. (2018). South Africa: Wealth inequality, South Africa, 1993–2017. *World Inequality Lab.* Retrieved from https://wid.world/ country/south-africa/

4

Hello Pretty, Hello Handsome!: Exploring the Menace of Online Dating and Romance Scam in Africa

Chiedu Eseadi, Chiamaobi Samuel Ogbonna, Mkpoikanke Sunday Otu, and Moses Onyemaech Ede

Introduction

In one of the episodes of the television series *Scorpion*, Leonard, a CIA agent, was arrested for secretly communicating and sending certain potential poisonous gas to his girlfriend, Sima (pseudo name). Sima was a terrorist specialised in romance scams with several security agents as her victims. She tricked Leonard to fall in love with her and then made him steal the gas from the CIA and deliver them to her. Sima convinced him that she is an aid worker with the Yemen government and that the gas

C. Eseadi (✉) • M. S. Otu • M. O. Ede
Department of Educational Foundations, University of Nigeria, Nsukka, Nigeria
e-mail: chiedu.eseadi@unn.edu.ng; mkpoikanke.otu@unn.edu.ng; moses.ede@unn.edu.ng

C. S. Ogbonna
Department of Arts Education, University of Nigeria, Nsukka, Nigeria

© The Author(s), under exclusive license to Springer Nature Switzerland AG 2021
H. C. O. Chan, S. Adjorlolo (eds.), *Crime, Mental Health and the Criminal Justice System in Africa*, https://doi.org/10.1007/978-3-030-71024-8_4

would be used to make pesticide for poor Yemeni farmers. Leonard fell for her love and lies. The love was so real to Leonard that he could not believe he was being played even after being shown overwhelming evidence (Santora, Pearlstein, O'brien, & Moore, 2015). This is usually the sorry state of romance scam victims who usually find it difficult to believe that a relationship they had invested so much in and the trust they strove to build was all a scam. Very few victims of such scam recover from the debilitating psychological challenges.

According to Maslow (1954), our actions are motivated by our desire to satisfy certain needs. The most basic need of man according to Maslow after the physiological needs (food, shelter, air, sleep and others) and the safety needs is the need to love and be loved (not necessarily in a sexual way). This need propels humans to seek for relationships where they will be loved, appreciated and taken care of. Fortunately, the advancement of information and communication technology has provided far greater opportunity and means of meeting our love needs. In contemporary times, people are no longer restricted to their small circle of friends and community to find romantic relationships and partners. There are now social platforms, websites and virtual communities where people could seek out for and easily meet potential dates. This practice has indeed become popular. As noted by Mateo (2020), data from Statista suggested that online dating audience is expected to grow to 37.5 million users by 2023. Also, as predicted by eHarmony, 70% of couples will have started their relationships online by the year 2040.

Unfortunately, with the increasing popularity of online dating, online relationship scammers are equally on the rise. These scammers create fake accounts in the different dating sites as potential relationship seekers. They make their victims believe that they are genuinely in need of a relationship. Then, they try to gain their victim's trust only to have him/her duped eventually. The Federal Trade Commission (FTC) (2019) reported that 21,000 cases of romance scams were recorded with a cumulative financial loss totalling $143 million in the United States in 2018. On the average, each victim lost about $2600, which is seven times higher than any other reported consumer fraud. In 2019, the FTC reported that the total financial loss due to romance scam was $210 million. This represents a six-time increase in financial loss since 2015 (FTC, 2019). Apart from the huge financial loss on the part of the victim, victims are left with the emotional bruise of having lost an apparent real relationship (Whitty & Buchanan, 2012). They may also suffer social stigma for getting involved in such scams (Koon & Yoong, 2013). Although online romance scam is a global phenomenon, however, it does appear that a greater number of these romance scammers originate from Africa (Edwards et al., 2018; Kopp, Layton, Sillitoe, & Gondal, 2015; Park, Jones, McCoy, Elaine Shi, & Jakobsson, 2014). They target lonely, vulnerable and romantic people mostly from Europe and America who are looking for love and companionship. Just recently, *The Nation* newspaper in Nigeria reported that the FBI has declared six Nigerian nationals wanted for alleged internet-related fraud (romance scam) that caused American citizens and businesses over $6 million losses (Abiola, 2020).

On the part of the perpetrators of these crimes, they are driven by greed, the desire to make quick and easy money, and lack of love and empathy. On the part of the victims, they suffer huge financial loss, betrayal, disappointment, stigmatisation, depression, fear and other emotional and psychosocial challenges. This chapter discusses the concept of online dating and romance scam, outlines some platforms for online dating and romance, X-rays the menace of online dating and romance scam, and some mental health challenges experienced by victims of online dating and romance scam. The chapter also pays attention to the tricks used by online romance scammers, strategies for curbing online dating and romance scam, and proffers recommendations for research and policy.

Concept of Online Dating and Romance Scam

Ideally, online dating may be seen as a complement of face-to-face, offline dating. A relationship could be initiated online by two individuals who share common relationship interest. Thanks to dating websites, social media dating apps and even the conventional social media, there are many alternative platforms for people to meet and hit things off romantically, thus breaking the barriers of geographical boundaries. Online dating provides an avenue where people could connect with those they admire (by viewing their profile information) on the internet through dating websites or social networking websites. In the process, a feeling of love and intimacy is developed through frequent chats (and communication), which leads to building a relationship with someone the individual has not physically seen (Jimoh & Kyass, 2018). Such relationships started online could be eventually moved to offline in a situation where the lovers decide to meet in person. On the other hand, lovers who began a relationship offline could sustain their relationship via online dating platforms in a form of 'distance relationship' when it is not possible to meet physically and when physical distance poses a barrier. With online dating often hijacked by scammers, people looking for romantic partners are taken advantage of, often via dating websites, apps or social networking sites by pretending to be potential partners. Their sole intention is to exploit their victims' vulnerabilities and get them to provide money, gifts or personal details. This type of scam is known as romance scam or *catfishing* (Scamwatch, 2020).

How Do Online Romance Scammers Operate?

Scammers normally create fake online profiles on dating websites, but scammers may also use social media profiles or email to make contact designed to lure their victims. These profiles usually have fabricated names, or stolen identities of real, trusted people such as models, military personnel, aid workers or professionals working abroad (Sorell & Whitty, 2019). Having created a catchy profile, they lie in wait for a potential victim. Once a victim is acquired, online dating and romance scammers will express strong emotional feelings for their victims in a relatively short period of time, and will propose to move the relationship away from the dating website to a more private channel, such as phone call and text messaging, email or instant messaging, often with the claim that they want an exclusive relationship with the victim (Whitty, 2013a). At this initial time, scammers maintain frequent and often intense communication with their victims, over periods spanning weeks, months or even years. There is also the possibility of scammers disguising their voices using special phone apps. The overall aim at this stage is to prime their victims, gain the victims' trust and make the victims develop strong emotions and feelings towards the relationship. With time victims are deceived to give away intimate details about themselves, thereby further developing a trusted relationship with the criminal. With time, the other party eventually falls in love with the scammer. To increase their victim's trust, scammers may send the victim gifts to persuade them that the relationship is real. At this point, the scammers may decide to apply the testing-the-water strategy (Whitty & Buchanan, 2015). This strategy involves the scammer requesting for small gifts such as perfume, mobile phone or laptop. When such requests and gifts are granted and received, they present a sign that the victim has developed deep love and trust for the scammer; the scammer will then make requests for small amounts of money, and will proceed to increase to larger amounts of money if the requests are granted.

To continuously extort and scam their victims, scammers will pretend to need the money for some sort of personal emergency. For example, they may feign to be hospitalised or claim to have a severely sick family member who requires urgent medical attention such as an expensive operation, or they may claim some financial misfortune due to an unfortunate run of bad luck such as a failed business, fire disasters or being arrested by security agents. Sometimes, the scammer may also claim that they want to travel to visit the victim, but cannot afford it. Then they request that the victim lend them money to cover flights or other travel expenses. When such money is sent by the victims, the scammers usually invent other stories why they could not travel. These stories are meant to appeal to the victim's emotions who at this point has developed trust, love and strong feelings for the criminal. While some victims may suspect fraud at this point, some remain unsuspecting. The fraud ends only when the victims become aware that they have been scammed and stop to give money. Some victims at this point may suffer a second wave of re-victimisation. According to Whitty (2013a), the second wave occurs when the scammers find new ways to defraud the victim after the victim becomes aware that the relationship was a scam and the criminal is equally aware that the victim knows he/she has been duped.

To depict online romance scammers' operation and how they succeed in scamming their victims, Whitty (2013a) proposed the *scammers persuasive technique model* illustrated below.

In the model presented above, relationship seekers are motivated by the need to find an ideal lover/partner. Scammers prey on this to create profiles that mirror the ideals and desires of these relationship seekers. When victims fall for scammers' phony profiles, they are subsequently groomed; this is the stage that involves getting the victims to fall in love with the scammers. This is followed by the application of the 'foot-in-door technique' or testing the water strategy. Here, the scammer requests for small gifts from the victims. If the victims oblige this request, the scammers enter the crises stage where they cook up emergency situations that would require their victims parting with substantial sum of money. If grooming was very successful, scammers might skip the 'foot-in-door technique' and move on to the crises stage. Victims may be re-victimised or abused sexually in the final stage. The Scammer Persuasive Technique Model was updated in Whitty (2019) to include a 'Human detection of scam vs genuine profiles' stage. This stage comes immediately before the grooming stage. It involves a decision period when potential online scam victims decide whether a particular profile is genuine or fake (belonging to scammers).

Analysis of Some Platforms for Online Dating and Romance

As noted by Orchard (2019), online dating and romance is a computer-mediated dating system to help people find love, and has been in existence since as early as the 1960s and 1970s when computer technology was still at its early stage, mostly in the United States and parts of Northern Europe. With the current advancement in ICTs, several online dating platforms have come into existence and provide platforms where relationship seekers could meet and hook up with potential dates easily. Such platforms include dating websites and relationship application and social networking websites such as Facebook, Skype and LinkedIn (Whitty, 2019). With over 8000 online dating sites globally, and 2500 based in the United States alone as at 2013 (Tracy, 2013), one can only imagine the prevalence and proliferation of online dating and romance today. Because of the popularity of smartphones, many online dating sites provide app-based version of their services for users to access on their smartphones and similar mobile devices.

There are basically two methods through which one can find a romantic partner via online dating platforms (Orchard, 2019). First, users can browse the profiles of potential partners on the site after which they contact the person(s) they find appealing. Second, users may be provided with forms where they are meant to enter their demographic details and preferences, and an algorithm processes this information to generate potential partners. Similar to helping love seekers find potential partners, Finkel et al. (2012) also noted that online dating sites (or apps) generally provide some combination of three broad classes of services: access, communication and matching. Finkel et al. (2012) explain that online dating sites offer users *access* to (exposure to and opportunity to evaluate) potential romantic partners whom they are otherwise unlikely to meet. This is because dating sites basically accumulate thousands and sometimes millions of profiles of potential partners that users can browse, far exceeding what anybody can have access to in the offline world. *Communication* service refers to the choice and opportunity users have to deploy diverse forms of computer-mediated communication (CMC) to interact with specific possible partners on the dating site before meeting physically. Although modes of communication vary reasonably across the different dating sites, generally it is usually asynchronous forms of communication or real-time, synchronous forms of communication, such as chats (either text-based or video). *Matching* service refers to the use of a mathematical algorithm by the dating site to analyse potential partners and suggest a likely compatible pair to a user (see Finkel et al., 2012, for details of the assumptions underlying these matching algorithms). Access and communications services are commonly offered in most dating sites while a few sites provide matching service to their users. Below is a description and categorisation of some platforms for online dating and romance (adapted from Finkel et al., 2012; see Table 4.1).

Table 4.1 Types of dating sites and their distinctive features

Type of site	Distinctive feature	Example sites
General self-selection sites	Users browse profiles of a wide range of partners	Tinder, Coffee Meets Bagel, Badoo, Bumble (female users make the first contact), mamba, etc.
Niche self-selection sites	Users browse profiles of partners from a specific population	Her (for lesbians), Christian Connection, Adam4Adam (for gays), Christian Mingle, Muzmatch (for Muslim women), CompartibleParntners, Gaydar, Manhunt, Jdate (for people with Jewish background), Jswipe, etc.
Family/friend participation sites	Users' family/friends can use the site to play matchmaker for them	Kizmeet, HeartBroker, Ship, etc.
Video-dating sites	Users interact with partners via webcam	SpeedDate, Video dating, WooMe, CooMeet, The Intro, Fliqpic, Meet4u, Mico, etc.
Virtual dating sites	Users create an avatar and go on virtual dates in an online setting	OmniDate, Weopia, VirtualDateSpace
Matching sites using self-reports	Sites use algorithms to create matches based on users' self-report data	EliteSingles, Eharmony, Silver Single, OkCupid, Chemistry, etc.
Matching sites not using self-report	Sites use algorithms to create matches based on non-self-report data	Moonit, Match.com, Our Time, Telegraph Dating, Lumen, Hinge, GenePartner, ScientificMatch, FindYourFaceMate, Ashley Madison, etc.
Sites for arranging group dates	Users propose get-togethers with a group of strangers	Zoosk, Match, Cliq, 3Fun, Cheers, Squad, Instnt, etc.
Sex or hook-up sites	Users meet partners for casual sexual encounters	OnlineBootyCall, iHookup, Tinder, Match, OkCupid, Pure, Clover, 99 Flavor,Cams.com, AdultFriendFinder, etc.

(continued)

Table 4.1 (continued)

Type of site	Distinctive feature	Example sites
Social networking sites	Users can meet friends of friends	Facebook, QQ, Instagram, Twitter, Viber, Sina Weibo, Vkontakte, LinkedIn, etc.
Smartphone apps	GPS-enabled apps inform users of partners in the vicinity	Zoosk, Badoo, Grindr, Happn, Taimi, etc.

Online Dating Process

Ideally, online dating involves multiple processes before two partners would commence a romantic relationship. Finkel et al. (2012) proposed a nine-step prototypical, idealised online dating process. In step 1, a relationship seeker seeks information about one or more online dating site (ODS). Then, in step 2, he/she registers in one or more ODS. In step 3, he/she creates a profile. After this step, he can either browse other users' profiles (step 4). This enables him/her to initiate contact with potential partners in the ODS (step 5) or he receives contact through the ODS (step 6). Step 7 involves engaging in mutual communication (chats) with interested partner. In step 8, the two partners would decide to meet face to face and could finally develop an offline relationship should they find each other desirable (step 9). In the online dating process, relationship seekers could move forward in sequential and logical manner or backwards to previous steps if need be. Although an individual can drop out along the line; this was not captured in the steps.

Menace of Online Dating and Romance Scam

Given the prevalence of online dating and romance scam, it is particularly worrisome since these scams are usually perpetrated using communication channels such as private messaging and emails which may be difficult to trace. This is after victims are usually lured away from the dating sites to a more private platform so as to cover scammers' tracks.

Also, romance scams are on the rise because it is very difficult or almost impossible to detect a fake profile—possibly created by a scammer—in online dating sites. According to a study by Whitty (2019), it was found that in general, online romantic relationship seekers find it difficult to detect scams especially by viewing potential scammers' profile. This makes it easy for the scammer to continue to perpetrate their heinous activities unhindered. Similarly, dating sites appear equally at a loss as to the possible means of curbing the activities of online romance scammers in the dating sites. As reported in *The Telegraph*, many online dating sites are slow to identify the menace of romance scams and are not doing much to prevent their occurrence. Even when scammers are reported, the sites are slow to take action, and often scam accounts are not taken down (Hunt, (2020). It is also very easy for scammers to create a new account under a new identity in case a previous account is blocked. These reasons make the menace of online dating and romance scams real with a number of severe consequences.

First, online relationship scam attacks the very foundation of human relationships, which is based on trust and commitment by breeding mistrust and suspicion among online daters. A relationship seeker who has been scammed in a previous online relationship may find it difficult to trust and love someone (especially on relationship and financial basis) (AnKee & Yazdanifard, 2015; Joomratty, 2019). Such individuals may not be committed to future relationships as they may tend to hold back their feelings and emotions for fear of experiencing another heartbreak or scam. In all, romance scam victims find it difficult maintaining healthy future relationships given the trauma and troubles associated with romance scams (Khader & Yun, 2017). Second, online dating scams may have led to proliferation of (fake) dating sites and apps and possible surge in reported number of (users) accounts in these dating sites. As of 2013, Online Dating Magazine estimated that there are over 2500 online dating services in United States alone, with about 1000 new online dating services opening every year (Zwilling, 2013). It is not impossible that scammers could be creating new dating sites to foster their fraudulent activities (AnKee & Yazdanifard, 2015) in response to the likelihood of switching between dating sites by relationship seekers in search of true lovers. Similarly, the large number of registered accounts found in most dating sites may be due to fraudsters who open multiple accounts to increase their chance of getting victims. This puts genuine users at risk of falling prey to so many existing potentially fake profiles. For example, a popular dating site Badoo (badoo.com) has at present over 479 million registered users worldwide. It is not impossible that a significant number of the user profiles in the site belong to scammers.

Furthermore, the menace of online dating and romance scam has led to adoption of stringent measures for vetting users by some dating sites which may affect the activities of genuine users. For instance, online dating sites may validate users to ensure legitimate use of the service and minimise the ease with which scammers can create fake profiles. Vetting of users may involve the following: checking the language used in the profile, including identification of common phrases, usernames, passwords used by scammers and a preponderance of spelling/grammatical errors; checking of profile pictures to identify usual pictures used by scammers; checking of Internet Protocol (IP) addresses to identify users registering from places/countries linked to scam activity; checking the use of proxy servers and other methods to dodge IP checking; monitoring abnormal behaviour by users within the site, such as the volume of messages sent or responded to, amongst others (Australian Competition and Consumer Commission, 2016). However, vetting systems are not perfect and may sometimes indict genuine users. Such situation may deny the genuine user access to the services of the dating site.

Third, the menace of online dating and relationship scam also present a huge setback to the online dating industry. The online dating business has shown significant financial growth in recent years. In the United Kingdom for instance, the online dating market alone was worth £165 million in 2013, and was predicted to grow by 36.4% to £225 million by 2019 (Kopp, Sillitoe, Gondal, & Layton, 2016). However, investors in the online dating business are at risk of great financial loss as the activities of romance scammers in the dating sites continue to rise, as both present and future relationship seekers could be scared from patronising dating sites. Potential investors may equally be deterred from investing in the industry given the instability caused by online romance scammers.

Already, it is being predicted in some quarters that revenue growth in the industry would slow through 2022 (Brittany, 2018). This might be an indication of the impact of the menace of scammers in the online dating industry. Apart from the threatening financial loss on investors in the online dating industry as a result of the growing activities of online relationship scammers, such fraudulent activities also create an unsafe environment for online relationship seekers as they could be substantially defrauded financially and emotionally. Several research findings acknowledge this two-dimensional loss: financial loss and loss of a relationship, on the part of victims of online romance scam (Finkel et al., 2012; Kopp et al., 2016; Whitty, 2018; Coluccia et al., 2020; Edwards et al., 2018).

Since it appears that online relationship scammers are commonplace, genuine people seeking for love online may suffer discrimination. Studies have significantly linked African countries to online romance scams with target victims coming mainly from America and Europe (Edwards et al., 2018; Rege, 2009; Kopp et al., 2016). Such unsavoury record creates a stereotype which labels any young online love seeker with African background as potential scammer. Such situation encourages discrimination and makes it difficult for genuine love seekers to find a romantic partner in dating sites. This systemic discrimination may not be peculiar to individuals with African origin alone; other special populations or individual in certain profession may be avoided in online dating since scammers are known to pose as such. Moreover, online dating and romance scams perpetrated by some people are due to get-rich-quick syndrome and the eroding spirit of true industriousness. The severe punishment meted for perpetrators of such crimes have not deterred people from indulging in the crime. This is evident in alarming prevalence of the crime among African youths (Edwards et al., 2018). This is particularly worrisome as it showcases the extent African countries have failed to harness and maximise the talents of their youthful population for the growth and development of Africa.

Mental Health Challenges of Online Dating and Romance Scam Victims

Victims of crime in general have been noted to battle mental health challenges associated with the after-effect of the crime experience. In a survey conducted by Dinisman and Moroz (2017) among victims of various crimes, participants were presented with a set of questions on the impact of the crime on their life. They were asked to indicate whether they were negatively affected, positively affected or not affected. It was found that across all crime types, a majority of the participants (83.7%) reported a negative impact on their emotional or psychological wellbeing. Concerning financial fraud victims, Joomratty (2019) examined the impacts of fraud victimisation other than financial impact. The study found profound emotional and psychological impact post victimisation. Specifically, victims suffered shame and embarrassment, distress, sadness and anger. They described their experience as 'devastating', 'heartbreaking' and as a 'nightmare' Joomratty (2019, p. 1106).

Similarly, in their study which sought to examine the typical psychological characteristics of fraud victims in general, and of romance scam victims in particular, Buchanan and Whitty (2014) found that aside from financial loss, romance scam victims experienced significant emotional distress irrespective of whether they lost money or not. Furthermore, in a follow-up study, Whitty and Buchanan (2015) carried out a study titled *The online dating romance scam: The psychological impact on victims—both financial and non-financial*, and specifically examined the psychological impact of the online dating romance scam. The findings revealed that victims suffered a range of emotions such as shame, embarrassment, shock, anger, worry and stress (post-traumatic stress), fear and the feeling of being mentally raped. It was also observed that victims of online romance scam had negative perception about their self-worth, low self-confidence, felt less inclined to be social, and lost trust in other people (Whitty & Buchanan, 2015). Cross (2018) reported that some victims of online romance scam were so depressed that they considered suicide as the only viable option to end their suffering.

Given these findings from previous studies, it is obvious that victims of scams especially online dating and romance scams suffer severe mental health challenge. The present findings may be considered a tip of the iceberg when compared to the actual magnitude of the health challenge faced by victims of romance scams. This is because given the nature of the online romance scam, victim stigmatisation and victim blaming are rife (Joomratty, 2019; Sorell & Whitty, 2019). Some victims were used by the scammers to launder money (Whitty, 2013b), thus, discouraging many victims from speaking up. Therefore, cases involving online romance scams may be highly under-reported, resulting in many victims of romance scams suffering in silence. Also, it is possible that many victims who may be inclined to seek for help may not know where to and how to get such help; further leaving them at great risk. As researchers shine the light on the issue of online dating and dating scams, it is important to highlight the different tricks used by online romance scammers in defrauding their victims.

Some Tricks of Online Dating Scammers

To lure their victims, online romance scammers invent subtle but effective tricks. A common trick is to present ideal profiles reflecting a potential victim's idealised romantic fantasies. According to Whitty (2013a) and Shaari, Kamaluddin, Paizi, and Mohd (2019), scammers' profiles are usually set up using physically attractive and stolen pictures of people. For male (heterosexual) scammers, profile pictures often depict (European or American) men in professional jobs such as the military or a position normally associated with a high level of skill, education and/or status (Whitty, 2013a, 2013b; Shaari et al., 2019). They typically describe themselves as rich with bogus job titles such as 'Chief Engineer', 'Marine Engineer' and 'Electronics Technician' (Archer, 2017). Age in the profile may vary but usually male scammers chose age ranging from early 1940s to late 1950s and may be widowed and with a child (Whitty, 2013b). Such profile descriptions are intended to inspire trust and confidence in potential female victims who are typically attracted to men of high status and in position of authority (Whitty, 2013a). For female scammers, profiles typically contain physically attractive young women (usually not more than 30 years) in need of support; scammers may pose as a student or someone in a low-paying job (e.g. nurse, teacher) (Whitty, 2013b). This makes sense since it has been shown that men are more likely to be attracted by very beautiful ladies (Kenrick, Sadalla, Groth, & Trost, 1990).

Apart from setting up an ideal profile, scammers have also tricked their victims through making marriage proposals or constantly making allusion to the permanency of the relationship (Archer, 2017). This typically comes at a very early stage of the relationship. A possible reason for this tactic is to give the victim a feeling that the relationship has a 'future' and provide him/her with something to hold on to or an emotional prize to be won later in the relationship. Whitty (2013b) likened this to *visceral influences*; victims of scams often experience visceral triggers (provided by the scammers), such as when they focus on the prize and imagine positive future emotional states (Whitty, 2013b). Still at the onset of the relationship, scammers may try to identify existing commonalities between them and their victim and exploit this to gain their victims' trust (Archer, 2017). They may claim to share the same hobbies as the victim, grow up in the same neighbourhood, share the same ethnic nationality, share the same religious affiliation, love the same music or are fans of a particular sport as their victim. This trick works especially in the earliest stages of the relationship as the intention of the scammer at this stage is to build rapport and develop friendship and solidarity with the victim. According to Archer (2017), demonstrating common ground not only helps to achieve consensus between scammers and victims, but also reduce any form of cognitive dissonance between strangers.

Another trick employed by scammers to deceive their victims is the assumption of religious or pious disposition. In their study involving the analysis of 21 scammers-victim correspondence, Koon and Yoong (2013) reported that in order to establish themselves as people with good moral character, scammers tend to present themselves as being religious through the intentional use of religious discourse throughout the correspondence. In conversations, scammers deliberately use religious connotative words such as 'pray', 'praying', 'thank God', 'grace', 'God fearing' (Koon & Yoong, 2013). Therefore, by creating a persona that appears to profess devotion, belief in and fear of 'God', the scammer tricks his target to believe that he cannot perchance harbour evil intentions, hence allaying his target's fears of him being a stranger and possibly a danger (Koon & Yoong, 2013). Another trick scammers use is (fake) storytelling. Scammers are good storytellers. They are likely inclined to weave very emotional stories around their biographies. For instance, to justify why they are widowed they may link their widowhood to past tragedies crafted in an elaborate story depicting death of spouse in car accidents, due to terminal illness or during childbirth (Archer, 2017). These personal stories of the past life of the scammer are emotional traps. The scammers conveniently set these traps to get the victims to open up emotionally, get attached and even feel valued (sharing of personal stories with someone may suggest we value and trust them with our past experiences and secrets). This building of victim's emotion around the scammer is an important part of the victim's grooming process (Witty 2013a, 2013b).

Online relationship scammers can trick their victims into developing a strong emotional bond for them through deliberate and generous use of compliments. This makes the targets feel desirable and special (Koon & Yoong, 2013; Shaari et al., 2019). In their study, Koon and Yoong found that the scammer made effort to develop a strong emotional bond with his target by expressing keen attraction for the target, putting the target as the main priority in his life and also giving compliments to the target (p. 35). It has been shown in previous works (DeLameter & Myers, 2011; Pendell, 2002) that such acts of adoration—giving compliments and praises and by giving assurance that one is special and desirable, could lead to a general good feeling about oneself (the recipient) and could also bring about stronger emotional bond and intimacy between two partners. Therefore, scammers exploit this trick often to get their victims into an emotional trap where they would readily play the scammers' deceitful scripts.

Apart from lavishing praises on their victims, online dating scammers have been known to also trick their targets by presenting scarcity or an emergency or crises. In her study Whitty (2013b) found that for most of the victims who suffered financial loss, at some point during the scam, the scammer came up with an emergency situation which required the victim to send some amount of money urgently with serious consequences for the apparent lover (the scammer) if the victim did not comply with immediate effect. When the victim yields to the initial request for money, scammers continue to invent several crises stories to demand for more money until the victim stops sending any money. The following story presented in Archer (2017) represents a typical emergency situation created by a scammer as narrative by the victim:

[He was] leaving Iran and was flying to Calgary, via Dallas Fort Worth. Because he brought some of his equipment with him, customs in DFW detained him and said that he would need to pay them to bring the equipment to Canada as they said it was 'contraband'. I was given bank accounts in Canada to deposit money into – as the U.S. customs officer had friends in Canadian customs who would help him. Eventually he made it to Calgary and was detained again... He needed more money. After I had paid, a day or two later he contacted me to say they deported him as the money that was paid was not enough.

From the foregoing, we have attempted to highlight some of the tricks online dating and romance scammers employ in order to defraud their victims. The list is not exhaustive; however, they have provided common tricks as contained in existing literature.

Strategies for Curbing Online Dating and Romance Scam

Having identified some of the tricks online dating and relationship scammers employ to scam their victims, in addition to the mental health challenges these pose to their victims, it is important to highlight some possible strategies which could be adopted to curb the activities of online dating and romance scammers. To do this, insight could be drawn from the findings and recommendations of previous studies. For example, Whitty and Buchanan (2012) submitted that an important strategy for combating online dating and romance scam could be to provide more avenues for victims to report the crime or at least make victims more comfortable when doing so as this is necessary to determine the true impact of the crime. Presently, online romance scams are severely under-reported as a result of lack of enough avenues where people can seek redress in addition to the shame and embarrassment victims feel from others when they share their story. Finkel et al.'s (2012) suggestion might be helpful in curbing online romance scam as well. They proposed that a closer collaboration between scholars and online dating service providers is necessary as this would provide greater opportunity for researchers to test their theories and develop new ones with large samples of participants who are highly motivated to establish romantic relationships. Such collaboration will provide better insight into online dating experiences and information that could guide informed solution to online dating scams.

Since users of online dating sites bear a significant part of the responsibility for their safety, Khader and Yun (2017) advise that user awareness need to be intensified. Potential daters should be warned on the apparent danger they face as a result of possible scammers' activities on the dating sites. Such warning could include the possibility for dating sites to create a checklist of some of the tactics used by scammers (Khader & Yun, 2017). Such checklist should be made available to any new member who signs up on the dating site. Suarez-Tangil et al. (2019) developed a system for automatically detecting online dating fraud through profile analysis. The system is meant to identify fraudulent profiles at the creation stage. Such a system, if successfully developed, would go a long way in assisting online dating sites to curb the activities of online dating scammers. In their study, Edwards et al. (2018) found that West Africa in general accounts for over 50% of the source locations of online dating and romance scams. Therefore, if security agencies and dating site managers could monitor the IP addresses of dating site users from fraud-prone regions, it could help in early detection of fraudulent activities. Also, studies have identified possible psychological attributes that predispose users to romance scam victimisation (Whitty, 2018; Buchanan & Whitty, 2014). Such findings could be used by dating sites (especially those sites that administer personality trait questionnaires to new entrants) to design questionnaires for their (new) users. Users at risk of victimisation could be identified for target intervention. At present some countries have registry of accredited dating agencies (and websites), for example Singapore (Khader & Yun, 2017). Individuals are then encouraged to patronise only these accredited agencies for their own safety. Such accreditation if widely adopted could greatly minimise the existence of fake dating sites created by romance scammers.

Suggestions to Increase Research Attention in This Area

Online dating scams appear to be a very recent fraud which according to Whitty and Buchanan (2012) became apparent from around 2008. Its emergence is partly due to greater broadband and internet penetration which resulted in proliferation of social networking sites and online dating sites. The increasing availability and affordability of the internet, especially in developing countries, also fuels the present scourge of online dating scam. With the emergence of this unique type of fraud, many scholars have attempted to understand its nature from different disciplines. While it would not be denied that there has been significant achievement in this regard, it is also important to accept that much more still need to be done in understanding the different facets of online dating and romance scam for effective development of preventive strategies. Coluccia et al. (2020) in their scoping review suggested further studies using quantitative methodology to examine the epidemiological and cross-cultural characteristics of online dating scams. They also call for a determination of the dynamics and factors that may lead the victim to report fraud cases more often, and examination from a clinical perspective of the association between being victim/perpetrator and specific psychiatric disorders, for example dependent personality traits in the victims or antisocial personality (Mazzoni, Contena, Fanciullacci, & Pozza, 2018). Other suggestions include development of screening tools aimed at identifying at-risk individuals by analysing personality traits and relational vulnerabilities. In addition, Sorell and Whitty (2019) called for interdisciplinary research drawing on computer science, psychology and moral philosophy undertaken to obtain and assess possible criteria for competent decision-making in victims who suffer re-victimisation. The authors argue that findings of such a study could inform debates around algorithms triggering the blocking of suspect communications with or without the victim's permission. Finally, given the findings emerging from previous studies on the psychological impact of online romance scam on the mental health of victims, it is important to initiate further research to develop effective programmes, interventions and resources for assisting victims of this type of fraud to regain their mental health.

Need for Stronger Internet Security Regulations, Policy Formulation and Implementation in Africa

It is no doubt that there is a need for stronger internet security, regulation and policies to curb the activities of online dating scammers in vulnerable areas. The activities of these fraudsters bear severe financial and emotional consequences not just on the victims but also on the general population. Victims incur not just huge financial loss but loss of a relationship they have invested psychological and emotional resources to build. No wonder many victims need urgent psychiatric attention to restore their mental health after this experience. While some agencies, programmes and policies have been created or developed in different African countries to counter the activities and influence of these cyber fraudsters, it appears that these have not made significant impact given the continuous rise in the number of people reportedly involved in this crime. Since research has shown that majority of these online romance scams are perpetrated by criminals residing in Africa or have African origin, governments of African countries need to rise to the occasion and collaborate with their Western counterparts in finding effective and lasting solution to the rising prevalence of online dating fraud. Governments of African countries could seek collaboration with foreign agencies with proven capacity to combat online dating frauds. Such collaboration could afford African countries with greater resources to fine-tune their existing internet security regulations and policies to meet current realities and provide them with unique opportunity for formulation and/or implementation of these regulations and policies following international best practice for greater effectiveness. Such partnership may also guarantee greater information sharing among governments in Africa and foreign agencies for better monitoring of dating sites, tracking and arrest of romance scammers.

Conclusion

The incidence of online dating and romance scams has continued to rise across the globe. Online dating and romance scams may be rife and rising in African countries. This is a cause to worry not just to the African nations but indeed to the whole world. The activity of the fraudsters who pose as potential relationship partners in the different dating sites is a cause for worry because the scammers end up fleecing their victims as well as inflicting serious emotional and psychological wound. In this chapter, we attempted to examine online dating scam and the likely processes involved in such a scam. We also analysed common features of popular dating sites (and relationship apps), the menace of online dating scams, tricks employed by scammers and the possible strategies which could be adopted to curb the activities of online dating fraudsters. The need for more empirical studies focusing on developing effective ways of reducing fraud in online dating sites are highlighted. Finally, we recommended that governments of African countries should collaborate with their Western counterpart for more efficient information and resource sharing to guarantee a positive impact in combating online dating and relationship scam in this part of the world.

References

Abiola, P. (2020, June 27). FBI declares six Nigerians wanted over $6m scam. *The Nation*. Retrieved from http://community.thenationonline.net/forum/fbi-declares-six-nigerians-wanted-over-6m-scam

AnKee, A. W., & Yazdanifard, R. (2015). The review of the ugly truth and negative aspects of online dating. *Global Journal of Management and Business Research: E Marketing, 15*(4), M39.

Archer, A. K. (2017). *I made a choice: Exploring the persuasion tactics used by online romance scammers in light of Cialdini's compliance principles.* All Regis University Theses. 823. Retrieved from https://epublications.regis.edu/theses/823

Australian Competition and Consumer Commission. (2016). *Best practice guidelines for dating sites: Protecting consumers from dating scams.* Canberra: Australian Capital Territory: Commonwealth of Australia.

Brittany, W. (2018, March 3). *The "Harvard" of dating Apps: The League.* Retrieved from https://www-statista-com.ezp-prod1.hul.harvard.edu/outlook/372/100/online-dating/worldwide#market-revenue

Buchanan, T., & Whitty, M. T. (2014). The online dating romance scam: Causes and consequences of victimhood. *Psychology, Crime & Law, 20*(3), 261–283. https://doi.org/10.1080/1068316X.2013.772180

Coluccia, A., Pozza, A., Ferretti, F., Carabellese, F., Masti, A., & Gualtieri, G. (2020). Online romance scams: Relational dynamics and psychological characteristics of the victims and scammers. *Clinical Practice & Epidemiology in Mental Health, 16*, 24–35. https://doi.org/10.2174/1745017902016010024

Cross, C. (2018). (Mis)Understanding the impact of online fraud: Implications for victim assistance schemes. *Victims & Offenders, 13*, 757–776. https://doi.org/10.1080/15564886.2018.1474154

DeLamater, J. D., & Myers, D. J. (2011). *Social Psychology.* Belmont: Wadsworth.

Dinisman, T., & Moroz, A. (2017). *Understanding victims of crime: The impact of the crime and support needs.* Victim Support.

Edwards, M., Suarez-Tangil, G., Peersman, C., Stringhini, G., Rashid, A., & Whitty, M. (2018). The geography of online dating fraud. In *Workshop on technology and consumer protection (ConPro)* (Vol. 7). San Francisco: IEEE.

Finkel, E. J., Eastwick, P. W., Karney, B. R., Harry, T., Reis, H. T., & Sprecher, S. (2012). Online dating: A critical analysis from the perspective of psychological science. *Psychological Science in the Public Interest, 13*(1), 3–66. https://doi.org/10.1177/1529100612436522

Hunt, M. (2020, September 10). Revealed: the favourite dating websites used by scammers. Retrieved from https://www.telegraph.co.uk/money/consumeraffairs/revealed-favourite-dating-websites-used-scammers/ [Accessed December 5, 2020].

Jimoh, I., & Kyass, R. S. (2018). Is this love? A study of deception in online romance in Nigeria. *Covenant Journal of Communication (CJOC), 5*(1), 40–61.

Joomratty, Q. B. (2019). "Stripped wallets, ripped hearts" victims of financial fraud: An analysis beyond financial fraud. *People: International Journal of Social Sciences*, *4*(3), 1101–1112. https://doi.org/10.20319/pijss.2019.43.11011112

Kenrick, D. T., Sadalla, E. K., Groth, G., & Trost, M. R. (1990). Evolution, traits, and the stages of human courtship: Qualifying the parental investment model. *Journal of Personality*, *58*(1), 97–116. https://doi.org/10.1111/j.1467-6494.1990.tb00909.x

Khader, M., & Yun, P. S. (2017). A multidisciplinary approach to understanding internet love scams. *The Psychology of Criminal and Antisocial Behavior*, *2017*, 532–548. https://doi.org/10.1016/b978-0-12-809287-3.00018-3

Koon, T. H., & Yoong, D. (2013). Preying on lonely hearts: A systematic deconstruction of an internet romance scammer's online lover persona. *Journal of Modern Languages*, *23*(1), 28–40. Retrieved from https://jml.um.edu.my/article/view/3288

Kopp, C., Layton, R., Sillitoe, J., & Gondal, I. (2015). The role of love stories in romance scams: A qualitative analysis of fraudulent profiles. *International Journal of Cyber Criminology*, *9*(2), 205–217. https://doi.org/10.5281/zenodo.56227

Kopp, C., Sillitoe, J., Gondal, I., & Layton, R. (2016). The online romance scam: A complex two-layer scam. *Journal of Psychological and Educational Research*, *24*(2), 144–161. Retrieved from https://www.researchgate.net/publication/311794327_The_online_romance_scam_A_complex_two-layer_scam

Maslow, A. (1954). *Motivation and personality*. Harpers and Brothers.

Mateo, A. (2020, April 9). 13 of the best online dating Apps to find relationships. *The Opera Magazine*. Retrieved from https://www.oprahmag.com/life/relationship-love/a28726299/best-online-dating-apps/

Mazzoni, G. P., Contena, B., Fanciullacci, S., & Pozza, A. (2018). A comparative analysis of the MMPI-2 personality profiles between patients with borderline personality and prisoners with antisocial personality disorder. *RivisitaPsichiatria*, *53*(5), 267–273. https://doi.org/10.1708/3000.30006

Orchard, T. (2019). Online dating site. In A. D. Lykins (Ed.), *Encyclopedia of sexuality and gender*. Switzerland AG: Springer Nature. https://doi.org/10.1007/978-3-319-59531-3_18-1

Park, Y., Jones, J., McCoy, D., Elaine Shi, E., & Jakobsson, M. (2014). Understanding targeted Nigerian cams on craigslist. *System*, *1*, 2. https://doi.org/10.14722/ndss.2014.23284

Pendell, S. D. (2002). Affection in interpersonal relationships: Not just a "fond and tender feeling". In *Communication yearbook 26* (pp. 70–115). Lawrence Erlbaum.

Rege, A. (2009). What's love got to do with it? Exploring online dating scams and identity fraud. *International Journal of Cyber Criminology (IJCC), 3*(2), 494–512. Retrieved from https://www.researchgate.net/publication/228373590_What%27s_Love_Got_to_Do_with_It_Exploring_Online_Dating_Scams_and_Identity_Fraud

Santora, N., Pearlstein, R., O'brien, W. (Writers), & Moore, C. (Director). (2015, January 18). Charades (season 1, episode 14) [TV series episode]. *Scorpion*. CBS Production.

Scamwatch. (2020, May). Dating & romance. *Scamwatch*. Retrieved from https://www.scamwatch.gov.au/types-of-scams/dating-romance

Shaari, A. H., Kamaluddin, R. M., Paizi, F. W., & Mohd, M. (2019). Online-dating romance scam in Malaysia: An analysis of online conversations between scammers and victims. *GEMA Online® Journal of Language Studies, 19*(1), 97–115. https://doi.org/10.17576/gema-2019-1901-06

Sorell, T., & Whitty, M. (2019). Online romance scams and victimhood. *Security Journal, 32,* 342–361. https://doi.org/10.1057/s41284-019-00166-w

Suarez-Tangil, G., Edwards, M., Peersman, C., Stringhini, G., Rashid, A., & Whitty, M. (2019). Automatically dismantling online dating fraud. *IEE Transactions on Information Forensics and Security, 15,* 1128–1137. https://doi.org/10.1109/tifs.2019.2930479

The Federal Trade Commission. (2019, February). *Consumer protection data spotlight: Romance scams rank number one on total reported losses.* Retrieved from http://www.ftc.gov

Tracy, J. (2013). Another look: Starting an online dating service. *Online Dating Magazine.* Retrieved from https://www.onlinedatingmagazine.com/columns/industry/2007/startinganonlinedatingservice.html

Whitty, M. T. (2013a). The scammers persuasive techniques model: Development of a stage model to explain the online dating romance scam. *British Journal of Criminology, 53*(4), 665–684. https://doi.org/10.1093/bjc/azt009

Whitty, M. T. (2013b). Anatomy of the online dating romance scam. *Security Journal, 28,* 443–455. https://doi.org/10.1057/sj.2012.57

Whitty, M. T. (2018). Do you love me? Psychological characteristics of romance scam victims. *Cyberpsychology, Behavior, and Social Networking, 21*(2), 105–109. https://doi.org/10.1089/cyber.2016.0729

Whitty, M. T. (2019). Who can spot an online romance scam? *Journal of Financial Crime, 26*(2), 623–633. https://doi.org/10.1108/jfc-06-2018-0053

Whitty, M. T., & Buchanan, T. (2012). The online dating romance scam: A serious crime. *CyberPsychology, Behavior, and Social Networking, 15*(3), 181–183. https://doi.org/10.1089/cyber.2011.0352

Whitty, M. T., & Buchanan, T. (2015). The online dating romance scam: The psychological impact on victims—both financial and non-financial. *Criminology & Criminal Justice, 16*(2), 176–194. https://doi.org/10.1177/1748895815603773

Zwilling, M. (2013, March 1). How many more online dating sites do we need? *Gorbes.* Retrieved from https://www.gorbes.com/sites/martinzwilling/2013/03/01/how-many-more-online-dating-sites-do-we-need/amp/

5

An Exploratory Study on Kidnapping as an Emerging Crime in Nigeria

Alaba M. Oludare, Ifeoma E. Okoye, and Lucy K. Tsado

Introduction

Kidnapping is not a novel crime in human history. Many nations of the world have dealt with the crime at different levels of historical development. The history of kidnapping in contemporary Nigeria began as a

---

The original version of this chapter was revised. The correction to this chapter can be found at https://doi.org/10.1007/978-3-030-71024-8_18

A. M. Oludare (✉)
Department of Criminal Justice, Mississippi Valley State University, Itta Bena, MS, USA
e-mail: alaba.oludare@mvsu.edu

I. E. Okoye
Department of Criminal Justice, Virginia State University, VA, USA
e-mail: iokoye@vsu.edu

L. K. Tsado
Department of Sociology, Social Work and Criminal Justice, Lamar University, Beaumont, TX, USA
e-mail: ltsado@lamar.edu

H. C. O. Chan, S. Adjorlolo (eds.), *Crime, Mental Health and the Criminal Justice System in Africa*, https://doi.org/10.1007/978-3-030-71024-8_5

politically motivated incidence around the 1980s and continued into the early 2000s with ideologically motivated militant groups in the Niger Delta area kidnapping expatriate oil company workers. The perpetrators in these early incidents demanded environmental justice and control of natural resources (Akinsulore, 2016). The incidents attracted the attention of the government as well as the international communities ending in some compromises (Okengwu, 2011). Subsequent incidents of kidnapping erupted not only in the region but all over the country with demands that are apparently antithetical to environmental and social justice but directed towards personal, political and economic gains (Odoemelam & Omage, 2013).

This chapter adopts the rational choice theory and general strain theory as possible criminological perspectives to understand the recent proliferation of kidnapping in Nigeria. Tracing the history of kidnapping as a phenomenon experienced in many countries and continents of North America, Europe, the Oceanian subregion including New Zealand and Australia and Asia, there is an indication that Africa has experienced kidnapping at a rather large scale. Nigeria has experienced different waves of kidnaping motivated by several factors including political, ideological and economical insurgencies from the twentieth century to present times. The chapter also provides available data on kidnapping in Nigeria and discusses the responses of governments, and concludes with recommendations.

Defining Kidnapping and the Psychological Aspects of the Crime

Defining kidnapping is problematic because of variations in the legal and moral terrain of the geographical location as well as circumstances in which the crime occur. The definition of kidnapping changes from time to time and place to place based on the political, economic and social cultural environment for operationalising the meaning. According to the Black's Law Dictionary (2009), kidnapping involves the seizing or taking away of a victim by force or fraud; the unlawful seizure or confinement of a person typically in a secret place, while attempting to extort a ransom. *The Oxford English Dictionary* (2010) places emphasis on the act of taking someone away by force usually for ransom. Merriam-Webster (n.d.) describes kidnapping as the crime of seizing, confining, inveigling, abducting or carrying away of a person by force or fraud often with a demand for ransom or in furtherance of another crime. However, the common law describes kidnapping as the unlawful restraint of a person's liberty by forceful abduction or stealing, or the expression of force in order to send the victim into another country (Rementeria, 1939). Therefore, considering kidnapping in this light has to involve an element of unlawful seizure and removal of a person from his country or state against his will. Blackstone (2010) sees kidnapping as the "forcible abduction or stealing away of a man, woman, or child, from their own country, and sending them into another." The crime is punishable under the common law by fine, imprisonment and derision as a misdemeanour.

Following the American definition of kidnapping, the perpetrator does not necessarily have had to send or intend to send the victim out of his country. Kidnapping is a federal crime categorised as a felony by virtue of 18 U.S.C.A. No. 1201. The Model Penal Code also includes acts of terrorism and interference with government and political duties in the definition of kidnapping (Model Penal Code, No. 212.1). Following case law in Nigeria, the Supreme Court laid out the elements required for establishing a crime of kidnapping in the case of Okashetu v. State (2016):

1. That the victim was seized, and taken away by the accused person.
2. That the victim was taken away against his consent.
3. That the victim was taken away without lawful excuse.

In that case, the victim testified that he was abducted close to his hotel by two boys who forcefully put him in his car and drove off while the perpetrator followed behind with the car they came in. A prosecution witness also testified that he apprehended the appellant with the assistance of the police shortly after the incident. The Supreme Court cited R v. CORT (2004) to confirm that a person needed only to have been detained against his will for kidnapping to occur.

Scholars have attempted to distinguish kidnapping from other related violent crimes. Nnam (2013) describes kidnapping as the unlawful and coercive taking away of a person or group of persons without their own volition to an undisclosed hostile environment often in order to demand and obtain a ransom, or to settle a political score. The question is whether an involuntary taking of a victim to another destination though not necessarily hostile is sufficient to alleviate a perpetrator's act to kidnapping. According to Douglas, Burgess, Burgess, and Ressler (1992), it suffices that the perpetrator seizes, detains or removes his victim by unlawful force or fraud, often with the demand for ransom. The process of negotiating the victim's release can be used to distinguish kidnapping from hostage-taking. Generally, the family of the victim, government, business leaders and law enforcement may be involved in negotiating the kidnapped person's release. In the case of a hostage-taking, the victim is held and threatened by an offender who in turn blackmails or pressurise a third party to fulfil conditions for the release of the victim. Akpan (2010) also sought to make a distinction among the crimes of kidnapping, hostage-taking and hijacking. While in some countries kidnapping may include the abduction of minors, it is not so in other countries (United Nations Office on Drugs and Crime, 2015). Sometimes, abduction is used in a wider sense to define a crime of kidnapping that does not require the threat or use of force.

Psychological Aspects of Kidnapping

Generally, kidnapping is a traumatic experience for both victims and families. Research conducted by Oludayo, Usman and Adeyinka, (2019), on experiences of victims of kidnapping revealed that victims were tortured, threatened with violence and death, and often relocated to different camps to keep them in custody. The kidnappers used victims' telephones to contact family members so as to instill fear and create agonising emotions and ordeal. These experiences put relatives in panic to source for the demanded payoff. Victim's gender, family and social status, and level of cooperation influence the type of treatment the kidnappers meted out to victims. Some kidnappers go as far as recording videos of how the victim is being tortured; these videos are sent to the victim's families to induce the quick payment of ransom.

On the other hand, the psychological aspect of the kidnapping perpetrator's behaviour cannot be restricted to one psychological framework. Kidnappers may not be stereotyped into a personal profile, neither can they be typically classified as psychopaths. Mental illness is not a critical factor in understanding the behaviour of kidnappers. Research has shown that violent behaviour such as kidnapping is often planned and calculated towards observable goals. Perceived injustice, need for identity and belonging are common motives for kidnappers. They may hold ideologies and strong beliefs that propel and compel them to act violently towards others in society. Generally, the kidnapper believes that his action is justified even though it may not be legal (Anazonwu, Onyemaechi, & Igwilo, 2016).

Theoretical Framework

This chapter considers the rational choice theory and general strain theory as elements of criminological theories that have been influential in understanding the proliferation of kidnapping. The rational choice theory explains that offender's motivations to commit crime are determined by the potential cost of action and the anticipated benefits. Cornish and Clarke (1986) describe motivations to commit crime as an individual's effort to meet common personal needs and involves creating opportunities for meeting those needs. Individuals are expected to have the ability to weigh the pleasure to be gained against the likely punishment while considering committing an illegal behaviour and also have the ability to decide against the act. This theory assumes that all crime is intentional because of the calculated benefit to the offender. The theory is further characterised by free will and is consensus oriented; it understands that an individual who commits a crime intentionally decided to act contrary to the established order of society (Schmalleger, 2018).

Due to the fact that kidnapping is either politically or economically motivated for profit, most or all kidnapping incidences depend on rational choice. In an attempt to realise monetary benefits or needs, kidnappers decide to use acts of abduction or hostage-taking to easily actualise their objectives. Kidnapping is therefore considered a logical means to advance desired goals. In other words, kidnappers have the ability to calculate the potential cost of action against anticipated benefit and subsequently decide to disobey the law notwithstanding the certainty of punishment. For example, Muritala Umaru was one of the Fulani herdsmen involved in kidnapping who admitted realising over N100 million from kidnapping activities within four years. This affirmation indicates that the act of kidnapping is a lucrative business in which benefits outweigh the expected cost (Johnson, 2018). In addition, where kidnapping is politically motivated and ransoms are demanded, it is assumed that the kidnappers rationally chose to engage in such acts so as to further their political objectives or facilitate the kidnapper's political organisation notwithstanding the risk or cost involved.

Rational choice theorists like Beccaria (1738–1794) and Bentham (1748–1832) argued that the state should punish offenders just enough to offset the amount of pleasure gained from the offense. Bentham created the *felicific calculus*, a schedule designed to calculate the exact degree of punishment required to offset the gain derived from perpetrating the crime (Williams & McShane, 2010). In practical parlance, this burden of punishment should not only match the pleasure but also outweigh the derivable pleasure in some cases, which are supposedly covered under the Nigerian criminal law. Scholars have also recommended that policymakers should increase the perceived effort and risks involved in committing illegal acts and reduce the perceived benefits, thereby altering the offender's decision-making processes and consequent illegal behaviour (Bernard, Snipes, & Gerould, 2010).

The second fundamental theory that explicitly explains kidnapping in practical language is the general strain theory developed by Agnew (1985). This theorist did not base his theory solely on problems of achieving positively valued goals as did the traditional strain theories (Durkheim, 1951; Merton, 1938); rather, he added the concept of blocked avoidance of painful situations. Therefore, the possibility of an individual's goals being blocked can also lead to blocked abilities to avoid stressful life events or unwanted negative situations. He contended that both blocked opportunities and inability to avoid stressful circumstances creates strain.

Such negative situations can trigger anger and frustration and thus put pressure on individuals, particularly youths with weak coping mechanisms. For instance, contemporary Nigerian standards define goals and values that entail material possession, power, wealth and class stratification without providing corresponding legal means for achieving those goals. Members of the society who are not able to realise these Nigerian dreams through legal means become frustrated and seek for unconventional ways of meeting societal goals, hence resorting to crimes such as kidnapping.

Apart from the desire to realise the societal dream, Agnew (2006) categorised other sources of strain as (a) failure to achieve positively valued goals because of a disjunction between aspirations and expectations, a disconnection between expectations and actual achievements, or a dislocation between reasonable results and actual results; (b) the presentation of negative stimuli, such as feeling economically and socially humiliated or criminal victimisation; and (c) the removal of positive stimuli, such as the death of a loved one or removal of educational benefits. Notably, the degrees of strain and the different ways individuals perceive and tolerate negative situations contribute to the level of pressure on an individual to act out. For example, youths or adults with a very low level of self-control who lack attachment to significant others and are aggressively treated and intimidated are more likely to involve in criminal activities.

Brief History of Kidnapping in Nigeria and Other Countries

Kidnapping is a global security threat that affects countries all over the world. The practice of kidnapping is an age-long lucrative business for organised criminals like drug cartels, human traffickers, terrorists, criminal gangs and others. Kidnapping is not a new phenomenon in Nigeria; presently, it is one of the biggest security challenges nationally. Plethora of literature have characterised the historical advancement of kidnapping in various parts of the world, and others have outlined the stereotypical typologies of kidnappings such as kidnapping for ransom, express kidnapping, virtual kidnapping, tiger kidnapping, political, instrumental or ideological kidnapping (Khan & Sajid, 2010; Ochoa, 2012; Webster, 2007 & Wilson, 1994).

Kidnapping started as early as the 75 BC mostly in the south-eastern part of Europe and later spread to North America, Australia, Central Asia, some parts of Middle East, Austria, Rome, Britain and New Zealand. Most victims of kidnapping were held as captives with the objective of extorting large sums of money for ransom or in exchange for release of prisoners. Turner (1998) documented that kidnapping started in seventeenth century in England where children were "kidnapped" and often sold as slaves or agricultural workers to colonial farmers. In ancient Rome, Emperor Constantine (AD 315) ordered the death penalty as punishment for kidnapping because of the high incidences of kidnapping in Rome at the time (Schiller, 1985). According to *Encyclopaedia Britannica*, kidnapping started in earlier times in America, when kidnappers were involved in the unlawful conveyance of persons away from one country to another country for involuntary servitude, forcefully impressing males into military service, abducting young women for prostitution or marriage and abducting young children for ransom (Augustyn et al., n.d.). Kidnapping children for ransom became common in the United States during the 1920s and 1930s, and this prompted legislation against kidnapping with punishment of death penalty for transporting a kidnapped victim from one state to another (Augustyn et al., n.d.).

Africa is one of the continents that has experienced kidnapping in large scale. In precolonial Africa, significant number of children were kidnapped in the course of the trans-Atlantic slave trade from the fifteenth through nineteenth centuries in West Africa, and in the Eastern and Central African Arab-Swahili slave trade (Kanogo, 2020). Both children and adults were kidnapped and sold into slavery to other continents like Europe and America. Most perpetrators of kidnapping at that time were international merchants, slave traders, intermediaries and European partners. In addition, children were also kidnapped as war hostages during the early postcolonial period to supplement limited adult soldiers in civil wars against other localities. In some parts of Africa, both rebel forces and governments perpetrate the abductions of children during civil wars. According to the report, these children were abducted to serve as domestic servants, concierges, messengers, camp followers, sex slaves for the soldiers and combatants. Some of the abducted children were forced to commit atrocities on other children such as rape, killings, violence and so on. Children were also abducted for religious ritual sacrifices and forced into early marriages (Kanogo, 2020).

African countries like South Africa, Nigeria, Somalia, Uganda, Mali, South Sudan, Libya and Cameroun have historically experienced spates of kidnapping mostly due to high levels of crime, corruption, unemployment, inadequate policing, long history of political instability and ethnic conflagrations ravaging these countries. Hence, kidnapping in these countries are often seen as more profitable and yielding quick resources than genuine lawful businesses. The growth of this phenomenon can be interpreted as the rational strategy used by criminals who seek new unlawful opportunities to make quick profits. Notwithstanding that kidnapping is a growing crime problem in sub-Saharan Africa, research projected that 80% of all kidnappings for ransom occur in Latin America (Pharoah, 2005).

Other kidnapping hubs in East Africa includes Somalia known for capturing foreign hostages such as journalists, aid workers, emissaries and tourists. At some point, Somalia was tagged the "kidnapping red zone" because of the nefarious activities of Somalian pirates. From 2006 till the present time, kidnapping of foreigners for ransom has continued to thrive in Somalia, and this became more prominent since the start of the Ethiopian intervention in the Somalia civil war. The Somali Islamist umbrella group used kidnapping as a tactics in retaliating against the armed conflict involving Ethiopian and Somali Transitional Federal Government forces and Somali troops. Many foreign nationals were kidnapped in the process. Some of the notable kidnapped victims since the 2006 involved Canadian and Australian journalists, British nationals, British environmentalists, French security consultants and other French nationals, Spanish aid workers, Kenyan nationals, Italian nationals and so on ("Somalia: Shaabab Displays", 2012; Heaton, 2017; Mullin & Petkar, 2018).

According to reports, most of the kidnappers were Somalian pirates and militants with the Al-Shabaab Islamist group ("Africa piracy: Foreigners being held hostage", 2011). Consequently, some of the hostages escaped after months of being held captive; some were killed and raped; others were released in exchange for monetary ransom and/or other special conditions ("French hostage Marie Dedieu", 2011; Mullin & Petkar, 2018). While the Somali pirates made demands for huge sums of money from victims' families and respective governments, the insurgents, in addition to ransom, demanded for cessation of foreign army support from the Somali authorities and the complete withdrawal of the African Union Mission from Somalia.

Recent developments in South Africa have projected the country as one of the African countries experiencing this dangerous crime wave, where abductors demand millions in ransom. Before the 2000s, targets were mostly wealthy individuals but recent increase indicated shift to citizens, teenagers, children, tourists, foreigners and so on. The South African Police Service (2014) reported 4101 kidnappings in the year 1994 and 1995 financial year and recorded 4100 kidnappings during the 2013 and 2014 financial year. By population size, kidnapping rates declined from 10.6 per 100,000 people in the 1995 to 6.5 in the 2004 period. Statistics from the United Nations Office on Drugs and Crime (2015) Survey of Crime Trends and Operations of Criminal Justice Systems indicated that South Africa has the fourth highest kidnapping rate globally after Kuwait, Belgium and Canada at 6.8 per 100,000 population. According to the indicator provided by TheGlobalEconomy.com, South Africa had the highest record of kidnappings in Africa in 2017, 2016, 2015 at 9.6, 8.9, 9.1 kidnappings per 100,000 population, respectively ("Kidnapping rate in Africa", n.d.). Official police statistics indicated that kidnapping in South Africa skyrocketed by 139% between 2008 and 2018 ("Watch: Kidnappings on the rise", 2019). South Africa was reported in the top ten countries with the highest number of kidnappings globally from 2015 to 2017 ("Kidnapping rate in Africa", n.d.). This further reiterated the seriousness of kidnapping in Africa.

Nigeria has largely encountered kidnapping since the middle of the twentieth century. Kidnapping then was mostly for political reasons ranging from government's repatriation of political leaders for embezzlement of public funds to using kidnapping as a political weapon to attack political enemies. This later developed into unlawful profit-making business that involved dissidents, criminal groups, police officers, politicians, entrepreneurs, gatemen and other members of the society. This form of criminality could be attributed to the high level of unemployment wrecking Nigerian youths, poverty, greed, vengeance, rituals, monetary and political gains. In the past decades, kidnapping ravaged mostly the south-western and south-eastern part of the country but, presently, kidnapping has presented serious national security challenge. With insurgent groups like the Boko Haram, Niger Delta militants and Fulani herdsmen committing these acts of injustice against innocent members of the society. The Boko Haram terrorist group made headlines in 2014 globally, when it kidnapped 276 Chibok school girls in an attempt to attract government and the public attention.

The first recorded case of political kidnapping in Nigeria was perpetrated by the Nigerian government in conjunction with the Israeli secret service Mossad who conspired to kidnap the Nigerian ex-minister, Umaru Dikko in 1984. The attempt was to repatriate the ex-minister from London to Nigeria to face charges of corruption brought by his political enemies in Lagos. According to reports, his abductors handcuffed him, drug-stupefied him and stuffed him into a wooden crate with a doctor by his side ensuring that he kept breathing. Though this plot was foiled by British customs officials at the point of departure, it provoked diplomatic crisis between Britain and Nigeria (Weber, 2014).

The next wave of political kidnapping started in the Nigeria's oil-rich Niger Delta region in the early 2000s when the Niger Delta militants took hostage of oil workers to protest the inequality and economic marginalisation in the region. The agitations were against environmental degradation caused by the exploration activities of multinational oil companies in the area (Ogbuehi, 2018). The abduction started with the kidnapping of expatriates, government officials and foreign nationals. Expatriates working with these multinational oil giants were taken hostage in order to force oil companies operating in the region to compensate the community through community development projects and to force negotiation with government for economic benefits to the region (Okafor, Ajibo, Chukwu, Egbuche, & Asadu, 2018). According to reports, Niger Delta militants started operations around 1998 when they kidnapped foreign nationals from the United States, South Africa and Britain working with Chevron, Shell and Texaco. Between 2003 and

2006, the militants kidnapped over 280 oil workers, including seizure of oil rigs in the region and blowing up pipelines (Ngwama, 2014). The militants were also involved in kidnapping of foreign humanitarian workers and military personnel on mission to guard the region. Through negotiations and payment of ransom, some of those abductees regained their freedom, while others died in the process (Ogbuehi, 2018). The kidnappings continued until 2009 when government granted amnesty and unconditional pardon to the militants and introduced socio-economic empowerment programmes.

Apart from the kidnappings perpetrated by the Niger Delta militants, the Boko Haram terrorist group has continued to kidnap, men, women, children, school girls, religious leaders and government officials in the north-eastern part of Nigeria since 2009 (Global Terrorism Database, 2019). As earlier mentioned, the sect held the world to a standstill with the news of kidnapping over 270 Chibok, schoolgirls in Borno Northeast Nigeria in 2014 (Umar, 2014). This malevolent act led to the campaign "Bring Back Our Girls Movement" in Nigeria, and subsequently some of the girls were released in exchange for certain conditions from the Nigerian government. Few years later, in 2018, the Islamist terrorist sect abducted about 110 girls from a government-owned secondary school in Dapchi, Yobe State, Nigeria, (Bolaji, 2018). The Ansaru group, a faction of the Boko Haram sect, was also responsible for some of the kidnappings in Northern Nigeria involving foreign nationals (Bayagbon, 2013).

The Fulani herdsmen known for their recent incessant killings in various parts of Nigeria especially in the south-eastern and south-western Nigeria are also involved in the atrocious acts of kidnapping. Since 2017 till the present time, they have continued to kidnap men, women, children and police officers (Godwin, 2018). This group operates mostly by laying ambush against their victims or disguising as security operatives on duty. In exchange for the release of their captives, they usually demand for ransom from victims and victims' family members. In 2017, the group succeeded in kidnapping a Delta monarch who was travelling with some of his relatives in a private car. After they demanded for money and other personal items from the victims, they attacked them with machete and eventually took the monarch as captive and made demands for ransom in exchange for his release ("Fulani Herdsmen kidnap Delta Monarch", 2018).

Presently, kidnapping has metamorphosed into lucrative business ventures in Nigeria. While other countries may be experiencing various types of kidnapping, kidnapping for ransom is one of the biggest organised crime in Nigeria. The terror of kidnapping is usually violent, and delays in greasing the pockets of those bandits with the ransom money or resistance from victims usually result in the death of victims. The current upsurge of kidnapping in Nigeria makes every person a potential target regardless of gender, nationality, social class or economic status. Many Nigerians have fallen victims of this malady, and some had to pay millions of naira in ransom for their freedom (Ngwama, 2014). The action which started as a political weapon and government tactics to expatriate wanted persons has moved against religious leaders and their children, politicians and their family members, grandparents, commuters and so on. Kidnappers also target government officials, traditional rulers, and members of the executive, legislative and the judicial branch of government and their family members despite the level of security surrounding these groups (Ngwama, 2014). While Nigerian law enforcement officers are making efforts to curtail these abominable acts, inadequate policing in Nigeria is a big problem.

Statistics and Incidents of Kidnapping in Nigeria

Incidents of kidnapping have continued to increase in Nigeria, costing citizens their lives and family members millions of dollars. In this chapter, we will present the statistics from SBM Intel that depict the seriousness of the problem and why it must be addressed. We used this secondary source because there are no reliable official data on kidnappings in Nigeria available for analysis. SBM Intel is a research and communications consulting firm that collects and analyses data, using the findings to influence change in Africa.

Between June 2011 and March 2020, kidnapping cost victims and their families about $18.34 million, with $11 million spent between 2016 and 2020 alone. The rapid rise in the crime shows how lucrative it has become in recent years. Even more alarming are the 1331 fatalities reported (SBM Intel, 2020). The report states that kidnappings in Nigeria have triggered the use of the military in response to incidents of kidnapping in almost all of the country's 36 states except the Federal Capital Territory (FCT) and Kebbi State.

As of 2020, the ten states with the highest incidences of kidnapping are detailed in Table 5.1. Rivers State topped this group with 120 incidences, closely followed by Kaduna State with 117 incidences. Delta, Bayelsa and Borno States follow with 96, 85 and 82 incidences, respectively.

However, when the data is analysed by the number of fatalities, Borno, Kaduna and Katsina States jump ahead of Rivers State with 489, 209 and 147 fatalities, respectively (see Table 5.2). In addition, other states that do not have high numbers of incidence but have high fatality rates are worthy of closer scrutiny. States such as Adamawa, Niger and Zamfara, all in the northern part of the Nigeria, show higher numbers of fatalities, even though they are not featured in the top ten states for a high number of incidences.

Finally, when the ratio of the number of fatalities to the number of incidents is computed, the most dangerous states for kidnapping are revealed, with Borno State in the lead with almost six deaths per incident. Other states with a notably high death-to-incidents ratio are Katsina and Adamawa with almost three, Zamfara with two and Kaduna and Niger

Table 5.1 Top ten states with the highest number of kidnapping incidents between 2010 and 2020

State	Number of kidnapping incidents
Rivers	120
Kaduna	117
Delta	96
Bayelsa	85
Borno	82
Kogi	59
Edo	55
Ondo	54
Katsina	52
Taraba	47

Note: Adapted from SBM Intel, 2020.

Table 5.2 States with the highest number of fatalities between 2010 and 2020 and greatest fatality-to-incidence ratio

State	Fatalities during kidnap attempts	Number of kidnap incidents	Top ten states in kidnap attempts	Fatality by incident ratio
Borno	489	82	YES	5.9
Kaduna	209	117	YES	1.7
Katsina	147	52	YES	2.82
Rivers	131	120	YES	1.09
Adamawa	91	35	NO	2.6
Niger	62	32	NO	1.93
Delta	58	96	YES	0.60
Zamfara	58	29	NO	2.0
Taraba	56	47	YES	1.19
Edo	30	34	YES	0.88
Total	1,331	644		2.06

Note: Adapted from SBM Intel, 2020.

with almost two deaths per incidence. The southern states, namely Rivers, Edo and Delta, though having higher numbers of incidences, do not have high fatality ratios. These results are not surprising, especially as we observe that in previous decades the southern states' kidnapping incidents were higher, but this insecurity threat has gradually moved north. The rise in terrorism in the north, especially by Boko Haram over the last decade, is also a major influencer because the terrorist organisation is heavily involved in kidnapping (SBM Intel, 2020).

Causes of Kidnapping in Nigeria

Factors precipitating kidnapping in Nigeria may be conceptualised as array of observable, economic, political and social influences reasonable enough to motivate perpetrators into acts of kidnapping. Understanding some of the conditions underlying the decision to resort to the use of abduction or hostage-taking to achieve economic objectives is sine qua non to the repertoire of actions necessary to quell the state of kidnapping in Nigeria, as effective solutions to a problem cannot be met without an understanding of the "whys" and "hows" of the problem. The underlying causes of kidnapping are discussed in this section; the radial diagram in

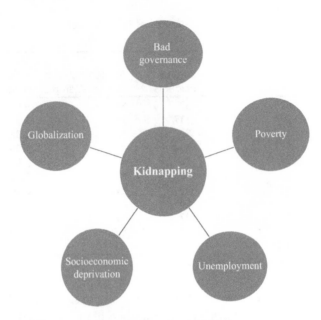

Fig. 5.1   Factors contributing to kidnapping in Nigeria.

Fig. 5.1 visually shows the interconnectedness of the various factors that contribute to kidnapping.

Bad Governance

Extant literature on the factors precipitating kidnapping indicates that general bad governance resulting from government inefficiency, neglect, oppression, domination, exploitation, deprivation, victimisation, discrimination, marginalisation, nepotism and bigotry contributes to kidnapping and other criminal activities (Ogundiya & Amzat, 2008; Salawu, 2010). Other scholars have also identified the inability of the Nigerian government to manage diversity, corruption, class inequality, environmental degradation and gross violations of human rights as causes of criminal activities (Kwaja, 2009). The most practical explanation for criminal activities lies with the failure of government, which has led to inefficiency, lack of transparency, poverty, corruption, and a nonchalant attitude towards the suffering of the people.

Also, weak political will in terms of a government's inability or unwillingness to prevent kidnapping and the absence of effective security in communities, ineffectiveness of the internal security service and intelligence failures in the criminal justice system contributes to kidnapping. The lack of seriousness towards the safety and security of the nation, lack of apparatus to protect the homeland security and the failure of government at all levels to prioritise the welfare of the citizens are threats facing the Nigerian people. Hillary Clinton, former U.S. secretary of state, captured the problem associated with the rise of conflict in Nigeria by noting that the failure of governance at the federal, state and local levels contributed to the rise of groups that embrace criminal activities and reject the authority of the state.

The Nigerian government and its executive branch, especially the law enforcement agencies, have not yet established realistic and proactive strategies to fully address the problem of kidnapping. Neither has the government created the preconditions for the elimination of kidnapping through measures such as creation of employment, effective home-grown poverty alleviation programmes, socio-economic equality, provision of infrastructure, affordable and quality education, preservation of true democracy, eradication of corruption at all levels, protection of life, pursuit of justice and so on. The government's inability to revitalise the country's declining industries or revamp the economy have also contributed to low employment rate in Nigeria; hence, young, enterprising graduates resort to easy ways to live their Nigerian dreams.

Poverty

Nigeria is the most populous African country with an approximate population of 202 million and has one of the largest populations of youth in the world (the World Bank, 2019). Nigeria is Africa's biggest oil exporter but recent oil price instability continues to influence Nigeria's growth performance and subjects the country to more poverty crises. In early 2000s, Nigeria's gross domestic product (GDP) grew at an average rate of

Table 5.3 Relative poverty trend in Nigeria, 1980–2010 (in %)

Year	Poverty incidence (%)	Estimated total population (in millions)	Poverty population (in millions)
1980	28.1	65	17.7
1985	46.1	75	34.7
1992	42.7	91.5	39.2
1996	65.6	102.3	67.1
2004	54.7	126.3	69.09
2010	69.0	163	112.47

Note: Adapted from Nigerian National Bureau of Statistics (2010).

7% per year; however, the oil price collapse in 2014–2016 resulted to a growth rate drop of 2.7% in 2015. The country recorded its first recession in 25 years in 2016 leading the economy to shrink by 1.6% (the World Bank, 2019). Since then, economic growth has continued to regress downwards and remained stable at 2% in 2019. Presently, majority of the population is trapped in abject poverty as a result of bad governance, defective economic policies, the government's unsustainable poverty alleviation programmes and economic marginalisation of certain parts of the country (Country Watch, n.d.; Nwagwu, 2014) (Table 5.3).

Relative poverty is defined by the living standards of a majority of people in a given population. According to the Nigerian National Bureau of Statistics (2010), there was slight fluctuation of poverty incidence from 1980 to 2004, as Table 5.1 shows. While poverty incidence was 28.1% in 1980, it increased to 46.1% in 1985, decreased to 42.7% in 1992, then increased to 65.6% in 1996, which meant that 67.1 million people lived in poverty. Poverty decreased to 54.7% in 2004, but with an increased poverty population of 69.09 million due to population growth. The above statistics indicated that the percentage of poverty increased from 54.7% in 2004 to 69.0% in 2010. The report also shows that the proportion of those living on less than $1 per day in 2004 was 51.6% but that figure increased to 61.2% in 2010 and even worse in 2019 (National Bureau of Statistics, 2010).

Poverty has become domesticated in Nigeria and is prevalent in the north-eastern part of Nigeria where frustration stemming from lack of access to the basic needs of life has made many Nigerian youth to take solace in criminal activities. Nigeria is the fifth-largest producer of oil in the world but the vast majority of the population lives below the poverty line of $1 a day. It is obvious that the teaming population of poor and unemployed youths, especially in the urban centres, take full advantage of the opportunities provided by poverty crises to wreak havoc on the innocent masses and economic institutions of the state. In this sense, there is a correlation between poverty and kidnapping as various groups emerge and use criminal activities as an avenue to unleash their frustration on innocent citizens.

Unemployment

As noted above, Nigeria has one of the largest populations of youth in the world. Notwithstanding the slow pace in expanding the economy in some sectors, employment creation is not sufficient to engage the fast-growing labour force that graduates out of Nigerian universities every year. This situation has resulted in high unemployment rate; in 2018, Nigeria had 23% unemployment rate and 20% underemployed labour force (the World Bank, 2019). According to National Bureau of Statistics, 7.53 million out of 85.08 million Nigerian labour force were unemployed in 2018 (Ahiuma-Young, 2018). This level of unemployment is alarming and is considered a threat to national development.

The present level of unemployment in Nigeria confirmed the crisis of governance and underdevelopment in Buhari's administration. While unemployment is continuously increasing at a disturbing rate, the victims of unemployment continue to resort to ways of making quick cash despite all odds. These victims become more susceptible as agents of election fraud and political kidnapping. They become militarised into the election process as arms and ammunitions are readily made available to them by political godfathers. Obviously, unemployed youths are easily enticed as political weapons to perpetrate kidnapping against political enemies. After elections, this group serendipitously emerged as full-time organised criminals and continued the trend in criminal activities, thus choosing to escalate their training in kidnapping of citizens for profit-making ventures.

Socio-economic Deprivation

Crenshaw (1981) and Adeoye (2005) asserted that economic imbalances, deprivation of socio-economic amenities, inflation and poverty provide a breeding ground for criminal activities. This position could lead to what Durkheim (1951, as cited in Williams & McShane, 2010) referred to as state of anomie where economic crises, forced industrialisation and commercialisation lead to a breakdown in the rules and order of the society. Merton (1938, as cited in Williams & McShane, 2010) expanded the theory of anomie by emphasising that when there is inequality in achieving legitimate financial success, those deprived of the legitimate means to achieve goals may search for illegitimate ways of succeeding. Thus, social inequality or blocked legitimate opportunities deprive certain groups of people, particularly the lower social class and minorities, of the opportunity to pursue the goal of financial success. The resultant effect of strain is a state of lawlessness, or anomie.

Furthermore, the socio-economic causes of kidnapping can be traced back to Karl Marx's ideology that conflict in society results from scarcity of resources and historical inequality in the distribution of those resources (Lynch & Michalowski, 2010). According to Marx's argument, the impact of the capitalist economic system results in the creation of class struggles between the proletariat (the working class) and the dominant bourgeoisie (the non-working owners of wealth; (Lynch & Michalowski, 2010). The class conflicts and socio-economic deprivations thus give rise to a sort of collective and individual aggression that erupts into organised criminal activities.

Solomon (2014) also argued that the emergence of armed militants in Nigeria such as the Boko Haram and Niger Delta militants' resurgence resulted from socio-economic marginalisation, poor governance, resource control, deprivation of social amenities, impoverishment of citizens, declining economic opportunities, limited educational opportunities and unemployment. Despite the fact that Nigeria oil revenues within 1980–2013 was about US$74 billion per annum, many regions of the country have no access to social amenities such as water, electricity and educational opportunities (International Crisis Group, 2014; Sergie & Johnson, 2011).

Globalisation

Globalisation has also created opportunities that have made countries more vulnerable to organised criminal activities through global network of communications, easy transportation and urbanisation, all of which make targets easily accessible. The global trend in technology has made citizens more vulnerable to kidnapping and hostage-taking due to the easy access to internet and the use of smart mobile phones and instant messaging. The ease of transporting goods and free trade associated with globalisation has enabled kidnappers such as drug cartels, human traffickers, terrorist groups and criminal gangs to reach across international borders just like businesspeople. Free movement across borders has enabled criminal groups to perpetrate kidnapping very easily. Globalised information technology has promoted greed and insatiable wants among men and women of Nigeria. Internet and fluent network of communications glamourised affluence, wealth, easy good life and fantasies, which persons with low internal self-control try to emulate such expensive lifestyle, hence resorting to quick money-making strategies.

Response to Kidnapping and Lessons Learned

Generally, in hostage situations, the policy adopted by most Western countries including the United States is that of no negotiation (Meyer, 2017). This policy is predicated upon the assumption that payment of ransom is not a guarantee that the kidnapped person will be returned safe, and the belief that payment is an incentive to embolden future incidents of kidnapping for gain, and that as long as governments can stand their ground, terrorists or kidnappers would be discouraged, knowing that there will be no financial gain from their criminal enterprise. Despite this policy, many nations have been criticised for negotiating with hostage-takers (Powell, 2017). Italy, France, Germany and Switzerland are more receptive to negotiating and paying terrorists than Britain, Canada and the United States. Sometimes, political leaders in the most exacting jurisdictions indulge in secret negotiation with terrorists (Meyer,

2017). For example, in 2014, President Obama was criticised for securing the freedom of Sergeant Bowe Bergdahl in exchange for the release of five Taliban prisoners from Guantanamo (Bolton, 2014). In the mid-1980s, the government of President Reagan came under fire for a convoluted case of trading hostages for dealing in munitions with Iran (Kornbluh & Byrne, 1993). The governments of Israel, Spain and the United Kingdom have all been criticised at one time or the other for secret negotiations with kidnappers (Neumann, 2007). Two Japanese hostages were killed by ISIL when Japan refused to yield to paying $200 million for their release. The Al-Qaeda is claimed to have received over $125 million from European governments as ransom money masked as development aids (Callimachi, 2014; Pearl, 2015).

The punishment for kidnapping among the Hebrews is death (Arewa, 2011). Under the Nigerian criminal law, kidnapping is considered a felony punishable by imprisonment for ten years and fine; and under Sect. 274, where a perpetrator kidnaps or abducts any person in order that such victim may be killed or disposed of as to be put in danger of being killed, such perpetrator shall be punished with imprisonment for a term extending up to 14 years and fine (Umego, 2019).

The governments of different states in Nigeria have legislated to deal with kidnapping. In 2009, six eastern states, Abia, Akwa-Ibo, Anambra, Ebonyi, Enugu and Imo, prescribed the death penalty for kidnapping offences. In 2010, Ondo State prescribed the death penalty for kidnapping only where the crime has led to the death of the victim and life imprisonment where the victim is still alive. The Ondo state law further prescribes punishment for those who harbour or procure kidnapping. Ondo also establishes pecuniary liability for corporations that have aided kidnapping. The fine for corporate liability is a sum not less than 20 million naira and not more than 50 million naira. The law also punishes "attempt to kidnap" with 20 years' imprisonment and aiding and abetting with life imprisonment with no option for fine in both instances. Where a kidnapping victim has been found to facilitate his own kidnap, he will be punished with a term of 15 years' imprisonment with no option for fine. In 2013, Bayelsa, Edo and Delta states passed anti-kidnapping laws prescribing the death penalty for all manner of kidnapping irrespective of whether death is involved or not (Akinsulore, 2016). In Lagos State, the law prescribes a life imprisonment for kidnappers and death penalty where the victim dies. The law also punishes any person who threatens to kidnap another person through telephone calls, email and text messages or any other form of communication with a term of imprisonment for 25 years. A term of imprisonment for 14 years is prescribed for anyone who knowingly or wilfully allows the use of his premises or belongings over which he has control to be used for the purpose of facilitating the kidnapping of any victim. Anyone who knows that a person has been kidnapped, or abducted, and conceals such information or confines such a person is also punishable with three years' imprisonment (Umego, 2019).

Other states have also prescribed the death penalty for kidnapping, including Bauchi, Enugu, Cross River, Kogi, Rivers, Ogun and Oyo. In 2017, the Kidnapping Abduction Act was promulgated by the National Assembly prescribing a punishment of 30 years' imprisonment for anyone colluding with an abductor to receive ransom money and death sentence where the victim dies.

It is now standard practice across the states to prescribe capital punishment for kidnapping. At least 15 states have enacted laws with the death penalty for kidnapping and related violent offences particularly where the death of the victim occurs. Earlier laws on kidnapping and related offence prescribed less serious punishments. For example, under the Terrorism Act of 2011 the prescribed punishment is limited to a term of ten years' imprisonment for anyone who takes another person hostage. By virtue of Sect. 20 of the Trafficking in Persons (Prohibition Law Enforcement and Administration Act, 2003), anyone who kidnaps, abducts or lures any person away to be killed was liable to life imprisonment. Arguably, the stricter penalties will serve as deterrence to result in a downward trend in the spree of kidnapping across the country.

In the United States, kidnapping is punished under 18 U.S. Code § 1201. That law prescribed imprisonment for any term of years or for life and, death or life imprisonment if there is loss of life involved during the kidnapping of a victim who is a foreign official, an internationally protected person or an official guest on performance of official duty. There is a presumption that the victim has been transported in interstate or foreign commerce if he is not released by the FBI into the case before the expiration of 24 hours. Kidnapping is also punished as first-degree or aggravated assault where there is bodily injury, sexual assault or a demand of ransom.

Conclusion: Recommendations and Policy Implications

Violent crimes including kidnapping and abduction pose serious threats and undermine the quality of life in local communities and entire nations. Kidnapping and violent crimes threaten the national security and the existence of Nigeria as a federation. These crimes can be controlled not only by adopting a holistic national security policy approach but also addressing the core national values of Nigeria as a community of people within a democracy bound by a social contract. It has become highly imperative to preserve and protect the core national values and interests of the country enshrined in Chapter IV of the Nigerian Constitution (1999), which provides for the right to life, dignity of the human person, personal liberty, freedom of movement, private and family life amongst other rights. Basic national values, goals and interests must emphasise the promotion of prosperity and employment, the provision of security within a broad global framework and the projection of fundamental values and culture. Therefore, a dogmatic perspective of national security in terms of safety and perpetuation of the state and state actors should no longer be the order of the day (Arewa, 2011). It is recommended that the government of Nigeria must work on the following key points:

1. Encourage public safety behaviour and awareness crusades by security agencies and government highlighting contemporary strategies being used by kidnappers that could reduce kidnapping in Nigeria (Oludayo et al., 2019).
2. The use of an integrated and holistic national security policy framework must be predicated upon the following: the protection and preservation of core national values, goals and interests such as democracy,

the rule of law, good governance, human liberty; freedom from the erosion of the political, economic and social values which are essential to the quality of life in Nigeria; preservation of Nigeria's political identity and institutions; fostering an international political and economic order which complements the essential interests of Nigeria and its allies; preservation of human rights, particularly the protection of socio-economic rights (Colucci, 2008).

3. Expand the national core values, goals and interests to effectively embrace the economic empowerment, employment and security of all citizens. In order to control the high rate of unemployment, the government should diversify the economy, and encourage local production of commodities, manufacturing and mechanised farming to create more jobs (Arewa, 2011).

4. Extant local efforts directed at controlling crime should be complemented by the federal government through the provision of needed resources and funding. Training should be provided for law enforcement and security agents at all levels, and there should be fair distribution of resources to all the regions to include those who feel cheated (Umego, 2019). The best approach for locating a kidnapped person is routine police investigation. The government should employ and train hardworking investigators to help resolve kidnapping cases.

5. Provide youth empowerment programmes and policies in the effort towards national development. Youth engagement is imperative to crime reduction and national advancement.

6. Propagate social justice to limit the gap between the upper class and lower class in society. This will involve the provision of social services to those in need including food, social security to the aged and ageing population, unemployment benefits and workforce services to unemployed youth, shelters for the homeless, counselling and treatment centres for those dealing with health, drug, depression and similar life issues.

7. Equal opportunities under the law for all citizens to afford a decent living, doing away with the system where few extremely rich citizens control resources while the deprived resort to kidnapping and demanding for ransom to get even.

8. Revisit the public school system to a system that works to provide quality and affordable education to all children, uninterrupted by incessant strikes, lack of effective oversight and accountability (Nnam, 2013).

References

Adeoye, M. N. (2005). Terrorism: An appraisal in the Nigerian context. In *Issues in Political Violence in Nigeria*. Hamson Printing Communications.

Africa piracy: Foreigners being held hostage. (2011, October 14). Telegraph. https://www.telegraph.co.uk/news/worldnews/piracy/8824953/Africa-piracy-foreigners-being-held-hostage.html

Agnew, R. (1985). A revised strain theory of delinquency. *Social Forces, 64*, 151–167. https://doi.org/10.2307/2578977

Agnew, R. (2006). *Pressured into crime.* Los Angeles: Roxbury Publishing Company.

Ahiuma-Young, V. (2018). *Nigeria's unemployment rate, a national threat—labour.* Vanguard. https://www.vanguardngr.com/2018/01/nigerias-unemployment-rate-national-threat-labour/

Akinsulore, A. (2016). Kidnapping and its victims in Nigeria: A criminological assessment of the Ondo State criminal justice system. *ABUAD Journal of Public and International Law, 2*, 180–209. https://www.researchgate.net/publication/311202422_KIDNAPPING_AND_ITS_VICTIMS_IN_NIGERIA_A_CRIMINOLOGICAL_ASSESSMENT_OF_THE_ONDO_STATE_CRIMINAL_JUSTICE_SYSTEM

Akpan, N. (2010). Kidnapping in Nigeria's Niger Delta: An exploratory study. *Journal of Social Sciences, 24*(1), 33–42. https://doi.org/10.1080/09711892 3.2010.11892834

Anazonwu, C. O., Onyemaechi, C. I., & Igwilo, C. (2016). Psychology of kidnapping. *Practicum Psychologia, 6*(1) https://journals.aphriapub.com/index.php/PP/article/view/144

Arewa, J. A. (2011). Core national values as determinant of national security and panacea for the crime of kidnapping and abduction in Nigeria. *Law and security in Nigeria, 1*, 127–139. https://www.researchgate.net/publication/311202422_KIDNAPPING_AND_ITS_VICTIMS_IN_

NIGERIA_A_CRIMINOLOGICAL_ASSESSMENT_OF_THE_
ONDO_STATE_CRIMINAL_JUSTICE_SYSTEM

Augustyn et al. (n.d.). Kidnapping: Criminal offence. In *Encyclopedia Britannica.* https://www.britannica.com/topic/kidnapping

Bayagbon, M. (2013, February 18). *Ansaru claims kidnap of 7 foreigners in Nigeria.* Vanguard Newspaper. https://www.vanguardngr.com/2013/02/ansaru-claims-kidnap-of-7-foreigners-in-nigeria/

Bernard, T. J., Snipes, J. B., & Gerould, A. L. (2010). *Vold's theoretical criminology* (6th ed.). Oxford: Oxford University Press.

Black's Law Dictionary. (2009). (9th ed.). West Publishing Co.

Blackstone, W. (2010). *Commentaries on the Law of England* (Forgotten Books), 955-956.

Bolaji, S. (2018, March 28). *Dapchi girls' abduction: Some unanswered questions.* Punch.   https://punchng.com/dapchi-girls-abduction-some-unanswered-questions/

Bolton, A. (2014, June 3). *Prisoner swap blows up White House.* The Hill. https://thehill.com/policy/defense/208163-prisoner-swap-blows-up-on-the-white-house

Callimachi, R. (2014). Paying ransoms, Europe bankrolls Qaeda terror. *The New York Times.*

Colucci, L. (2008). *Crusading realism: The Bush doctrine and American core values after 9/11.* University Press of America, passim.

Cornish, D., & Clarke, R. V. (1986). *The reasoning criminal: Rational choice perspectives on offending.* Berlin: *Springer- Verlag.*

Country Watch. (n.d.). Nigeria. http://www.countrywatch.com.ezproxy.apollolibrary.com/cw_country.aspx?vcountry=12

Crenshaw, M. (1981). The causes of terrorism. *Comparative Politics, 13*(4), 379–399. https://doi.org/10.2307/421717

Douglas, J. E., Burgess, A. W., Burgess, A. G., & Ressler, R. K. (1992). *Crime classification manual: A standard system for investigation and classifying violent Crimes.* New Jersey: John Wiley & Sons.

Durkheim, E. (1951). *Suicide.* London: Routledge.

French hostage Marie Dedieu held in Somalia dies. (2011, October 19). *BBC News.* https://www.bbc.com/news/world-africa-15365469

Fulani herdsmen kidnap delta monarch. (2018, June 5). *PM News.* https://www.pmnewsnigeria.com/2018/06/05/gunmen-kidnap-delta-monarch/

Global Terrorism Database. (2019). *About the GTD.* https://www.start.umd.edu/gtd/about/

Godwin, A. C. (2018, February 10). *Fulani Herdsmen Strike again in Benue, Kidnap four Policemen.* Daily Post. https://dailypost.ng/2018/02/10/fulani-herdsmen-strike-benue-kidnap-four-policemen/

Heaton, L. (2017, May 31). *The Watson files.* Foreign Policy News. https://foreignpolicy.com/2017/05/31/the-watson-files-somalia-climate-change-conflict-war/

International Crisis Group. (2014). Curbing violence in Nigeria (11): The Boko Haram insurgency. *Crisis Group Africa Report, 216*(1–54) https://d2071andvip0wj.cloudfront.net/curbing-violence-in-nigeria-II-the-boko-haram-insurgency.pdf

Johnson, A. (2018). Fulani herdsman has made over N100 million from Edo abductions. *Pulse.ng.* https://www.pulse.ng/gist/business-man-fulani-herdsman-has-made-over-n100m-from-edo-abductions/gln8ewg

Kanogo, T. (2020). *Abduction in modern Africa.* Encyclopedia. https://www.encyclopedia.com/children/encyclopedias-almanacs-transcripts-and-maps/abduction-modern-africa

Khan, N. A., & Sajid, I. A. (2010). Kidnapping in the North West Frontier Province (NWFP). *Pakistan Journal of Criminology, 2*(1), 175–187. https://www.researchgate.net/publication/268821034_Kidnapping_in_The_North_West_Frontier_Province_NWFP

Kidnapping rate in Africa. (n.d.). The Global Economy. https://www.theglobaleconomy.com/rankings/kidnapping/Africa/

Kornbluh, P., & Byrne, M. (1993). *The Iran-Contra scandal: The declassified history.* New York: The New Press.

Kwaja, C. M. A. (2009). Strategies for rebuilding state capacity to manage ethnic and religious conflict in Nigeria. *The Journal of Pan African Studies, 3*(3), 105–115. https://go.gale.com/ps/anonymous?id=GALE%7CA306598784&sid=googleScholar&v=2.1&it=r&linkaccess=abs&issn=08886601&p=LitRC&sw=w

Lynch, M. J., & Michalowski, R. (2010). *Primer in radical criminology: Critical perspectives on crime, power & identity* (4th ed.). Boulder: Lynne Rienner Publishers Inc.

Merriam-Webster. (n.d.). Kidnapping. In Merriam-Webster.com legal dictionary. https://www.merriam-webster.com/legal/kidnapping

Merton, R. K. (1938). Social structure and anomie. *American Sociological Review, 3*(5), 672–682. https://doi.org/10.2307/2084686

Meyer, J. (2017). *Why the G8 pact to stop paying terrorist ransoms probably won't work—and isn't even such a great idea.* Quartz. https://qz.com/95618/

why-the-g8-pact-to-stop-paying-terrorist-ransoms-probably-wont-work-and-isnt-even-such-a-great-idea/

Mullin, G., & Petkar, S. (2018, August 9). *Living hell: Journalist kidnapped and raped in Somalia details horrific 15-month ordeal and reason why she decided not to kill herself amid torture*. The Sun. https://www.thesun.co.uk/news/6966500/journalist-amanda-lindhout-kidnapped-raped-somalia/

Neumann, P. R. (2007, January 1). *Negotiating with terrorists*. Foreign Affairs. https://www.foreignaffairs.com/articles/2007-01-01/negotiating-terrorists

Ngwama, J. C. (2014). Kidnapping in Nigeria: An emerging social crime and the implications for the labor market. *International Journal of Humanities and Social Science, 4*(1), 133–145.

Nigerian National Bureau of Statistics. (2010). *Nigeria Poverty Profile, 2010*. http://www.tucrivers.org/tucpublication/NigeriaPovertyProfile2010.pdf

Nnam, U. (2013). *Kidnapping and kidnappers in the South Eastern States of Nigeria: A sociological analysis of selected inmates in Abakaliki and Umuahia prisons*. A postgraduate seminar presented to the Department of Sociology and Anthropology, Ebonyi State University, Abakaliki, Ebonyi State, Nigeria.

Nwagwu, E. J. (2014). Unemployment and poverty in Nigeria: A link to national insecurity. *Global Journal of Politics and Law Research, 2*(1), 19–35. https://rcmss.com/2013/1ijpamr/Unemployment%20and%20Poverty_%20Implications%20for%20National%20Security%20and%20Good%20Governance%20in%20Nigeria.pdf

Ochoa, R. (2012). Not just rich: New tendencies in kidnapping in Mexico City. *Global Crime, 13*(1), 1–21. https://doi.org/10.1080/17440572.2011.632499

Odoemelam, U., & Omage, M. (2013). Changes in traditional cultural values and kidnapping: A case of Edo State. *British Journal of Arts and Social Sciences, 16*(1), 1–4. https://www.academia.edu/29335485/Changes_in_traditional_cultural_values_and_kidnapping_The_case_of_Edo_State

Ogbuehi, V. N. (2018). Kidnapping in Nigeria: The way forward. *Journal of Criminology and Forensic Studies, 1*(3), 1–8. https://chembiopublishers.com/JOCFS/JOCFS180014.pdf

Ogundiya, S., & Amzat, J. (2008). Nigeria and the threat of terrorism: Myth or reality. *Journal of Sustainable Development in Africa, 10*(2), 165–189. https://www.researchgate.net/publication/266883526_NIGERIA_AND_THE_THREATS_OF_TERRORISM_MYTH_OR_REALITY

Okafor, A. E., Ajibo, H. T., Chukwu, N. A., Egbuche, M. N., & Asadu, N. (2018). Kidnapping and hostage-taking in Niger Delta Region of Nigeria: Implication for social work intervention with victims. *International Journal of Humanities and Social Science, 8*(11), 94–100. https://doi.org/10.30845/ijhss.v8n11p11

Okengwu, K. (2011). Kidnapping in Nigeria: Issues and common sense ways of surviving. *Global Journal of Education Research, 1*(1), 1–8. http://www.globalresearchjournals.org/journal/gjer/archive/july-2011-vol-1(1)/kidnapping-in-nigeria:-issues-and-common-sense-ways-of-surviving

Oludayo T., Usman A.O. & Adeyinka A. A. (2019). 'I Went through Hell': Strategies for Kidnapping and Victims' Experiences in Nigeria, Journal of Aggression, Maltreatment & Trauma, https://doi.org/10.1080/1092677 1.2019.1628155

Pearl, M. (2015, January 27). *Where exactly is the rule that says governments can't negotiate with terrorists?* Vice. https://www.vice.com/en_us/article/9bzp5v/where-exactly-is-the-rule-that-says-you-cant-negotiate-with-terrorists-998

Pharoah, R. (2005). Kidnapping for ransom in South Africa. *South Africa Crime Quarterly, 14*, 23–28. https://doi.org/10.17159/2413-3108/2005/v0i14a1007

Powell, J. (2017). *We must negotiate with terrorists: The dirty secret our government does not want to admit.* Salon. https://www.salon.com/2015/07/12/we_must_negotiate_with_terrorists_the_dirty_secret_our_government_does_not_want_to_admit/

Rementeria, D. (1939). Criminal law-kidnapping-ransom and reward. *Oregon Law Review, 19*, 301.

Salawu, B. (2010). Ethno-religious conflicts in Nigeria: Causal analysis and proposals for new management strategies. *European Journal of Social Sciences, 13*(3), 345–353. https://gisf.ngo/wp-content/uploads/2014/09/0071-Salawu-2010-Nigeria-ethno-religious-conflict.pdf

SBM Intel. (2020, May). Nigeria's kidnap problem: The economics of the kidnap industry in Nigeria. https://www.sbmintel.com/wpcontent/uploads/2020/05/202005_Nigeria-Kidnap.pdf

Schiller, D. T. (1985). The European experience. In *Terrorism and personal protection* (pp. 46-63). Butterworth.

Schmalleger, F. (2018). *Criminology today: An integrative introduction* (9th ed.). London: Pearson Education Inc..

Sergie, M. A., & Johnson, T. (2011). *Boko Haram.* Council on foreign relations. http://www.cfr.org/africa/boko-haram/p25739

Solomon, H. (2014). *Nigeria's Boko Haram: Beyond the rhetoric.* Policy & Practice Brief Knowledge for Durable Peace. Accord.

Somalia: Shaabab displays four abducted Kenyans. (2012, January 13). *Daily Nation*. https://allafrica.com/stories/201201140015.html

South African Police Service. (2014). Crime Situation in South Africa. https://www.saps.gov.za/resource_centre/publications/statistics/crimestats/2014/crime_stats.php

Turner, M. (1998). Kidnapping and politics. *International Journal of the Sociology of Law, 26*(2), 145–160. https://doi.org/10.1006/ijsl.1998.0061

Umar, H. (2014, April 21). *Up to 233 teenage girls were kidnapped from this Nigerian school*. Business insider. https://www.businessinsider.com/233-teenage-girls-kidnapped-from-chibok-nigeria-school-2014-4?IR=T

Umego, C. (2019). *Offence of kidnapping: A counter to national security and development*. SSRN. https://papers.ssrn.com/sol3/papers.cfm?abstract_id=3337745

United Nations Office on Drugs and Crime. (2015). International classification of crime for statistical purposes (ICCS)—Version 1.0.W.O. https://www.unodc.org/documents/data-and-analysis/statistics/crime/ICCS/ICCS_English_2016_web.pdf

Watch: Kidnappings on the rise in South Africa. (2019, November 20). https://www.enca.com/news/watch-kidnappings-rise-south-africa

Weber, B. (2014, July 8). *Umaru Dikko, Ex-Nigerian official, who was almost kidnapped, dies*. The New York Times. https://www.nytimes.com/2014/07/08/world/africa/umaru-dikko-ex-nigerian-official-who-was-almost-kidnapped-dies.html

Webster, M. (2007). Kidnapping: A brief psychological overview. In O. Nikbay. & S. Hancerli, (Eds.), *Understanding and responding to the terrorism phenomenon: A multi-dimensional perspective* (pp. 231-241). National Criminal Justice Reference Service. https://www.ncjrs.gov/App/Publications/abstract.aspx?ID=247116

Williams, F. P., & Mcshane, M. D. (2010). *Criminological theory* (5th ed.). London: Pearson Education Inc..

Wilson, C. (1994). *Freedom at risk: The kidnapping of free Blacks in America, 1780–1865*. Kentucky: University Press of Kentucky.

Cases

Okashetu v. State. (2016). ALL FWLR (Pt.861) 1262 S.C.

R v. CORT. (2004). 4 All ER 137.

6

An Overview of Serial Murder and its Investigation in South Africa

Gérard Labuschagne

Introduction

Serial murder occurs throughout the world (Gorby, 2000). Cases of serial murder have been documented in Australia (Gorby, 2000), Austria, Brazil (Lubaszka, Shon, & Hinch, 2014), Canada (Campos & Cusson, 2007), Germany (Harbort & Mokros, 2001), Hungary (Lubaszka et al., 2014), Israel (Kallian, Birger, & Witztum, 2004), Italy (Campobasso et al., 2009), Japan (Aki, 2003), Norway (Lubaszka et al., 2014), Russia (Myers et al., 2008), Sweden (Sturup, 2018), Switzerland (Lubaszka et al., 2014), United Kingdom (Jenkins, 1988), United States (Jenkins,

G. Labuschagne (✉)
L&S Threat Management, Johannesburg, South Africa

Department of Forensic Medicine and Pathology, University of the Witwatersrand, Johannesburg, South Africa

African Association of Threat Assessment Professionals, Johannesburg, South Africa
e-mail: doc@forensic-psychologist.co.za

© The Author(s), under exclusive license to Springer Nature Switzerland AG 2021   **121**
H. C. O. Chan, S. Adjorlolo (eds.), *Crime, Mental Health and the Criminal Justice System in Africa*, https://doi.org/10.1007/978-3-030-71024-8_6

1989), Zimbabwe (Lubaszka et al., 2014) to name a few. Egger (2002) reported cases from China, Colombia, Ecuador, France, Nepal, Nigeria, Peru, Thailand, Singapore, and Turkey. The author himself has assisted with investigations in Namibia (the 'B1 Butcher' series), in India (the 'Nithari serial murderer') and a murder series in Swaziland (Labuschagne, 2010).

This chapter will examine serial murder in the South African context. The goal is to illustrate how serial murder presents itself in terms of offenders, victims and modus operandi. It will also inform readers how the South African Police Service (SAPS) adapted to identify and investigate these crimes. It will begin by discussing the definition of serial murder, followed by an examination of certain myths about serial murder, then review the local research on serial murder, and conclude by discussing the SAPS' response to managing this crime. South Africa has not been immune to such cases, with a significant number of murder series throughout its recent history; most cases came to law enforcement's attention in the mid-1990s. It is reported that the post-apartheid, the levels of serial murder increased by 900% (Hodgskiss, 2004). By 2007, the SAPS had identified 131 murder series, of which 74% had been solved (Labuschagne & Salfati, 2015). By 2015 it had increased to 160 murder series (Labuschagne, 2017). The earliest series for which there are official records dates back to 1936, using a modus operandi that is uncannily similar to modern murder series (Labuschagne, 2006). The majority of murder series in South Africa are sexual in nature, as evidenced by victims having been found in various degrees of undress, forensic evidence of sexual violation, or confessions by the offender as to the sexual aspects of their crimes.

Defining Serial Murder

Serial murder has been defined in various ways by academics, clinicians, researchers and law enforcement agencies over the years. In 2005 the FBI hosted a multinational serial murder symposium in San Antonio, Texas, where issues central to serial murder were discussed among delegates. One of the main goals of the symposium was to come to a consensus about certain often-debated issues in the field, among them the definition of serial murder. In most definitions there is some overlap, but also many differences with respect to certain criteria. Most definitions include three elements: the number of victims, the time frame of the murders, and motivation.

One of the most common shortcomings regarding definitions is when *criteria* are confused with *characteristics*. For example, a criterion for serial murder would be the number of victims. A characteristic would be that offenders are *often* male, or that the murders are *typically* sexual murders, or the victims are *usually* strangers. Words like 'often', 'usually', 'typically' or 'frequently' tend to refer to characteristics and not to an essential criterion or element, and caution should be used when including them in a definition of serial murder. When a characteristic is elevated to a criterion, it often limits the application of a definition.

At the 2005 FBI Serial Murder Symposium, an effort was made to reach consensus on the definition for serial murder. Delegates were divided into groups and asked to formulate a single definition, designed primarily for use by law enforcement agencies (Morton & Hilts, 2005). The integrated outcome of this was a definition formulated as 'the unlawful killing of two or more victims by the same offender(s) in separate events' (Morton & Hilts, 2005). This definition is consistent with the one used by the SAPS to classify a murder series, which was reflected in the *Policy on the Investigation and Management of Serial Rape and Serial Murder* (Civilian Secretariat for Police, 2016) as: 'murders perpetrated on at least two separate occasions by the same offender(s)' (p.7). This definition allows for one or more offenders, two or more victims, and that at least two of the incidents should occur at separate events. The time period of separate events also distinguishes serial murder from mass murder. The definition does not include motives for the murders. While the FBI symposium did address the motives for serial murder, motive was not made part of the criteria, and wisely so. Motive can, however, be added on as a specifier to categorise the type of serial murderer.

Some researchers (Fridel & Fox, 2017) have criticised the criterion of two victims, indicating that including such offenders drastically skews the population. They state that those in the two-victim group, the three-to-seven group, and the eight-victims-or-more group differ in key areas such as presence of a co-offender, use of torture, motive and totem-taking. They recommend reverting to the three-victim criterion. The problem with this is that an eight- or more victim serial murderer started out as a two-victim serial murderer and progressed through the three-to-seven victim category to end up in the eight or more category. This progression may take years, resulting in an ever-changing classification of the same series as it progresses. Similarly, someone who had the intention to have eight or more victims may have been apprehended by law enforcement after two victims. Therefore, the practicality of applying this evolving definition, especially in active law enforcement cases, is limited, and would only have academic use after a suspect has been arrested and convicted. And while serial murderers in the different groups mentioned above may qualitatively display different behaviours, they are still serial murderers. It appears that law enforcement tends to prefer a two-victim number, while academics and researchers tend to prefer three-or-more victims as the criteria for the victim count. A two-victim criteria allows for law enforcement to activate serial murder resources sooner rather than later. Similarly, most persons in society don't ever murder someone, thus those that murder one person are already in a small, unique group, with those that murder two persons being in an even smaller group, bearing in mind that murder is always, by definition, an intentional act, not an accidental one.

Other researchers argue that the defining feature should be intentionality, and not the actual number of victims (Adjorlolo & Chan, 2014). A South African example would be someone like Jose da Silva, who murdered an interior decorator at his home after luring her there with a false request for a quotation. He hit her with a blunt object, then later killed her with a hand-axe, kept her body in his house for a few days before leaving the victim naked along a highway. Prior to this murder, and after her murder, he had made appointments with numerous real-estate agents, using a false name, with the pretence of being interested in purchasing an expensive property. He did not offend against any of these real-estate agents that he did end up meeting. Shortly before the murder of the interior decorator described above, he lured the first interior decorator to his house but did not harm her. Upon interviewing this interior decorator shortly before da Silva's arrest, she commented that there had been a hammer on the en suite bathroom basin which made her feel uncomfortable and she ended the consultation shortly thereafter. In court da Silva also said he saw himself as a serial murderer who would not have stopped, and chastised the police for taking 6 weeks to arrest him. His continuation to meet with estate agents after the first murder also raises concerns for the repeat of a similar pattern that led to the initial murder. In summary, da Silva engaged in trial runs by luring victims with a con-story which is often noted in murder series, murdered his first victim, disposed of her naked body, and claimed he would have done it again had he not been caught. He referred to all of these actions as his 'game' in which the women he approached had to play the part of making him feel good and treat him well during their interactions. Should this be ignored because he was caught after his first victim due to good police work? From a risk assessment point of view, da Silva should be treated as having the same risk level as any other convicted serial murderer.

Another example, where a speedy arrest seems to have cut short the career of two serial murderers, would be that of Chané van Heerden and Maartens van der Merwe. This romantic couple hailed from the small Free State Province mining town of Welkom. This couple met and lured an unsuspecting male victim by means of an instant messaging chat service, to the local graveyard on the outskirts of the town, under the pretence of a romantic date. Shortly after arrival, the victim was killed in the graveyard and his body was dismembered. They buried the torso and some limbs in the graveyard in a shallow grave, and took the head and other parts home.

The following day the female offender skinned the face of the victim, taking photographs on her cell-phone as she did so. The male offender had a murder fantasy, while the female offender had fantasies of skinning a victim. The female offender had a history of skinning animals since childhood. Prior to the murder, they had attempted to kill and skin a dog but did not proceed because they felt sorry for the dog. They eventually killed and skinned a cat shortly before the murder, which was also photographically recorded. Both were fascinated with serial murderers, were avid fans of the TV series 'Dexter', and the female offender was fascinated with dismemberment, as evidenced by their online activity and books in their home. A quick arrest occurred within days of the murder, having traced the offenders via their cell phone. Both said they would have killed again had they had not been apprehended, and this was a consensus shared by the various experts for both the defence and the prosecution, including the current author, that testified at the trial. By means of the strict two-victim limit, these offenders would not be regarded as serial murderers; if one includes intentionality and looks at the behaviours preceding the initial murder, a good argument can be made that these were serial murderers.

Sometimes jurisdictional or political issues can influence a serial murder definition. The federal law passed by the US Congress in 1988, titled the *Protection of Children from Sexual Predators Act*, defined serial murder as:

> three or more killings, not less than one of which was committed within the United States, having common characteristics such as to suggest the reasonable possibility that the crimes were committed by the same actor or actors.

This definition is limited in that it requires at least three murders, and that one murder must have been committed in the USA. It also illustrates how political considerations and jurisdictional issues (federal v state) can influence a definition.

According to Egger (1984),

> serial murder occurs when one or more individuals ... commits a second murder and/or subsequent murder, is relationship less (victim and attacker are strangers); occurs at a different time and has no connection to the initial (and subsequent) murder; and is frequently committed in a different geographic location ... Victims share in common characteristics of what are perceived to be prestigeless, powerless, and/or lower socioeconomic groups (that is, vagrants, prostitutes, migrant workers, homosexuals, missing children, and single and often elderly women.

Egger's definition is problematic with regard to the following:

- Victim and attacker are strangers: It is not uncommon for serial murderers to murder people known to them. In South Africa this would include serial murderers like Stewart Wilken ('Boetie Boer') who murdered his own daughter and a neighbour's son and then a succession of street children and sex workers. Robin Cloete from the Northern Cape murdered his fiancée and years later, after his release from prison, he murdered his girlfriend and her mother in a single incident. Brydon Brandt from Port Elizabeth murdered a neighbour and other stranger sex-worker victims. Willem Grobler from Louis Trichardt murdered two girls known to him. Heinie van Rooyen from Knysna murdered two girls known to him over the space of one month. Johannes Van Rooyen and Dumisani Makhubela from Mhluzi township in Mpumalanga murdered a family known to them and a girlfriend of an acquaintance, as well as strangers. Gcunumuzi Makwenkwe, the Moffat Park serial murderer from Johannesburg, murdered his girlfriend and also stranger victims. The Donnybrook serial murderer, Christopher Zikode, murdered a female known to him amongst his other victims. Tommy Williams from Kimberley in the Northern Cape murdered three acquaintances over a 21-year period, including a neighbour's daughter and a friend.
- Murders are frequently committed in different geographic locations: In South Africa and internationally, serial murderers are known to have geographic comfort zones where they prefer to approach and/or murder their victims. South African examples include the Quarry serial murderer, Richard Nyauza; the Brighton Beach Axe serial murderer, Phindile Ntshongwana; the Newcastle serial murderer, Themba Anton Sukude, and the Johannesburg Mine Dump serial murderer, Sipho Dube. All of these offenders, and others, had clearly identifiable geographical areas of operation.
- Victims are perceived to be from prestigeless, powerless, and/or lower socioeconomic groups: In reality, victims are not necessarily from such groups and many are average everyday citizens.

Another example of a problematic definition is Schlesinger's (2000) which states:

... serial homicide consists of three fundamental components: (1) sexual sadism, (2) intense fantasy, and (3) a compulsion to act out the fantasy.

While some serial murderers do display such features, to state that one of the fundamental components is sexual sadism greatly limits our understanding of serial murder. Numerous serial murderers did not engage in any sexual behaviour with their victims, let alone sadistic activities. Similarly, determining whether an offender reaches the threshold or criteria for sexual sadism, or quantifying how intense the fantasy is, is problematic for consistency of application of the definition and may be difficult to apply in practice during a law enforcement investigation. Additionally, how does one objectively prove the existence of a fantasy and determine its intensity in a way that can be applied consistently by other researchers or law enforcement?

Ultimately, due to the limitations highlighted in many of the definitions discussed above, the 2005 FBI Symposium definition is the most inclusive, allowing for a wide range of sub-types of serial murders. To accommodate these wide ranges within the definition, the FBI typology that accompanied the symposium publication can be used to qualitatively group similar types of serial murderer scenarios.

Serial Murder Myths

The FBI Serial Murder Symposium identified seven myths in relation to serial murders which are discussed below (Morton & Hilts, 2005).

Myth 1: Serial Murderers are all Dysfunctional Loners

In South Africa, most serial murderers are not reclusive misfits who live alone, a stereotype that is frequently portrayed in fictional tales. Often, they are well known, liked, and integrated members of their community. It is not uncommon for people to be shocked to hear that the offender has been arrested in connection with a series of murders, and possibly initially overlooked by investigators. Numerous serial murderers are married or are involved in romantic relationships, have homes and some form of employment at the time of their murders. A study conducted in South Africa reported that 60% out of the 33 serial murderers had been in a relationship at the time of their arrest (Salfati, Labuschagne, Horning, Sorochinski, & De Wet, 2015b).

In South Africa, the following serial murderers had girlfriends, boyfriends, or wives at the time of their arrest, or an accomplice to their crimes:

- Richard Jabulani Nyauza—Quarry serial murderer, Centurion, Gauteng
- Dumisane Mthobeni—Soweto, Gauteng
- Elias Chauke—Highwayman serial murderer, Centurion, Gauteng
- Antonie Wessels and Jean-Pierre Havenga—Knysna serial murderers, Knysna, Western Cape
- Samuel Jacques Coetzee and Johan Frank Brown—East Rand crossdressing serial murderers, East Rand, Gauteng
- Heinie van Rooyen—Knysna serial murderer, Knysna, Western Cape
- Johannes van Rooyen and Dumisani Makhubela—Mhluzi serial murderers, Mhluzi, Mpumalanga
- Nicholas Ncama—Eastern Cape serial murderer, KwaZakele, Eastern Cape
- Kobus Geldenhuys—Norwood serial murderer, Johannesburg, Gauteng
- Cedric Maake—Wemmerpan Serial Murderer, Johannesburg, Gauteng

Such information becomes relevant when reviewing possible suspects and illustrates that disregarding someone as a potential suspect because of their relationship status can have disastrous consequences.

Myth 2: Serial Murderers are all White Males

This myth stems from the initial serial murder research conducted in the USA (Hickey, 2006), which has subsequently been challenged (McClellan, 2019). However, even in the USA, 24.95% of serial murderers are Black (Aamodt, 2016). Another US study which looked at 413 serial murders between 1945 and 2004 found that 90 (22%) were African American (Walsh, 2005). In South Africa, 67% of convicted serial murderers are

Black, 24% are White and 10% are Coloured (Salfati, Labuschagne, et al., 2015b). The population group of serial murderers will usually be reflective of the general population groupings in that country.

Myth 3: Serial Murderers are all Sexually Motivated

While serial murder cases that spring to the public's mind, or are often portrayed in movies, tend to be those that have sexual elements, the symposium highlighted various motivations for committing serial murder. These include sexual, power/thrill, anger, ideology, psychosis, financial gain and criminal enterprise (drug, gang or organised crime related) motivations (Morton & Hilts, 2005). In South Africa, a sexual motivation is often an aspect of serial murders, and the overwhelming majority of the murder series have murders that were sexual in nature. However, there were serial murderers that had no obvious sexual motive for their murders, such as the so-called Saloon Serial Murderer or the Brighton Beach axe murders.

Myth 4: All Serial Murderers Travel

In reality, serial murderers, like many serial offenders, prefer a 'comfort zone' defined by geographic areas of operation to commit their crimes. This has been noted amongst serial murderers throughout the world. South African examples of murder series that had clearly defined comfort zones include:

- the Brighton Beach axe murders in Brighton Beach, KwaZulu-Natal
- the Quarry serial murders in Centurion, Gauteng;
- the Newcastle serial murders in Newcastle, KwaZulu-Natal;
- the Modimolle serial murders in Modimolle, Limpopo;
- the Moffat Park serial murders in Johannesburg, Gauteng;
- the Newlands East serial murders in Newlands, KwaZulu-Natal;
- the Butterworth serial murders in Butterworth, Eastern Cape;
- the Port Elizabeth sex worker murders in Port Elizabeth, Eastern Cape;

- the Norwood serial murders, in Johannesburg, Gauteng; and
- the Soweto serial murders, in Johannesburg, Gauteng.

In a country such as South Africa, where the average serial murderer does not own a vehicle, this seems to limit the geographical movement of the offenders even more so.

Myth 5: Serial Murderers will continue to Kill

Some serial offenders in South Africa had pauses in between murders ranging from 7 to 14 years. Almost 30 murder series appeared to have stopped without arrests, and it is unclear why the murders stopped. Explanations such as the death of the offender, incarceration for an unrelated crime, or the possibility that the offender stopped their murder career, are all possibilities. Others continue after pauses of many years. Northern Cape serial murderer Tommy Williams committed 3 murders over a 21-year period, one each in 1987, 2004 and 2008. He was convicted of all 3 murders.

Myth 6: Serial Murderers are Insane or Evil Masterminds

This myth is propagated primarily by the media, with characters such as Hannibal Lecter from *Silence of the Lambs* in the forefront. In reality, many serial murderers suffer from personality disorders, but few are ever found to be 'insane'. This is echoed in South Africa, where only one serial murderer brought to trial was found to be unfit to stand trial. This murderer was Francois Potgieter, dubbed the 'Roadside Serial Killer', who operated mainly in the Potchefstroom area. After arrest he was sent for 30-day forensic mental health observation at a psychiatric facility to determine his criminal capacity, and was found lacking criminal capacity due to a diagnosis of schizophrenia.

Even if mental illness is present, there must be a significant link between the mental illness and the criminal act for it to have bearing on the criminal capacity of the offender at the time of the incident. In South African law this would mean that the offender would be sent for forensic mental health observation in terms of the Criminal Procedure Act to determine his competency to stand trial and criminal capacity. In terms of criminal capacity, the test would be to determine if the accused person had the mental ability to distinguish right from wrong and act in accordance with this appreciation at the time of the incident (Snyman, 2008). In Durban, the Brighton Beach axe serial murderer Phindile Ntshongwana had a long-standing diagnosis of schizophrenia prior to his murders. While this issue was raised pre-trial, and later again during the trial, it was found that his crimes were not a result of his mental illness and he was convicted of four murders, two attempted murders, one assault with intent to commit grievous bodily harm, one kidnap and one rape, and sent to prison, where he continued to receive his psychiatric treatment. With regard to intelligence, a South African study by Labuschagne (1998) tested the Intelligence Quotient (IQ) of convicted serial murderers and found that their IQ ranged in the average category of intelligence.

Myth 7: Serial Murderers want to Get Caught

As with any activity that is repeated, the offender gains experience and confidence each time he commits his criminal act. Serial murder is still a fairly complex activity consisting of selecting and approaching a potential victim, then luring the victim to a location to commit the crime, controlling the victim, attacking and murdering the victim and leaving the crime scene. When the offender becomes increasingly successful at committing the crime undetected, they become overconfident, take shortcuts and make mistakes. These mistakes are the ones that can lead to their arrest. Similarly, in South Africa, many offenders are still unaware of the sophisticated methods available to police, such as DNA analysis, fingerprints and cellphone-tracing technology that can be used to identify and locate an offender. This leads to them leaving evidence that can result in their arrest and conviction.

Does South Africa Have An Excessive Number of Serial Murderers?

As previously mentioned, to date the SAPS has identified 160 murder series between 1936 and 2015 (Labuschagne, 2017), the majority of which have been identified since the mid-1990s. But does South Africa have a disproportionately high number of serial murders compared to other countries? To determine this would be very difficult; however, the *Radford University Serial Killer Information Center* database ranks South Africa as having the third most serial murderers, after the USA and the UK (Aamodt, 2016).

However South Africa might be a victim of its own success, as discussed later in this chapter. The SAPS is one of a handful of law enforcement agencies across the globe that can claim to have relatively accurate statistics of all the known murder series in its country. One significant reason for this is that the SAPS is a national police service, making communication about cases of this nature much easier, as well as working from a standardised understanding of what serial murder is, and how to approach it.

Furthermore, the SAPS is one of the few law enforcement agencies in Sub-Saharan African that has forensic DNA capabilities and one national DNA database for crime-related DNA. It also has a database management section that tracks DNA 'hits' or linkages when two or more DNA profiles match and sends out notifications to various role-players that there has been a link between cases. Changes in how DNA is processed, that took place in the late 2000s, meant that DNA went from being only an evidential tool to be used in court to link a suspect to a crime, and to an intelligence tool used to link solved and unsolved cases.

Furthermore, the SAPS has a unit that is dedicated to identifying, tracking and assisting in these types of investigations, namely the Investigative Psychology Section (IPS). This unit fulfils a similar role to the FBI's Behavioral Analysis Units; however, it differs in that it has the ability to insert itself into any investigation without invitation and can provide direct instructions in the investigation. It is also the only unit allowed to classify something as a murder series, using one definition of serial murder when making such a classification. Also, the SAPS, through the IPS, is the only law enforcement agency in the world that has regular training for its detectives and crime scene experts in the identification and investigation of serial murder cases, and other psychologically motivated crimes.

All of the above factors place the SAPS in an envious position to be able to identify, track and respond to murder series in a consistent and effective way, but also can create a false sense that South Africa has a higher rate of such cases.

A South African Perspective on Serial Murders

Most research and publications on the topic of serial murder are from outside the boarders of Africa. South Africa has a small but growing body of research (Barkhuizen, 2006; Collaros, 2019, Del Fabbro, 2006; De Wet, 2005; Du Plessis, 1998; Hodgskiss, 2001, 2004; Hook, 2003; Hurst, 2003a, b; Knight, 2006; Labuschagne, 1998, 2001, Labuschagne, 2006, 2007; Lemmer, 2003; Pistorius, 1996; Snyman, 1992), but with the advantage that much of the research involved direct access to offenders in prison.

Those that involved research participants who were incarcerated serial murderers were first Labuschagne (1998, 2001) who focused on a systemic interactional approach to understanding serial murderers based on interviews with offenders. Du Plessis (1998) used grounded theory approach to explore serial murder, based on interviews with offenders. Later Hodgskiss (2001, 2004) interviewed 13 serial murder offenders to examine offender characteristics and behaviours. De Wet (2005) used a psychosocial perspective when interviewing offenders and Barkhuizen (2006) used an intrapsychic object relations approach. Del Fabbro (2006) used a family systems paradigm to understand serial murder based on interviews with the offenders, and where possible, their family members. Finally, Collaros (2019) explored the psychogeography of 15 serial murderers in prison.

The largest South African serial murder study to date is a collaborative study between the South African Police Service's Investigative Psychology

Section and the Department of Psychology at John Jay College of Criminal Justice of the City University of New York. The sample consisted of 33 of the 54 solved murder series in South Africa between 1953 and 2007 and used police case files as the source of data. This sample accounted for 62% of the prosecuted and convicted series for that time period. The sample consisted of 33 offenders, 302 victims, and 254 crime scenes. Serial murder was defined in accordance with the 2005 FBI Serial Murder Symposium definition as discussed above (Morton & Hilts, 2005). Salfati's Homicide Profiling Index version 4 (HPIv4©) was used to code the data (Salfati, 2006). The results of this study were published in a special edition of the *Journal of Investigative Psychology and Offender Profiling* (Horning, Salfati, & Labuschagne, 2015; Labuschagne & Salfati, 2015; Salfati, Horning, Sorochinski, & Labuschagne, 2015a; Salfati, Labuschagne, et al., 2015b; Sorochinski, Salfati, & Labuschagne, 2015).

In terms of crime scene location, more than 78% of the crimes occurred outside in the open veld. This seems to be a unique feature of South African serial murder crime scenes in comparison to the US scenes, where most US crime scenes were in urban areas. South African serial murder offenders tend to come from low-income groups and are often not in possession of a vehicle. This lack of vehicle ownership or access affects their modus operandi and as a result they tend to lure victims with a con story, most frequently the promise of employment, to a single secluded location where the victim is murdered and the body disposed of (Labuschagne & Salfati, 2015). The use of this con story is highly effective due to South Africa's high unemployment rate, with many females being desperate for employment. Many victims use public transport and walk long distances in their daily routine, thus making them vulnerable to such approaches. This con story was used as far back as 1953 in the KwaZulu-Natal province, when serial murder offender Elifasi Msomi would travel to small villages and lure victims with an employment con story before murdering them (Labuschagne & Salfati, 2015).

Horning et al.'s (2015) study, which was part of the larger collaborative study, identified that 47% of incidents in the South African sample involved deception in the form of a con story. This was also found by Woodhams and Labuschagne (2012) in their South African serial rape study in which 77% of victims were lured by some form of con story, and an offer of employment was used in 48% of the serial rape cases. The patterns of behaviour between South African serial murderers and South African serial rapists are almost identical except the serial murderer typically kills his victim at the end of the incident.

As mentioned, most crime scenes (65.7%) in this serial murder study had a sexual component, but when examined per series, it was noted that at least 29 of the 33 series (i.e., 88%) included at least some sexual murders, usually expressed by naked and/or raped victims (Horning et al., 2015). When the victims were grouped into one data-pool, results indicated that a firearm was used in 30.2% of cases. Blunt force was used in 27.6% of cases, strangulation in 25.7% of cases, and 10.8% of victims were stabbed (Salfati, Labuschagne, et al., 2015b). However, when analysed per series, few serial murderers use firearms to kill their victims, but those that do, tend to have a high victim count in their series. An example would be the so-called Saloon Killer from Mpumalanga, Velaphi Ndlangamandla, who murdered 21 people and attempted to murder nine others, and his victims were a mixture of males and females. His typical modus operandi would be to confront victims walking along a dirt road in a rural area, or in their homes, and shoot them. The shootings appeared to be entirely unprovoked and unnecessary to commit the crime of robbery. Similarly, the Wemmerpan serial murderer, Maoupa Cedric Maake, murdered 32 victims and had 10 victims who survived. After initially using blunt force trauma to injure his victims, he came across a victim with a firearm. Thereafter, most of his victims (including the owner of the firearm) were shot using the firearm he had stolen from the victim. In total, 19 of his 42 victims were shot. The gunshot victims of these two series total 40 of the 302 victims in this study—in other words 13%—and nearly half of all gunshot victims.

South African serial murder victims tend to reflect the population dynamics of the country: 77.5% were Black, 7.7% were White, 11.7% were Coloured, 2.3% were Indian, and 0.7% were Asian (Salfati, Labuschagne, et al., 2015b). This differs from victims in the USA, where 50% to 70% of victims were White. In this South African study, the average victim age was 31.3 years, which is consistent with US and German serial murder studies (Hickey, 2010). Consistent with the con story mentioned above, 40.3% of victims were unemployed, 22.2% were labourers, 14.8% were students, 4.5% were sex workers, and 2.3% were professionals. It is interesting to note the low percentage of sex worker victims in South Africa, compared to US studies (22% of victims) (Salfati & Bateman, 2005). Sex workers are frequently targeted in the USA because of the nature of the work they do, which places them at high risk for victimisation, and they will accompany a stranger to a secluded place. Similarly, in South Africa unemployed, or low-socioeconomic category persons share similar risk factors, living in informal settlements and being desperate for employment to help support themselves and their families. To lift themselves out of poverty, they will accompany a stranger in the hope of finding work if they have none, or for better-paying work. It is the author's experience that White serial murderers are more likely to target sex workers, and in those series where all the victims were Black sex workers, the offender tended to be White (Labuschagne, 2020). Such an example would be the Port Elizabeth serial murderer, Riaan Stander, who murdered two sex workers approximately one month apart in August 2007, having picked each one up in a similar part of town and leaving their bodies 432m apart, at and nearby, his residence.

Approximately 18.2% of serial murder victims are not identified. In only five of the 55 unidentified cases was the lack of victim identification due to advanced decomposition. At the age of 16 years, most teenagers in South Africa are fingerprinted for the purpose of obtaining a national identity card, which is essential when applying for employment, opening a bank account, and other daily activities. One possible explanation for the 18.2% of unidentified bodies is the high rate of undocumented persons from other countries in South Africa. For victims who were identified, they tended to be strangers to the offender, with 73.3% not knowing their murderer, while 15.7% were acquaintances or friends to the offender. Only 6.8% were family, and 2.6% were in a relationship with the offender (Salfati, Labuschagne, et al., 2015b). This also challenges the belief that strangers only are targeted by serial murderers.

In this study, all the offenders were men. To date, no solo female serial murderers have been identified in South Africa in any of the series that have occurred. One series from the mid-1980s, that of Charmaine Phillips and Pieter Grundling, was one of the few where a female co-offender was involved. The average age of the offenders at the time of the first identified murder in the series was 29 years. The race of offenders in the sample was reasonably consistent with the population dynamics of the country. Black offenders accounted for 66.7% of the sample, followed by White offenders at 24.2%, and Coloured offenders at 9%. While White serial murder offenders accounted for 24.2%, White persons make up only 7.7% of the general population in South Africa, as such they are over-represented in the sample of serial murderers (Salfati, Labuschagne, et al., 2015b). Interestingly, however, prior to South Africa becoming a democratic country in 1994, and during the apartheid system, approximately 50% of all serial murderers arrested and convicted were White. After the changeover to a democratic society in 1994, the number of White serial murderers arrested dropped to a handful. This makes one wonder if the apartheid system, which empowered White people in all spheres of life, also empowered those who may have had serial murder tendencies to act upon those tendencies.

Most (60%) offenders in the study were in a romantic relationship at the time of the series and 36% were single (Horning et al., 2015). These figures are comparable to those observed with US serial murderers (Hickey, 2006). In terms of occupation, 55.2% were general labourers, employed in what is colloquially referred to as 'piece jobs': essentially opportunistic, short-term manual labour employment such as gardening, cleaning, construction work and the like. A further 34.5% were unemployed at the time of arrest. Educationally, 48.4% had junior school education (up to grade 7) whereas 39.3% had some measure of high school education (grade 8–12). Compared to their US counterparts, these offenders tended to be less educated, possibly due to the effects and legacy of the apartheid system in place until the mid-1990s, which had a negative influence of the education of persons who were not White.

Regarding criminal history before the murder series, 89.3% of offenders had a criminal history. Keeping in mind that some offenders had multiple arrests under different crime types, when analysed per crime type, 57.1% had an arrest for violent crimes against the person, 35.7% had a sexual offence arrest, 64.3% had a property-related arrest, and 35.7% had an arrest in the 'other' category.

The SAPS Response to Serial Murder

Due to the increase in serial murder cases coming to the attention of the South African Police Service in the late 1980s to mid-1990s with the likes of the Norwood Serial Murderer in Johannesburg, the Station Strangler in Cape Town, and Moses Sithole in Pretoria and Johannesburg, they realised that there was a need to create a capacity to deal with such cases. Initially Micki Pistorius, a psychologist in the SAPS, was called in to assist due to research she had previously conducted into serial murder during her academic studies.

The SAPS also made contact with retired FBI Profiler, Robert Ressler, who came out the South Africa in 1994 to assist with the Moses Sithole investigation. Ressler later came back to South Africa to train members of the SAPS in serial murder investigation. Ressler was one of the original FBI offender profiler pioneers and claims to have coined the term 'serial murder'. This initial training was adapted by the SAPS, including incorporating experiences from those early cases, into the Investigative Psychology courses, and later revamped and rebranded as the Psychologically Motivated Crimes Course in 2002.

As a formal structure in the SAPS, the Investigative Psychology Unit was created as a unit in 1997 with a mandate to assist in the investigation of psychologically motivated crimes, and later expanded to a Section (a larger organisational structure) in 2011. At the time of its creation, the main focus was on serial murder investigations due to a sharp increase in the detection of these types of cases between 1994 and 1997; however, the focus expanded over the years to include a wide variety of psychologically motivated crimes. These types of crimes are crimes that typically have no external (usually financial) motive. These include, but are not limited to, serial murder, serial rape, sexual murders, muti murders (a form of murder for human body parts linked to traditional medicine practices; see Labuschagne, 2012a), child sexual offenders, intimate partner murders, child abductions and kidnappings, mass murder, spree murder, cold cases, and equivocal death scenarios to name a few. This is a common pattern of development seen in such units as people turn to such units for advice and insight into a wide variety of unusual cases that investigators may never have seen before.

In its early days, the Unit was staffed only by members with a psychology background, after a few years a detective joined the Unit. Since then, detectives have been a permanent part of the Unit; in fact, currently the majority of staff are members of the service with a detective background. Typically, detectives with a background in sexual crime investigation and violent crime investigation are prime candidates for the unit. Later the Unit also included a research capacity, and criminologists.

The Unit was originally stationed within national Detective Service Head Office in Pretoria. The SAPS is a national police service with a mandate for all policing in South Africa, with the result that the IPU would assist throughout the whole of South Africa. In 2009 the Unit was relocated to the Forensic Services Division where it remains until today. The placement of the IPS in the National Head Office structure was advantageous in that it provided the Unit with the authority to intervene anywhere in the country, and with limited human resources, being centralised at the National Head Office thus made sense.

As mentioned, in 2011 the Unit became a Section, and between 2012 and 2013 the Section underwent a rapid expansion in terms of staff. At the beginning of 2012, the Section consisted of two support staff and five sworn police officers, all of whom were based at the National Head Office of the South African Police Service. By the end of 2013 the National IPS consisted of four members who were licensed psychologists, six detectives, two researchers, and two support staff with plans to employ more detectives and psychologists. Also, by mid-2013, the IPS had opened satellite units in each of the nine provinces, each staffed by a single detective. By 2020 there were 44 persons within the structure of the IPS, divided between a large head office component and decentralised units within each of the 9 provinces. Decentralisation became advantageous as the number of cases the Section was dealing with increased dramatically as the Section's services gained popularity and the SAPS DNA processing began to work more efficiently and more serials were being identified than previously.

Currently, with its overall complement of 44 members providing services related to offender profiling, major case management and the investigation of psychologically motivated crimes, this makes the IPS one of the largest such units in the world. One of the biggest challenges to date has been the recruitment and retention of Clinical Psychologists within the IPS environment. Unfortunately, salaries for psychologists, throughout the whole of the SAPS and not just in the specialised environment of the IPS, are far lower than other government departments, and significantly lower than the average income of private practitioners. This has led to a massive loss of institutional knowledge and experience over the years, and at times a situation where there were no psychologists in the IPS environment.

Along with the rapid expansion of staff came an increase in training for the existing and newly appointed members. Between 2012 and 2013 training was provided to the members by International Criminal Investigative Analysis Fellowship (ICIAF) accredited profilers from the Royal Canadian Mounted Police, Ontario Provincial Police in Canada and Los Angeles Sheriff's Department. Further training focused on threat assessment and management, medico-legal death investigation, forensic pathology, psychopathy assessment and diagnosis, sexual offences investigation, serial arson investigation, anatomy of sharp force injuries, homicide and death investigation, SCAN statement analysis, Bloodstain Pattern Analysis, Arson and Bomb Profiling, and Geographic Profiling. Essentially the training program for the IPS members follows that of the curriculum of the understudy program of the International Criminal Investigative Analysis Fellowship.

The SAPS is also the only law enforcement agency to date to have developed a nationally applicable policy on the investigation and management of serial rapes and serial murder. This policy, which reflected the culmination of experiences with these investigations over the years, was formally adopted in 2016. It covers issues such as the roles and responsibilities of the different structures of the SAPS in the investigation of serial cases on national and provincial levels. This includes the responsibilities of the following structures:

1. Provincial Police Commissioners: These commissioners have to facilitate the identification of serial rape and serial murder offenders, liaise with the IPS, ensure that forensic investigative leads are

investigated, and form a task team of appropriately trained and experienced detectives. Any existing serial investigations are to be monitored by the Provincial Commissioner and feedback must be given to the national office.

2. Detective Service Division of National Head Office, which must establish nodal points for the communication of information about serial related forensic investigative leads.

3. Family Violence, Child Protection and Sexual Offences (FCS) Units throughout the country are tasked with the investigation of rape series. FCS detectives involved in the investigation of rape series must have attended the training presented by the IPS.

4. Provincial Task Teams for investigating serial murder must be established once a murder series has been identified and priority is given to detectives trained on the Psychologically Motivated Crimes Course.

5. The IPS, which will be discussed in more detail below.

6. Provincial Coordinators for Psychologically Motivated Crimes, whose role it is to liaise with the IPS, monitor such investigations, and ensure that the day-to-day operations of serial investigations are running smoothly and detectives receive the resources they require.

7. Forensic DNA Database Management Section, which is responsible for communicating forensic DNA investigative leads to the relevant role players such as detectives.

8. DNA Serial Team of the Forensic Science Laboratory, which has the responsibility of managing and providing forensic DNA reports in serial cases, monitoring the processing of serial DNA and providing forensic DNA findings to detectives. Furthermore, they prioritise the processing of offender reference samples submitted for analysis.

9. Crime Scene Management Units, which should task crime scene experts who have attended the Psychologically Motivated Crimes Course to assist with such incidents.

10. Crime Intelligence Analysis Centres at police station level should analyse modus operandi in their areas to determine if serial offenders are active and use intelligence screening to try and identify suspects.

In the above policy the central role played by the Investigative Psychology Section is indicated as providing:

1. Assistance to investigating officers in the investigation of psychologically motivated crimes such as serial rape and serial murder.
2. Training to detectives and other SAPS members in the identification and investigation of these crimes.
3. Expert evidence during the prosecution and sentencing of such offenders.
4. Conducting research intended to further the understanding of psychologically motivated crimes.

The involvement is mandated in the policy where it states that the IPS will typically become involved in those cases where an investigating officer has requested assistance, or where there is at least one murder within a rape series, even if their assistance is not requested. It further states that the IPS involvement in the investigation of serial murders is automatic when such cases come to their attention.

The policy furthermore deals with how serial cases are initially identified by the police. It then highlights the investigative steps that must be taken when dealing with such cases. These steps include:

1. Identifying similar cases
2. Revisiting crime scenes
3. Crime scene and autopsy attendance
4. Forensic exhibit management
5. Cell phone investigations
6. Maintaining contact with living victims
7. Steps to be taken after arrest
8. Identity parades
9. Preparation for the trial
10. Sentencing

The SAPS' investment in the IPS has paid off with numerous successes in the investigation of psychologically motivated crimes, and the role of IPS members during the prosecution of such offenders, most notably in terms of linkage analysis evidence to link crimes without forensic evidence to a particular series, had made them a formidable tool in such prosecutions (Labuschagne, 2006; Labuschagne, 2012b; Labuschagne,

2014; Woodhams & Labuschagne, 2011). The IPS, and the existing policy which gives a framework for how serial murder and serial rape cases are to be managed, sets the SAPS apart from other law enforcement agencies in its response to this type of crime.

References

Aamodt, M. G. (2016, September 4). *Serial killer statistics*. Retrieved July 11, 2020, from http://maamodt.asp.radford.edu/serial%20killer%20information%20center/project%20description.htm

Adjorlolo, S., & Chan, H. C. O. (2014). The controversy of defining serial murder: Revisited. *Aggression and Violent Behavior, 19*(5), 486–491. https://doi.org/10.1016/j.avb.2014.07.003

Aki, K. (2003). *Serial killers: A cross-cultural study between Japan and the United States*. Unpublished Master's thesis, California State University.

Barkhuizen, J. (2006). *An exploration of the intrapsychic development and personality structure of serial killers through the use of psychometric testing*. Unpublished master's thesis, University of Pretoria, Pretoria, South Africa.

Collaros, D. (2019). *Exploring the psychogeography of serial murderers in South Africa*. Unpublished PhD Thesis, University of the Witwatersrand.

Campobasso, C. P., Colonna, M. F., Carabellese, F., Grattagliano, I., Candelli, C., Morton, R. J., et al. (2009). A serial killer of elderly women: Analysis of a multi-victim homicide investigation. *Forensic Science International, 185*(1-3), 7–11. https://doi.org/10.1016/j.forsciint.2008.12.023

Campos, E., & Cusson, M. (2007). Serial killers and sexual murderers. In *Sexual murderers: A comparative analysis and new perspectives* (pp. 99–105). Chichester: John Wiley & Sons.

Civilian Secretariat for Police. (2016). *Policy on the Investigation and Management of Serial Rape and Serial Murder*.

De Wet, J. A. (2005). *A psychological perspective on the personality development of a serial murderer*. Unpublished master's thesis, University of Pretoria, Pretoria, South Africa.

Del Fabbro, G. A. (2006). *A family systems understanding of serial murder*. Unpublished PhD thesis, University of Pretoria, Pretoria, South Africa.

Du Plessis, J. J. (1998). Towards a psychological understanding of serial murder. Unpublished master's thesis, University of Pretoria, Pretoria, South Africa.

Egger, S. (1984). A working definition of serial murder and the reduction of linkage blindness. *Journal of Police Science and Administration, 12*(3), 348–357. https://psycnet.apa.org/record/1985-09764-001

Egger, S. A. (2002). *The Killers Among Us. An Examination of Serial Murder and its Investigation* (2nd ed.). Upper Saddle River: Prentice Hall.

Fridel, E. E., & Fox, J. A. (2017). Too few victims: Finding the optimal minimum victim threshold for defining serial murder. *Psychology of Violence, 8*(4), 505–514. https://psycnet.apa.org/doi/10.1037/vio0000138

Gorby, B. (2000). *Serial murder: A cross-national descriptive study* (unpublished Master's thesis, California State University)

Harbort, S., & Mokros, A. (2001). Serial murderers in Germany from 1945 to 1995: A descriptive study. *Homicide Studies, 5*(4), 311–334. https://doi.org/10.1177/1088767901005004005

Hickey, E. W. (2006). *Serial murderers and their victims* (4th ed.). Belmont: Thomson Wadsworth.

Hickey, E. W. (2010). *Serial murderers and their victims* (5th ed.). Belmont: Wadsworth Group.

Hodgskiss, B. (2001). A multivariate model of the offence behaviours of South African serial murderers. Unpublished master's thesis, Rhodes University, Grahamstown, South Africa.

Hodgskiss, B. (2004). Lessons from serial murder in South Africa. *Journal of Investigative Psychology and Offender Profiling, 1*(1), 67–94. https://doi.org/10.1002/jip.2

Hook, D. (2003). Reading Geldenhuys: Constructing and deconstructing the Norwood killer. *South African Journal of Psychology, 33*(1), 1–10.

Horning, A. M., Salfati, C. G., & Labuschagne, G. N. (2015). South African serial homicide: A victim focused behavioral typology. *Journal of Investigative Psychology and Offender Profiling, 12*(1), 44–68. https://doi.org/10.1002/jip.1426

Hurst, A. (2003a). Killer in our midst: Part one. An analysis of court transcripts pertaining to the defence of Stewart Wilken in Die Staat Teen Stewart Wilken. *South African Journal of Philosophy, 22*(4), 289–305.

Hurst, A. (2003b). Killer in our midst: Part two. An analysis of court transcripts pertaining to the defence of Stewart Wilken in Die Staat Teen Stewart Wilken. *South African Journal of Philosophy, 22*(4), 306–326.

Jenkins, P. (1988). Serial murder in England 1940–1985. *Journal of Criminal Justice, 16*, 1–15. https://doi.org/10.1016/0047-2352(88)90031-1

Jenkins, P. (1989). Serial murder in the United States 1900–1940: A historical perspective. *Journal of Criminal Justice, 17,* 377–392. https://doi.org/10.1016/0047-2352(89)90048-2

Kallian, M., Birger, M., & Witztum, E. (2004). Reassessing "Jacob's case": A serial killer re-examined. *Medicine and Law, 23*(1), 59–71. https://pubmed.ncbi.nlm.nih.gov/15163076/

Knight, Z. G. (2006). Some thoughts on the psychological roots of the behaviour of serial killers as narcissists: An object relations perspective. *Social Behavior and Personality, 34*(10), 1189–1206. https://doi.org/10.2224/sbp.2006.34.10.1189

Labuschagne, G. N. (1998). *Serial murder: An interactional analysis* (unpublished Master's thesis, University of Pretoria.

Labuschagne, G.N. (2001). Serial murder revisited: A psychological exploration of two South African cases. Unpublished doctoral thesis, University of Pretoria.

Labuschagne, G. N. (2006). The use of a linkage analysis as evidence in the conviction of the Newcastle serial murderer, South Africa. *Journal of Investigative Psychology and Offender Profiling, 3*(3), 183–191. https://doi.org/10.1002/jip.51

Labuschagne, G.N. (2007). Foreign object insertion in sexual homicide cases: An exploratory study. Unpublished Master's thesis, University of Pretoria.

Labuschagne, G. N. (2010). The use of linkage analysis as an investigative tool and evidential material in serial offences. In *Serial offenders: Theory and practice* (pp. 87–125). Burlington: Jones & Bartlett Publishers.

Labuschagne, G. N. (2012a). Muti murder. In *Serial offenders in theory and practice* (pp. 145–161). Burlington: Jones & Bartlett Publishers.

Labuschagne, G. N. (2012b). The use of linkage analysis as an investigative tool and evidential material in serial offences. In *Serial offenders in theory and practice* (pp. 187–215). Burlington: Jones & Bartlett Publishers.

Labuschagne, G. N. (2014). The use of linkage analysis evidence in serial offence trials. In *Crime linkage: Theory, research and practice.* Boca Raton: CRC Press.

Labuschagne, G. N. (2017). Stewart "Boetie Boer" Wilken: Serial murder, necrophilia, and cannibalism: A South African case study. In *Understanding Necrophilia: A global multidisciplinary approach* (pp. 411–417). California: Cognella Academic Publishing.

Labuschagne, G. N. (2020). Psychologically motivated crimes. In *Principles and practices of forensic psychology and other related professions* (pp. 239–278). Cape Town: Juta and Co.

Labuschagne, G. N., & Salfati, C. G. (2015). An examination of serial homicide in South Africa: The practice to research link. *Journal of Investigative Psychology and Offender Profiling, 12*, 4–17. https://doi.org/10.1002/jip.1415

Lemmer, C. (2003). *A comparative study between South African serial killers and their American counterparts.* Unpublished master's thesis, Rand Afrikaans University, Johannesburg, South Africa.

Lubaszka, C. K., Shon, P. C., & Hinch, R. (2014). Healthcare serial killers and confidence men. *Journal of Investigative Psychology and Offender Profiling, 11*, 1–28. https://doi.org/10.1002/jip.1394

McClellan, J. (2019). *African-American serial killers: The neglected investigative profile.* Author.

Morton, R. J., & Hilts, M. A. (2005). *Serial murder: Multi-disciplinary perspectives for investigators.* San Antonio, TX, Symposium presented by the National Center for the Analysis of Violent Crime (NCAVC).

Myers, W. C., Bukhanovskiy, A., Justen, E., Morton, R. J., Tilley, J., Adams, K., et al. (2008). The relationship between serial sexual murder and autoerotic asphyxiation. *Forensic Science International, 176*, 187–195. https://doi.org/10.1016/j.forsciint.2007.09.005

Pistorius, M. (1996). *A psychoanalytic approach to serial killers.* Unpublished DPhil thesis, University of Pretoria, Pretoria, South Africa.

Salfati, C. G. (2006). The Homicide Profiling Index (HPI)- a tool for measurements of crime scene behaviors, victim characteristics, and offender characteristics. In *Homicide Research: Past, Present and Future: Proceedings of the 2005 Meeting of the Homicide Research Working Group.*

Salfati, C. G., & Bateman, A. (2005). Serial homicide: An investigation of behavioral consistency. *Journal of Investigative Psychology and Offender Profiling, 2*(2), 121–144. https://doi.org/10.1002/jip.27

Salfati, C. G., Horning, A. M., Sorochinski, M., & Labuschagne, G. N. (2015a). South African serial homicide: Consistency in victim types, and crime scene actions across series. *Journal of Investigative Psychology and Offender Profiling, 12*, 83–106. https://doi.org/10.1002/jip.1428

Salfati, C. G., Labuschagne, G. N., Horning, A. M., Sorochinski, M., & De Wet, J. (2015b). South African serial homicide: Offender and victim demographics and crime scene actions. *Journal of Investigative Psychology and Offender Profiling, 12*, 18–43. https://doi.org/10.1002/jip.1425

Schlesinger, L. B. (Ed.). (2000). *Serial offenders: Current thought, recent findings.* Boca Raton: CRC Press.

Snyman, C. R. (2008). *Criminal law* (5th ed.). New York: LexisNexis.

Snyman, H. F. (1992). Serial murder. *Acta Criminologica: African Journal of Criminology & Victimology, 5*(2), 35–41. https://journals.co.za/content/crim/5/2/AJA10128093_399

Sorochinski, M., Salfati, C. G., & Labuschagne, G. N. (2015). Classification of planning and violent behaviors in serial homicide: A cross-national comparison between South Africa and the US. *Journal of Investigative Psychology and Offender Profiling, 12*, 69–82. https://doi.org/10.1002/jip.1427

Sturup, J. (2018). Comparing serial homicides to single homicides: A study of prevalence, offender, and offence characteristics in Sweden. *Journal of Investigative Psychology and Offender Profiling, 15*(2), 75–89. https://doi.org/10.1002/jip.1500

Walsh, A. (2005). African Americans and serial killing in America. The myth and the reality. *Homicide Studies, 9*(4), 271–291. https://doi.org/10.1177/1088767905280080

Woodhams, J., & Labuschagne, G. (2011). A test of case linkage principles with solved and unsolved serial rapes. *Journal of Police and Criminal Psychology, 27*(1), 85–98. https://doi.org/10.1007/s11896-011-9091-1

Woodhams, J., & Labuschagne, G. N. (2012). South African serial rapists: The offenders, their victims and their offences. *Sexual Abuse: A Journal of Research and Treatment, 24*(6), 544–574. https://doi.org/10.1177/1079063212438921

7

The Constitutional Imperative, Common Law Position and Domestic Legislation in the Context of Mental Health Care Law in South Africa

Magdaleen Swanepoel

Introduction

The impact of the Constitution of the Republic of South Africa, 1996, on psychiatry, psychology and mentally ill patients is threefold: First, the Constitution is considered to be the supreme law in South Africa, and any legislation that is irreconcilable with it is invalid to the extent of the conflict. Second, according to section 39 of the Constitution, the Bill of Rights applies to all law and binds the executive, legislature, judiciary and all organs of state. Every court, tribunal or forum must promote the spirit and objects contained in the Bill of Rights in the interpretation of legislation and the development of the common law. Third, the Bill of Rights instructs the state to use the power that the Constitution provides for in ways that do not violate fundamental rights. The Bill of Rights declares many of the traditional human rights and has been praised as one of the

M. Swanepoel (✉)
Department of Jurisprudence, School of Law, University of South Africa, Pretoria, South Africa
e-mail: swanem@unisa.ac.za

© The Author(s), under exclusive license to Springer Nature Switzerland AG 2021
H. C. O. Chan, S. Adjorlolo (eds.), *Crime, Mental Health and the Criminal Justice System in Africa*, https://doi.org/10.1007/978-3-030-71024-8_7

best human rights instruments in the international context. South Africa has certainly made great strides in terms of its human rights awareness or at least in terms of the Constitution and policies that address human rights. There are specific fundamental human rights protected in the Bill of Rights that are applicable to the psychiatric profession and the mentally disordered patient. The first is section 36 of the Constitution—the general limitation clause. If a court determines that a law or the conduct of a respondent impairs a fundamental right, it must be considered whether the infringement is nevertheless a justifiable limitation of the right in question. Further rights include the right to dignified and humane treatment (section 10), freedom from discrimination in terms of access to all forms of treatment (section 9), the right to privacy and confidentiality (section 14), the right to protection from physical or psychological abuse and the right to adequate information about their clinical status (section 12). According to Zabow (2007, p. 384), these rights should ideally include efforts to promote the greatest degree of self-determination and personal responsibility of patients.

The overall aim of the Mental Health Care Act (Mental Health Care Act 17 of 2002) is the regulation of the mental health environment so as to provide mental health services in the best interest of the patient. The provision of care at all levels becomes the responsibility of the State. The Act promotes treatment in the least restrictive environment with active integration into general healthcare being required. Furthermore, respect for individual autonomy and decreased coercion procedures have been introduced in the management of the acute stages of illness.

The Act also addresses the potential and alleged malpractices in institutions and provides for prevention and detection. This is related to reports of human rights abuses of those with mental illnesses, which required attention. Psychiatric hospitals' stigmatisation of patients used to occur. This is an important aspect in terms of the Constitution, which requires that there be no discrimination toward persons with disabilities (Currie & De Waal, 2013). Mentally disordered people have the right to be treated under the same professional and ethical standards as any other ill person. Zabow (2007) states that this must include efforts to promote the greatest degree of self-determination and personal responsibility on the part of patients. He further states that admission and treatment should always be carried out in the patient's best interest. The National Health Act (The National Health Act 61 of 2003) further provides a legal framework, based on consent, for the regulation of mental health with regard to adults and children.

The Concept of Human Rights

At the centre of the concept of human rights vests the idea that every person should be accorded a sense of value, worth and dignity and that every person (including the mentally disordered person) should be protected from infringements and abuses of these fundamental rights, whether the infringements emanate from political states, authorities, or fellow human beings. In a general sense, human rights are understood as rights which belong to an individual as a consequence of being a human being and for no other reason.

Fundamental rights and freedoms, as protected in the Bill of Rights, may be limited or restricted, and are therefore not absolute. Section 36, the general limitation clause, sets out specific criteria for the restriction of the fundamental rights in the Bill of Rights. However, given the importance of the rights and the total and irremediable negation of it caused by an infringement, the justification for a limitation would have to be exceptionally compelling (Gobodo-Madikizela et al., 2005, p. 344). Therefore, where an infringement can be justified in an open and democratic society based on human dignity, equality and freedom, it will be constitutionally valid.

Section 10 of the Constitution: Human Dignity

In *Carmichele v Minister of Safety and Security* (1995) it was said that human dignity is a central value of the objective, normative value system. Chaskalson (2000, p. 193) in this regard wrote: "The affirmation of human dignity as a foundational value of the constitutional order places our legal order firmly in line with the development of constitutionalism in the aftermath of the Second World War." He continues to say that as an abstract value common to the core values of our Constitution, dignity informs the content of all the concrete rights and plays a role in the balancing process necessary to bring different rights and values into harmony. It too, however, must find place in the constitutional order. O'Regan J remarked in *S v Makwanyane and Another* (CCT3/94) [1995] ZACC 3: "that recognising a right to dignity is an acknowledgment of the intrinsic worth of human beings: Human beings are entitled to be treated as worthy of respect and concern. This right is therefore the foundation of many of the other rights that are specifically entrenched in the Bill of Rights."

Human Dignity and the Use of Physical Restraints for and Seclusion of Mentally Disordered Patients

It has been said that how a society treats its least well-off members says a lot about its humanity. Sometimes mentally ill people are treated with extreme measures that they do not want, for example, psychosurgery, electroconvulsive therapy and unwanted medication with very serious risks and side effects. In addition, their liberty and dignity are taken away—sometimes for many years. There are many mentally ill people who are treated, who do not want to be treated. The question then arises: When should we treat those who do not want to be treated and when should we respect their choices? (Saks, 2002, p. 123).

According to Levenson (2005), physical restraints and seclusion may be required for confused, medically unstable patients, especially when chemical restraint is ineffective or contraindicative. Confused medically ill patients often climb over bed rails risking falls, which may result in fractures and head trauma. The stringent legal regulation of physical restraints has increased during the past decade, yet courts have generally held that restraints are appropriate when a patient presents a risk of harm to themselves or others and a less restrictive alternative is not available. While it should be acknowledged that physical restraints have been overused in the past, some argue that there are times when these restraints are the safest and most humane option. A full range of alternatives for preventing harm in confused medically disordered patients, and for respecting their dignity, should be considered, keeping in mind that there are clinical and legal risks, both in inappropriately using and foregoing restraints.

With regard to the seclusion of mentally disordered patients, there are, according to Saks (2002, pp. 125–126) at least two theories of how seclusion is directly therapeutic: "First, the patient is separated from stressful interpersonal relations and is so permitted to reconstitute and to feel more settled. Second, seclusion is therapeutic because of the destimulation it provides." The idea is that patients, especially psychotic ones, have a real problem with overstimulation. They have, as it were, lost their ability to filter out unnecessary detail. Therefore, placing a patient in a bare room with no stimuli to distract, impinge on and overwhelm him or her, can be most therapeutic. It is submitted that should less restrictive means be available to achieve the same putative therapeutic ends, seclusion should not be justified as a means of therapy.

The rights and duties of persons, bodies or institutions are set out in Chap. 3 of the Mental Health Care Act and are in addition to any rights and duties that they may have in terms of any other law. According to section 8 of the Mental Health Care Act, the person, human dignity and privacy of every mental health care user must be respected. Every mental health care user must be provided with care, treatment and rehabilitation services that improve the mental capacity of the user to develop to full potential and to facilitate his or her integration into community life. A mental health care user must receive care, treatment and rehabilitation services to the degree appropriate to his or her mental health status.

In addition, the Ethical Code of Professional Conduct to which a Psychologist shall adhere stipulates that: "A psychologist shall respect the dignity and worth of a client and shall strive for the preservation and protection of fundamental human rights in all professional conduct." The right to life, as protected in section 11 of the Constitution, is the most basic human right on which all other rights are premised (*Makwanyane*). With the possible exception of human dignity, life itself is the most basic value protected by the Constitution. In addition, The *Universal Declaration of Human Rights* 1948 reads: "Everyone has the right to life, liberty, and security of the person. This right shall be protected by law. No one shall be arbitrarily deprived of his life." The right to life is, however, not absolute.

Section 12(1) of the Constitution: Freedom and Security of the Person and Section 35: Arrested, Detained and Accused Persons

Introductory Remarks

Section 12(1) states:

> Everyone has the right to freedom and security of the person, which includes the right: (a) not to be deprived of freedom arbitrarily or without just cause; (b) not to be detained without trial; (c) to be free from all forms of violence from either public or private sources; (d) not to be tortured in any way; and (e) not to be treated or punished in a cruel, inhuman or degrading way.

When a person is deprived of physical freedom, Section 12(1) guarantees both substantive and procedural protection. The substantive component requires the state to have good reasons for depriving someone of their freedom and the procedural component requires the deprivation to take place in accordance with fair procedures. O'Regan J described these components as follows:

> [T]wo different aspects of freedom: the first is concerned particularly with the reasons for which the state may deprive someone of freedom; and the second is concerned with the manner whereby a person is deprived of freedom. … [O]ur Constitution recognises that both aspects are important in a democracy: the state may not deprive its citizens of liberty for reasons that are not acceptable, nor when it deprives its citizens of freedom for acceptable reasons, may it do so in a manner which is procedurally unfair.

Section 35 states:

1. Everyone who is arrested for allegedly committing an offence has the right-

    a. to remain silent;
    b. to be informed promptly-

    i. of the right to remain silent; and

    ii. of the consequences of not remaining silent;

c. not to be compelled to make any confession or admission that could be used in evidence against that person;

d. to be brought before a court as soon as reasonably possible, but not later than-

    i. 48 hours after the arrest; or

    ii. the end of the first court day after the expiry of the 48 hours, if the 48 hours, expire outside ordinary court hours or on a day which is not an ordinary court day;

e. at the first court appearance after being arrested, to be charged or to be informed of the reason for the detention to continue, or to be released and;

f. to be released from detention if the interests of justice permit, subject to reasonable conditions.

2. Everyone who is detained, including every sentenced prisoner, has the right-

a. to be informed promptly of the reason for being detained;

b. to choose, and to consult with, a legal practitioner, and to be informed of this right promptly;

c. to have a legal practitioner assigned to the detained person by the state at state expense, if substantial injustice would otherwise result, and to be informed of this right promptly;

d. to challenge the lawfulness of the detention in person before a court and, if the: detention is unlawful, to be released;

e. to conditions of detention that are consistent with human dignity, including at least exercise and the provision, at state expense, of adequate accommodation, nutrition, reading material and medical treatment; and

f. to communicate with, and be visited by, that person's-

    i. spouse or partner;

    ii. next of kin;

iii. chosen religious counsellor; and

iv. chosen medical practitioner.

The influence of the Bill of Rights on the criminal justice system has been significant (*S v Nombewu* 1996). As mentioned above, it provides grounds for reviewing both the substantive and procedural content of the intricate web of laws shaping criminal justice as well as providing remedies for breaches of the Constitution. In doing so it has impacted on the content of law in addition to influencing the conduct of those who participate in the criminal justice system (Currie & De Waal 740).

In addition, the Ethical Code of Professional Conduct to which a Psychologist shall adhere to in South Africa stipulates that: "A psychologist shall never coerce a recipient of a psychological service into complying with the provision of such service nor shall he or she compel a client to give self-incriminating evidence via the use of psychological techniques or otherwise."

The Regulation of State Patients and Mentally Ill Prisoners in Terms of the Mental Health Care Act

Chapter 6 of the Mental Health Care Act regulates the position with regard to State patients (patients who cannot afford private medical treatment). In terms of section 41, the head of the national department must, with the concurrence of the relevant heads of the provincial departments, designate health establishments, which may admit, care for, treat and provide rehabilitation services to State patients. Where a court issues an order in terms of the Criminal Procedure Act for a State patient to be admitted for mental health care, treatment and rehabilitation services, the Registrar or the Clerk of the court must send a copy of that order to the:

1. Relevant official *curator ad litem*; and
2. officer in charge of the detention centre where the State patient is or will be detained.

In terms of section 46(1) of the Mental Health Care Act, the head of a health establishment where a State patient is admitted or if on leave of absence or conditional discharge must cause the mental health status of the State patient to be reviewed after six months from the date on which care, treatment and rehabilitation services were commenced, and every 12 months thereafter. The review must make recommendations on:

1. A plan for further care, treatment and rehabilitation service;
2. the merits of granting leave of absence; or
3. the discharge of the State patient.

Chapter 6 of the Act further regulates the transfer of State patients between designated health establishments; the position with regard to State patients who abscond; leave of absence from designated health establishments; the application for discharge of State patients; and the conditional discharge of State patients, amendments to conditions or the revocation of conditional discharge.

Chapter 7 of the Mental Health Care Act regulates the position with regard to mentally ill prisoners. In terms of section 49, the head of the national department must, with the concurrence of the heads of the provincial departments, designate health establishments which may admit, care for, treat and provide rehabilitation services to mentally ill prisoners. If it appears to the head of a prison through personal observation or from information provided that a prisoner may be mentally ill, the head of the prison must cause the mental health status of the prisoner to be enquired into by a psychiatrist or where a psychiatrist is not readily available, by a medical practitioner and a mental health care practitioner. The person conducting the enquiry must submit a written report to the head of the prison, and must specify in the report the mental health status of the prisoner, and a plan for the care, treatment and rehabilitation of that prisoner.

If the person conducting the enquiry referred to in section 50 finds that the mental illness of the convicted prisoner is of such a nature that the prisoner concerned could appropriately be cared for, treated and rehabilitated in the prison, the head of the prison must take the necessary steps to ensure that the required levels of care, treatment and rehabilitation services are provided to that prisoner.

Section 28 of the Constitution: The Protection of Children's Rights

Section 28 sets out a range of rights that provide protection for children, which are additional to the protection they are given by other sections of the Bill of Rights. However, as important as these rights are, children's rights do not have a special status in the Bill of Rights. In *De Reuck v Director of Public Prosecutions* 2003, Epstein AJ held that "a child's best interests ... is the single most important factor to be considered when balancing or weighing competing rights and interests concerning children. All competing rights must defer to the rights of children unless unjustifiable." This decision was overruled by the Constitutional Court in *De Reuck v Director of Public Prosecutions*. To say that section 28(2) of the Constitution "trumps" other provisions of the Bill of Rights is "alien to the approach adopted by this Court that constitutional rights are mutually interrelated and interdependent and form a single constitutional value system."

There are currently serious concerns about the placement, treatment and care of children in need of mental health care in South Africa. It is evident that there is a lack of guidelines, protocol and specialised expertise for the treatment of children in psychiatric institutions, leading to practices which are deeply concerning. Incidents of maltreatment and abuse of children admitted to psychiatric institutions are frequently reported. It has become clear that there are a wide variety of serious systematic problems at psychiatric institutions that require an urgent, holistic and comprehensive solution.

The above systematic problems relate, *inter alia*, to the following: (Special gratitude is due to the Centre for Child Law, University of Pretoria, for their assistance in identifying these relevant and current issues.)

1. The criteria for admitting children in psychiatric institutions as well as the procedures followed for admission;
2. Whether children admitted to psychiatric institutions for observation are separated from institutionalised children who are receiving care on a continuing long-term basis;
3. The staffing of the psychiatric wards, including:

   a. Whether staff members are specifically trained to care for children and young people;
4. Whether staff members in psychiatric wards are trained to care for children with special needs (such as autistic children); and
5. Whether staff members receive continued training on how to care for children with psychiatric and/or special needs.
6. The procedures followed by staff when an incident occurs, including:

   a. Internal investigations to determine the cause of the incident and the course of action to remedy the situation;
7. Disciplinary measures taken by staff to discipline children when they break the rules in a ward or cause an incident; and
8. Notification of parents and family of children involved and/or injured in an incident.
9. Safety measures to prevent children from absconding from the psychiatric institution and procedures followed by staff when children have absconded from the institution;
10. The procedures followed to re-admit children who have absconded from a psychiatric institution, including:

    a. Treatment of children by staff members when they are returned to the psychiatric institution;
11. Appropriate measures to manage the behaviour of the children as well as the circumstances in which it would be necessary and appropriate to implement such measures; and

    a. disciplinary measures for absconding, taken by staff against the children, with specific reference to placing children in seclusion.
12. The practice of placing children in seclusion with special reference to the following:

a. Guidelines for the staff and coherence to constitutional provisions on when and under which circumstances children may be placed in seclusion;

b. whether there is a register recording when children are placed in seclusion and if so, what information is entered in the register and whether such information is sufficient.

13. The authority of staff to discipline children and the extent of such authority, including which measures are allowed and under which circumstances.

With reference to the matters listed above, the concern arises in South Africa that there are no clear, written policies in place which are adequate and appropriate; and that, to the extent that certain policies are in place, they are not adhered to consistently in practice, and that no measures or insufficient measures are taken when such policies are breached.

Child psychiatry training programmes have further encountered a number of administrative problems resulting from efforts to recognise, without isolating or submerging, the unique aspects of child psychiatry within existing departments of psychiatry. The intention is to question the validity of the concept of general psychiatry, which may be responsible for many of these administrative dilemmas. The author advances that child psychiatry actually represents a distinct field of practice, where training programs for children suffering from mental disorders should be integrated within departments of psychiatry through divisional administrative lines (Westman, 1978, p. 195). In terms of section 9 of the Children's Act (35 of 2008), the care, protection and well-being of a child in all matters concerning the standard that the child's best interest is of paramount importance, must be applied.

The Ethical Code of Professional Conduct to which a Psychologist shall adhere also safeguards the rights of children and stipulates that: "A psychologist shall be cognisant that a child's best interests are of paramount importance in every professional matter concerning direct or indirect psychological services to children." Further, a psychologist must take special care when dealing with children fourteen years of age and younger, and must at the beginning of a professional relationship, inform a child or a client who has a legal guardian or who is otherwise legally dependent, of the limits the law imposes on the right of confidentiality with respect to his or her communications with such psychologist.

Electroconvulsive Therapy

> There had been times when I'd wandered around in a daze for as long as two weeks after a shock treatment, living in that foggy, jumbled blur which is a whole lot like the ragged edge of sleep, that gray zone between light and dark, or between sleeping and waking or living and dying, where you know you're not unconscious any more but don't know yet what day it is or who you are or what's the use of coming back at all—for two weeks. (Kesey, 2002, p. 27)

When electroconvulsive therapy is mentioned in conversation, it invokes strong reactions from scientists and laypeople alike. A swirl of controversy has always surrounded the use of shock treatment. Electroconvulsive therapy has undergone many changes since its creation in the early 1930s in Europe (Newell, 2005). However, despite scientific innovations and legislative actions, South Africa and many other countries are not sufficiently protecting the mentally disordered patient's constitutional right to refuse, such an invasive and controversial treatment.

The use of electroconvulsive therapy is not a highly regulated and legislated treatment in South Africa. Up until the introduction of the Mental Health Care Act, legislation and monitoring of the use of electroconvulsive therapy in South Africa had been conspicuous by its absence. Fortunately, the Mental Health Care Act has a potential impact on the practice of electroconvulsive therapy in a variety of ways. One of the major limitations of electroconvulsive therapy is the neurocognitive side-effects that accompany its administration. However, with recent research on the effects of changes in electrode placement and dosing strategies, it is possible to minimise these side effects in the majority of patients. Despite these recent advances in the practice of electroconvulsive therapy, it should remain a highly regulated and legislated treatment modality in South Africa. According to Segal and Thom (2006), it has been shown that the more legislated the procedure becomes, the less frequently it is used. Their argument is that paternalistic psychiatrists are conducting electroconvulsive therapy on patients whose rights they are violating by utilising inadequate procedures for obtaining informed consent, thus undermining autonomy. This treatment is also potentially harmful, thus not adhering to the tenets of non-maleficence. Further, the increasing risk of litigation in the field of medicine played a role in the aforementioned phenomenon, both as cause and effect. On the contrary, Jorgensen (Jorgense 2008, http://works.bepress.com/mike_jorgensen/1) argues that the stigma that electroconvulsive therapy suffered due to prior barbaric type applications in the past are largely historical, and most medical professionals should agree that electroconvulsive therapy is safe today, has very minimal side effects, is not inherently abusive, and has no long-term detriments. Yet, with the increase in popularity and safe applications, electroconvulsive therapy is still treated archaically under certain laws and legislative restraints will cause an indigent, elderly population to be deprived of this useful and sometimes solely effective treatment.

Individuals requiring electroconvulsive therapy fall within groups or categories. The group that is most non-controversial are those who have mental capacity and may either refuse or request electroconvulsive therapy. Such individuals have statutory, common law and constitutional protections of autonomy and self-determination. The more controversial group are those patients who are mentally incapacitated and either refused electroconvulsive therapy, requested electroconvulsive therapy or who have not expressed a decision either way.

In *Rompel v Botha* 1953, Neser J made the following statement: "There is no doubt that a surgeon who intends operating on a patient must obtain the consent of the patient … I have no doubt that a patient should be informed of the serious risks he does run. If such dangers are not pointed out to him then, in my opinion, the consent to the treatment is not in reality consent—it is consent without knowledge of the possible injuries. On the evidence defendant did not notify plaintiff of the possible dangers, and even if plaintiff did consent to shock treatment he consented without knowledge of injuries which might be caused to him. I find accordingly that plaintiff did not consent to the shock treatment."

It is clear from the above that lawful medical interventions require the informed consent of the patient apart from the specific exceptions mentioned above. Therefore, a medical intervention without the required informed consent amounts to a violation of a person's physical integrity, and may amount to criminal assault, civil or criminal *injuria*, or result in an action for damages based on negligence.

A group of concern are those patients who were competent, but are now incapacitated. When these individuals enjoyed capacity, they may have either created medical advance directives that did not provide for mental health care decisions or they failed to provide directives at all. The category includes those who may have consented to electroconvulsive therapy before or who may have refused the treatments prior to losing capacity. Procedures are needed, which will protect the vulnerable individuals from the misuse of electroconvulsive therapy and at the same time continue to protect the incapacitated individual's rights and self-determination.

Institutionalisation of the Mentally Disordered

Far from providing a supportive environment, institutional care settings for the mentally disordered are often where human rights abuses occur. This is particularly true in segregated services including residential psychiatric institutions and psychiatric wings of prisons. Persons with mental disorders are often inappropriately institutionalised on a long-term basis in psychiatric hospitals and other institutions. While institutionalised, they may be vulnerable to being chained to soiled beds for long periods of time, violence and torture, the administration of treatment without informed consent, unmodified use of electro-convulsive therapy, grossly inadequate sanitation, and inadequate nutrition. Women are particularly vulnerable to sexual abuse and forced sterilisations. Persons from ethnic and racial minorities are often victims of discrimination in institutions and care systems. A lack of monitoring of psychiatric institutions and weak or nonexistent accountability structures allow these human rights abuses to flourish away from the public eye (Hunt & Mesquita, 2006).

In terms of the Mental Health Care Act, a health care provider or a health establishment may provide care, treatment and rehabilitation services to or admit a mental health care user only if:

1. the user has consented to the care, treatment and rehabilitation services or to admission;
2. it was authorised by a court order or a review board;
3. due to mental illness, any delay in providing care, treatment and rehabilitation services or admission may result in the death or irreversible harm to the health of the user; or
4. the user can inflict serious harm to himself or herself or others; or cause serious damage to or loss of property belonging to him or her or others.

Any person or health establishment that provides care, treatment and rehabilitation services to a mental health care user or admits the user in circumstances referred to in subsection (1)(c) of the Mental Health Care Act must report this fact in writing in the prescribed manner to the relevant review board, and may not continue to provide care, treatment and rehabilitation services to the user concerned for longer than 24 hours unless an application in terms of Chap. V is made within the 24-hour period.

Chapter V of the Mental Health Care Act regulates voluntary, assisted and involuntary mental health care. Subject to section 9(l)(c), a mental health care user may not be provided with assisted care, treatment and rehabilitation services at a health establishment as an outpatient or inpatient without his or her consent, unless a written application for care, treatment and rehabilitation services is made to the head of the health establishment concerned and he approves it; and at the time of making the application there is a reasonable belief that the mental health care user is suffering from a mental illness or severe or profound mental disability, and requires care, treatment and rehabilitation services for his or her health or safety, or for the health and safety of other people; and the mental health care user is incapable of making an informed decision on the need for the care, treatment and rehabilitation services.

An application referred to in section 26 may only be made by the spouse, next of kin, partner, associate, parent or guardian of a mental health care user, but where the user is under the age of 18 years on the date of the application, the application must be made by the parent or guardian of the user. If the spouse, next of kin, partner, associate, parent or guardian of the user is unwilling, incapable or not available to make such an application, the application may be made by a health care provider. The applicants referred to in paragraph (a) must have seen the mental health care user within seven days before making the application.

Such application must be made in the prescribed manner, and must set out the relationship of the applicant to the mental health care user; if the applicant is a health care provider, state the reasons why he is making the application; and what steps were taken to locate the relatives of the user in order to determine their capability or availability to make the application; set out grounds on which the applicant believes that care, treatment and rehabilitation services are required; and state the date, time and place where the user was last seen by the applicant within seven days before the application is made.

On receipt of the application, the head of a health establishment concerned must cause the mental health care user to be examined by two mental health care practitioners. Such mental health care practitioners must not be the persons making the application and at least one of them must be qualified to conduct physical examinations. On completion of the examination, the mental health care practitioners must submit their written findings to the head of the health establishment concerned on whether the circumstances referred to in section 26(b) are applicable; and the mental health care user should receive assisted care, treatment and rehabilitation services as an outpatient or inpatient.

A mental health care user must be provided with care, treatment and rehabilitation services without his or her consent at a health establishment on an outpatient or inpatient basis if:

1. An application is made in writing to the head of the health establishment concerned to obtain the necessary care, treatment and rehabilitation services and the application is granted;
2. at the time of making the application, there is reasonable belief that the mental health care user has a mental illness of such a nature that the user is likely to inflict serious harm to himself or herself or others; or

3. care, treatment and rehabilitation of the user is necessary for the protection of the financial interests or reputation of the user; and at the time of the application the mental health care user is incapable of making an informed decision on the need for the care, treatment and rehabilitation services; and is unwilling to receive the care, treatment and rehabilitation required.

Conclusion

Even though there is quite a lot of discrimination against mentally ill patients, a lot of steps have been taken to secure their human rights. The Constitution of the Republic of South Africa makes provision for equal treatment, dignity rights, the right to life, security of the body and access to health care services. The Mental Health Review Boards were also created to be the watch dog over mental health in South Africa. This research aimed to point out what is still needed to improve mental health care rights. It would be very beneficial if the health care system can improve in a manner where more patients who cannot afford private medical care can be accommodated. The Review Boards see to the maintenance of psychiatric institutions but they don't have the capacity to fix everything as the review board only comprise of a few board members. But strides are definitely made towards better health care services in South Africa.

References

Carmichele v Minister of Safety and Security 2001 (4) SA 938 (CC).

Chaskalson, A. (2000). Human dignity as a foundational value of our constitutional order. *South African Journal on Human Rights, 16*(2), 193–205. https://doi.org/10.1080/02587203.2000.11827594.

Children's Act 38 of 2005 of the Republic of South Africa?

Constitution of the Republic of South Africa, 1996.

Currie, I., & De Waal, J. (2013). *The bill of rights handbook* (6th ed.). Cape Town, South Africa: Juta.

De Reuck v Director of Public Prosecutions, Witwatersrand Local Division 2004 (1) SA.

Gobodo-Madikizela, P., & Foster, D. (2005). Psychology and human rights. In C. Tredoux, D. Foster, & A. Allan (Eds.), *Psychology and law* (pp. 343–383). Cape Town, South Africa: Juta.

Hunt, P., & Mesquita, J. (2006). Mental disabilities and the human right to the highest attainable standard of health. *Human Rights Quarterly, 28*(2), 332–343.

Jorgensen, M. E. (2008). Is today the day we free electroconvulsive therapy? Retrieved from https://works.bepress.com/mike_jorgensen/1/

Kesey, K. (2002). *One flew over the cuckoo's nest*. New York, NY: Penguin Books.

Levenson, J. L. (2005). Legal issues in the interface of medicine and psychiatry. *Primary Psychiatry, 12*(12), 19–22. Retrieved from https://www.researchgate.net/publication/289206043_Legal_issues_in_the_interface_of_medicine_and_psychiatry

Newell, E. R. (2005). A mentally ill prisoner's right to refuse invasive medical treatment in Oregon's criminal justice system. *Lewis & Clark Law Review, 9*(4), 1019–1022.

"Professional Board for Psychology: Rules of conduct pertaining specifically to the profession of psychology" published in GN R717 in *GG* No 29079, 4 August 2006 s 10(1).

Rompel v Botha 1953 (T) unreported.

Saks, E. R. (2002). *Refusing care: Forces treatment and the rights of the mentally ill.* Chicago, IL: The University of Chicago Press.

Segal, J., & Thom, R. (2006). Consent procedures and electroconvulsive therapy in South Africa: Impact of the Mental Health Care Act. *African Journal of Psychiatry, 9*(4), 206–215. https://doi.org/10.4314/ajpsy.v9i4.30219

Westman, J. C. (1978). Administrative issues in child and adult psychiatry training programs. *Child Psychiatry and Human Development, 8*, 195–203. https://doi.org/10.1007/BF01463551.

Zabow, T. (2007). The mental health care act. In *Primary health care psychiatry: A practical guide for South Africa* (pp. 569–584). Juta and Company Ltd.

8

Suicide Attempt and "Social Suffering": Disrupting Dangerous Binary Discourse and Fostering Kinship between the Mental Health and Legal Systems in Ghana

Johnny Andoh-Arthur
and Emmanuel Nii-Boye Quarshie

Introduction

The World Health Organisation (WHO) (2014) defines suicide as "the act of deliberately killing oneself" (p. 17) and suicide attempt as "intentional self-inflicted poisoning, injury or self-harm which may or may not

J. Andoh-Arthur (✉)
Department of Psychology, University of Ghana, Accra, Ghana

Center for Suicide and Violence Research (CSVR), Accra, Ghana
e-mail: jandoh-arthur@ug.edu.gh

E. N.-B. Quarshie
Department of Psychology, University of Ghana, Accra, Ghana

Center for Suicide and Violence Research (CSVR), Accra, Ghana

School of Psychology, University of Leeds, Leeds, UK

© The Author(s), under exclusive license to Springer Nature Switzerland AG 2021
H. C. O. Chan, S. Adjorlolo (eds.), *Crime, Mental Health and the Criminal Justice System in Africa*, https://doi.org/10.1007/978-3-030-71024-8_8

169

have a fatal intent or outcome" (p. 17). Globally, suicide accounts for over 800,000 deaths annually equating to about a death every 40 seconds, with the highest suicide mortality reported from low- and middle-income countries (LMICs) (WHO, 2014). A history of suicide attempt represents the single-most important risk factor for suicide across all age groups in the general population. WHO (2014) estimates that of those who attempt suicide, one-third go on to repeat the behaviour within a year and nearly 10% eventually die by suicide. The higher prevalence estimates of suicide attempt across the globe appear not to have yet attracted the full attention of some national governments to invest in prevention efforts and intervention programmes. Perhaps, unlike suicides in which systematic clinical guidelines have been developed for classifying and recording, the lack of common guidelines and surveillance systems for recording suicidal attempts may have either led to gross underestimation, under-representation of suicide attempts or misclassification of suicide attempts within countries. Indeed, the "WHO itself does not routinely collect data on suicide attempt" (WHO, 2014, p. 36). National and regional rates of suicide attempts have been obtained mainly from either self-reports of suicidal behaviours in surveys of (representative) community samples or medical records about clinical presentations and treatment of suicide attempt or self-harm (WHO, 2014, 2016).

Epidemiology and Patterns of Suicidal Behaviours

Epidemiological data from most Western countries suggests the phenomenon of "gender paradox" in suicidal behaviours where gender differences exist in suicide morbidity and mortality (Canetto & Sakinofsky, 1998). That is, comparatively, whereas more females report suicide attempts, more males die by suicide. This gender paradox, however, is not clear in other countries, particularly, LMICs, where suicide mortality and morbidity records show no clear cut gender differences or a higher mortality and morbidity figures for either males or females (Glenn et al., 2020; Mars, Burrows, Hjelmeland, & Gunnell, 2014; Naghavi et al., 2019;

Quarshie et al., 2020a; Uddin, Burton, Maple, Khan, & Khan, 2019). Many years of research have consistently showed underlying psycho-socio-economic factors in most attempted suicides and suicides across the globe. From the famous work of Emile Durkheim (1897), which posited social integration and regulation as explainable factors in suicide, mental illness, substance use and abuse, marital and interpersonal conflicts, financial and job constraints, change in social status, including religious and spiritual factors have been some other reported triggering factors to both suicide and suicide attempt across gender and age within the general population (Franklin et al., 2017; Hawton, Saunders, & O'Connor, 2012; Klonsky, May, & Saffer, 2016; Quarshie et al., 2020a).

Ghana is one such setting where estimates of both suicide and suicide attempts are higher for males (Adinkrah, 2011; Der, Dakwah, Derkyi-Kwarteng, & Badu, 2016; Quarshie, Osafo, Akotia, & Peprah, 2015). Age-specific precursors have included lack of parental warmth, relationship crisis, family conflict for adolescents and young people (Quarshie et al., 2015; Quarshie et al., 2020a), marital, economic/financial, spiritual and health challenges (chronic physical and mental), substance use and abuse, and social status loss for adults and older persons (Adinkrah, 2018; Akotia, Knizek, Hjelmeland, Kinyanda, & Osafo, 2019; Andoh-Arthur, Knizek, Osafo, & Hjelmeland, 2018; Andoh-Arthur et al., 2020; Osafo, Akotia, Andoh-Arthur, & Quarshie, 2015; Quarshie, Asante, Andoh-Arthur, Asare-Doku, & Navelle, 2018).

Crisis or Crime?

Paradoxically, even though suicide attempt is conceived both in the scientific literature and popular discourses as a global public health concern, the behaviour is still criminalised in many countries, including Ghana. The Black Law Dictionary defines suicide as the act of taking one's own life; thus, self-killing, self-destruction, self-murder, "felo-de-se",[1] or death by one's own hand (Black et al., 1999). From the definition, attempting suicide is seemingly likened to an "inchoate; offence" (Lubaale, 2017),

---

[1] "Felo-de-se" is an Anglo-Latin term for "one guilty of self-murder".

even though its "substantive", self-killing (suicide), is not an offence and therefore not prosecuted. Why suicide attempt is criminalised against the background of underlying psychiatric and psychosocial precursors continues to bewilder many people. The situation has led to strident arguments for and advocacy towards decriminalisation of suicide attempts. Nonetheless, some other persons have committed tacitly to ensuring that the status quo remains. The next section highlights some historical antecedents of anti-suicide laws, its current state and some arguments for and against decriminalisation, from both international and Ghanaian perspectives.

Criminalisation of Suicide Attempt: History, Current State, Arguments for and Against

Anti-suicide laws have their origins from Europe when St Augustine declared self-killing as a sin between 354 and 430 CE. This declaration put suicidal acts within a politico-religious purview, which created a fertile context for shaping the legal stance against suicidal attempts (Ranjan, Kumar, Pattanayak, Dhawan, & Sagar, 2014). In England, the anti-suicide laws are said to have undergone five distinct phases: from the incorporation of Augustine's damnation of self-killing into canon law in the seventh century; tenth-century forfeiture of suicide goods occasioned by the involvement of the secular state; proposal that suicide was neither a sin nor a crime within the enlightenment rationalism in the seventeenth and eighteenth centuries; attempted suicide becoming a crime due to widespread societal change in the control of deviancy in the nineteenth century; and finally, era of medicalisation, which drained morality from deviance as a result of growing interest in positivism and determinism (Moore, 2000). These developments led to the repeal of the anti-suicide laws in 1961 in England and Wales (Neeleman, 1996). The years after the French revolution, along with the socio-cultural changes that permeated the whole of Europe in the nineteenth and twentieth centuries, also birthed a watershed moment for dramatic changes in the way suicide was viewed and handled (Sareen & Trivedi, 2009; Trivedi, 1997).

A global review of the criminal codes of 192 countries shows that that suicide is currently illegal in 25 countries, whereas an additional 20 countries follow Islamic or Sharia law where jail sentences may be handed to suicide attempters (Mishara & Weisstub, 2016). The study further indicated that decriminalisation has taken place in 59 countries, with the whole of Europe, North America, and much of South America also expunging these laws. The story is different in majority of the countries in South Asian and most part of Africa, including Kenya, Malawi, Nigeria, Rwanda, Tanzania, Ghana, and Uganda where attempted suicide remains a crime.

Criminalisation of suicide attempt has been argued from several perspectives including one that is anchored in the religious belief that the right to life termination is the sole prerogative of God. Usurpation of this divine right, according to the view, constitutes a transgression, which thus gives grounds for punishment. This argument is often also linked to the Judeo-Christian injunction in the Bible (Exodus 20:13[2]) against murder. Usually, an extension is drawn from this injunction against the "right" to kill oneself. That is, God abhors the killing of others, and invariably frowns against the act of taking one's life. Seeking the retention of anti-suicide laws from such arguments reflects a deontological ethical position, which primarily presumes that suicide and suicidal attempt are bad because they do not adhere to the divine rule on self-preservation.

By far, the deterrence argument for the maintenance of the anti-suicide laws has been the most pervasive. Some people hold the view that retaining the anti-suicide laws has the potential of deterring others from suicidal acts. A utilitarian ethical argument is forcefully made to retain the law on the presumption that the "parens patriae"[3] powers of the state needs activation to punish offenders as a means of modifying the offenders' behaviours, and more importantly, to deter citizens from engaging in activities that threaten individual and collective existence. Consequentialist arguments have also been put forward to support the criminalisation agenda. These are grounded on views that suicidal actions leave adverse

---

[2] Exodus 20:13—"You shall not murder." (New International Version Bible).

[3] Parens patriae: This principle provides that the state has the legal duty to protect citizens who are unable to help or protect themselves.

174 J. Andoh-Arthur and E. N.-B. Quarshie

consequences not only for the offenders but also their close relations and society as a whole.

Several reasons have been given in support of the call to repeal the anti-suicide laws, One of which is situated within the bio-medicalised logic, which pushes suicide attempt away from the force of the law and morality into the realm of biomedical science. Within this logic, suicide is viewed either as comorbid with and/or a consequence of underlying psychiatric illness and that mental illnesses, particularly depression, accounts for about 90% of all suicides (Shahtahmasebi, 2013). The insanity plea that is often activated to seek clemency for suicide attempters is usually grounded on this biomedical logic. Thus, for clemency to be granted "offenders" of the anti-suicide law the "Mens Rea"[4] element must be necessarily rendered inconsequential, although the "Actus Reus"[5] can be firmly established. Though most popular in the decriminalisation discourses, the biomedicalised argument appears to have provided a strong basis for increased advocacy towards a consideration of other non-medical underpinnings of suicide, most of which have been psychosociocentric in nature—financial distress, marital problems, chronic illness, and existential matters. The psychosociocentric argument is that, apart from being untenable, the resort to suicide or suicide attempt in the face of psychosocial crises in itself, requires some urgent enquiry into the psychological health towards treatment, but not punishment. From this perspective, the anti-suicide law is conceived as producing an *ironic effect* in the sense that punishment will aggravate, rather than resolve, the underlying problem and thereby increase the potential for (repeated) suicidal behaviour, particularly, in vulnerable persons and groups. Arguments are also rife from within the libertarian discourses. Here, views on decriminalisation of suicide attempt rest on the assumption of individual rights and freedoms of choices. The right to death discourses, which have shaped mercy killing (Euthanasia) in many Western societies, appears to be utilised to support the repeal of anti-suicide laws. For those who do not see the sense in prosecuting an "inchoate" offence, as the "substantive" offense of

---

[4] A fundamental principle of criminal law consisting of a person's awareness of the fact that his or her conduct is criminal (i.e. the mental element).

[5] The principle of the act itself (the physical element).

suicide is non-prosecutable, the justification for keeping the law is palpably tenuous and hard to sustain. In Ghana and many former British colonies, the anti-suicide law is anachronistic, given that the British Empire, which introduced the law in most of its colonies, has since 1961, repealed the law in response to an improved understanding of the problem (Neeleman, 1996).

Views on the Anti-suicide Laws

Some recent studies from parts of Africa (including Ghana) have explored the views of key professionals on the anti-suicide law.[6] Views of these professionals were examined on the law because the nature of their work interfaces with persons who attempt suicides. In Uganda, a study examining the views of mental health workers on the criminalisation of suicidal behaviour found almost two-thirds of mental health workers seeking the abolishment of the law, while some wanted the law to be retained. A few ambivalent views were also recorded (Hjelmeland, Kinyanda, & Knizek, 2012). These professionals' main arguments for and against the law were respectively hinged on views that criminalisation serves a deterrent purpose and suicide is a mental health issue that needs treatment. Similarly, a study among clinical psychologists, emergency ward nurses, and police officers in Ghana emphasised mental health issues and deterrence as reasons against and for the continuous existence of anti-suicide laws in Ghana's penal codes. Again, the majority of the professionals did not agree with the law criminalising attempted suicide in Ghana, while a few emergency ward nurses and two police officers agreed with the law (Hjelmeland, Osafo, Akotia, & Knizek, 2014). Another study in Ghana that investigated the views of lawyers and judges, as well as police officers, followed similar trend with the majority in support of the view that suicidal behaviour has underlying mental crisis requiring help and not punishment for persons who attempt it (Osafo, Akotia, Andoh-Arthur,

---

[6] The *Criminal Code of Ghana* (*Act 29 of Ghana, Section 57; Subsection II, 1960*) stipulates that, "whoever attempts to commit suicide shall be guilty of a misdemeanour". Thus, persons in the country who attempt suicide must be apprehended and prosecuted, and upon conviction, receive criminal penalties ranging from hefty fines to prison terms between 1 and 3 years.

Boakye, & Quarshie, 2018; Osafo, Akotia, Quarshie, Boakye, & Andoh-Arthur, 2017).

The view that suicide is a personal health crisis and not a crime, prompting calls for help and not punishment is gradually becoming popular among these professionals. For instance, a recent study among physicians and nurses showed physicians viewing suicide as a personal crisis needing help, while views of nurses appear to be transiting from suicide as a moral infraction to suicide as a health crisis requiring help for the patient (Osafo, Akotia, Boakye, & Dickson, 2018). Among the factors implicated in the transition of nurses' views towards health crises were education, suicidal experiences, and religion. Notwithstanding these developments, there appears to be a pervasive generalised negative view of suicide as a moral infraction, and a crime among the larger populace. Recently in Ghana's Parliament, a senior Member of Parliament vehemently opposed calls for the decriminalisation of attempted suicide in the country; he argued that any attempt to take one's life was an unacceptable behaviour that must be punished and deterred (Agyeman, 2019).

Dangerous Binary Discourses

Thus far, arguments for and against anti-suicide laws have emerged from what we call *binary discourses*, which we perceive to portend danger for any context-driven approach to suicide prevention and intervention in Ghana. The danger in the binary discourse (crisis vs. crime) is seen in the fact of its lack of appreciation of the sociocultural context within which suicide is generally construed, which might inform a context-driven approach to prevention. Laws are generally believed to reflect the social and cultural ethos of a people, implying recourse to the ethos and values of the people whenever laws are ripe for repeal. Among many ethnic groups in Ghana, suicide is understood from within the ontology of life and death. Among the Akans, for instance, life is seen as a gift from the supreme God, and that life does not end with death but continues in another realm where one achieves a venerated position as an ancestor with a responsibility to serve the living. There exist, however, strict meritorious criteria for becoming an ancestor, one of which is related to the way a person dies (Adinkrah, 2015; De Witte, 2001). Harsh reactions towards suicide and suicidal persons stem from views that suicide is a "bad" death and an extraordinary moral evil which is believed to have dire consequences for family and community as well (Andoh-Arthur, Knizek, Osafo, & Hjelmeland, 2019). From this viewpoint, one can reason that the harsh reactions towards suicidal attempt are rooted mainly in the consequential effects of suicidal acts—dire consequences on others. There is thus no consideration for the antecedents of the acts and/or the wellbeing of the actor. The anti-suicide law thus appears to take its spirit from this globalised discourse. The implication is that a call for a repeal of the anti-suicide law ought to consider the perceived consequences of suicide for the people, while not neglecting the antecedents of the acts and the wellbeing of the suicidal actors. For instance, can calls for the decriminalisation of suicide attempt be tenable within a context where existing mental health services for suicide attempters continue to be hugely stigmatised, and there are no postvention services (formalised psychological support service for persons bereaved by suicide)? In many cases where suicidal antecedents are considered within the decriminalisation discourses, there appears to have been a tendency to focus almost exclusively on mental illness as underlying crises but not on other psychosocial underpinnings of suicide.

The focus on mental illness in the decriminalisation agenda looks appealing from the onset, because the role of agency is then shifted from the person to causes beyond the person's control, a situation that makes plea for insanity plausible and also likely to engender empathetic societal reactions. But, however appealing this is, overly focusing on perceived underlying mental illness in decriminalisation efforts has the potential also to misdirect prevention and intervention efforts, within the context of Ghana. That is, there will be the tendency to limit suicide prevention and intervention to biomedicine, against the background of abundant evidence suggesting mainly psychosocial and existential underpinnings of suicide attempts in Ghana, which are rooted in religio-spiritual, interpersonal, familial, social welfare and justice concerns (Adinkrah, 2012; Akotia, Knizek, Kinyanda, & Hjelmeland, 2014; Akotia et al., 2019; Asare-Doku, 2015; Quarshie et al., 2020b). Limiting suicidal behaviour to the individual and viewing it either as an individual crime or crisis hinder the importance of examining suicide from a public health perspective, which may prompt population-based social and economic measures towards prevention, particularly, in LMICs, including Ghana (Jacob, 2017).

Apart from the stigmatisation of mental illnesses (Semrau, Evans-Lacko, Koschorke, Ashenafi, & Thornicroft, 2015), there are also serious challenges with the mental health sector in most LMICs, in terms of limited human resources, ring-fenced budget and low resources (Chisholm et al., 2019; Jack, Canavan, Ofori-Atta, Taylor, & Bradley, 2013; Roberts, Mogan, & Asare, 2014). So, even though it might be appealing to plead the insanity clauses to get persons who attempt suicide out of the legal system, we may likely cause dehumanisation and intense stigma for such persons, if we do not also seek massive social and health reforms, including improving the mental health care delivery system and public attitudes towards mental health. Our works with other colleagues in Ghana (e.g., Osafo et al., 2015) have shown many cases of suicidal attempters going ahead to eventually kill themselves due to social taunts, stigma, and discrimination they suffered from community members after their first attempt. The pervasive stigma related to seeking psychiatric treatment in Ghana (Barke, Nyarko, & Klecha, 2011) for instance, has been found also to underlie poor help-seeking behaviours and intentions in the society among various vulnerable groups, including students (Andoh-Arthur, Asante, & Osafo, 2015; Badu, O'Brien, & Mitchell, 2018). A lack of reforms and attitude change in the sector will mean that persons in suicidal crises, for fear of stigma, might be discouraged from seeking professional help, a situation which might impede suicide prevention efforts.

Another reason for which a contextualised decriminalisation drive ought to be considered is provided for by the element of agency in some suicides. Through our own research and abundance of evidence on suicides in and outside Ghana, there is the issue of agentic suicides (Broz & Münster, 2015); suicides which appear to have arisen from conscious decisional choices based on careful analysis of one's condition. For such behaviours, the insanity plea may be hard to sustain as libertarian argument on right to freedom and choice to die cannot also survive in the communal societies including Ghana. This is because the strong communal systems existing in Africa provide the knowledge and values that are noted to enlighten one and one's choice (Ikuenobe, 2017). Accordingly, when one chooses suicide for whatever reason, that choice is seen as not emerging from among the acceptable options that the community makes available (Ikuenobe, 2017), hence the proscription of the act and condemnation of the actor. Thus, whereas in the West arguments for decriminalisation of anti-suicide laws can also be made from libertarian perspectives just like in Euthanasia, similar arguments can ruffle collective sensitivities in most African societies including Ghana. An opinion piece published widely in defence of the law on suicide in Ghana is an indication of how some persons (presumably for lack of understanding of suicidal behaviour) can push the libertarian argument to counter genuine decriminalisation efforts in Ghana (Korang, 2013). This implies that calls for decriminalisation should be evidenced based and situated within the local particularities of the nature and patterns of suicide, as well as the social and cultural realities of the people.

Narrow binary definitions of the act as individual crime and a mental health crisis may limit progress if they do not take into consideration the sociohistorical and cultural context within which suicide and suicide attempts are embedded. Such definitions foster a *dichotomisation* instead of *kinship* among two of the most important systems for dealing with suicides in Ghana, that is, the mental health and the legal systems. In this regard, we propose an alternative perspective that situates suicide and suicide attempt within a broader notion of *social suffering*. This perspective also offers promise for promoting a *kinship* between the mental health and the legal systems and incorporates social justice matters in the way we view and address suicidal matters in Ghana.

Social Suffering: An Alternative Perspective for Viewing and Addressing Suicide and Suicide Attempt in Ghana

The concept of social suffering in its original formulation reflects the assemblage of human problems that have their origins and consequences in the devastating harm that social forces can inflict on the human experience (Kleinman, Das, & Lock, 1997). According to Kleinman et al.

(1997), "Social suffering results from what political, economic, and institutional power does to people and, reciprocally, from how these forms of power themselves influence responses to social problems" (p. ix). The categorisations of social suffering include "conditions that are usually divided among separate fields, conditions that simultaneously involve health, welfare, legal, moral, and religious issues" (p. ix).

The concept of social suffering has been studied through various dimensions across many disciplinary perspectives. For instance, in medicine, the study of social suffering is related to disease, debility and illness-centric: suffering exudes from and is embodied by disease and illness in social networks (Kuah-Pearce, Kleinman, & Harrison, 2014). As an interrelated term, social suffering is an omnibus term that incorporates a variety of issues from several life domains including health, social, economic, political, subjective and spiritual problems. "By lumping these somewhat different human conditions together, the term is meant to reverse the intellectually problematic trend of academic splitting of human problems into ever more narrowly reduced disciplinary-bound, methodologically-defined objects of enquiry" (Kuah-Pearce et al., 2014, p. 4).

Our quest to situate suicide and suicide attempt within the notion of social suffering is intended to achieve four-pronged aims: (1) to counter narrow perceptions of the acts, which often leads to conceptualisation of suicide prevention programmes in universal, apolitical and decontextualised terms, giving them a one-size-fits-all quality (White, Marsh, Kral, & Morris, 2015); (2) to disrupt the binary discourses in the decriminalisation agenda: (3) foster a kinship, rather than dichotomies, among the legal and the mental health systems; and (4) to allow for a more social justice approach to managing suicides and attempted suicides within the Ghanaian society.

In both popular and social scientific arenas, suicide is recognised as a multidimensional phenomenon, which "takes place in a powerful social context" (Kral, 1998, p. 221). In his Western definition of suicide, Shneidman (1998) asserted that suicide is a conscious act of self-induced annihilation, best understood as a multidimensional malaise in a needful individual who defines an issue for which the suicide is perceived as the best solution. From the definition, the agentic element of suicide and its context specificity are implied. A deeper understanding of the phenomenon will be realised, therefore through frameworks incorporating the dialectic of a person and social and cultural context (Hjelmeland & Knizek, 2010; Kral, 1998; Rogers & Soyka, 2004; White et al., 2015). As a multidimensional malaise, suicidal behaviour needs to be approached from broader and multiple perspectives and situated in contexts, in order to avoid a one-size-fits-all framework for prevention. As indicated earlier, the binary discourse on decriminalisation of suicide attempt that is framed predominantly from mental illness (insanity) and crime (culpability) perspectives often misdirects prevention and intervention efforts, as biology is often prioritised over the underlying socioeconomic, cultural, and political factors. The biomedical concentration is said to be short-term focused and has almost the singular aim of getting the suicidal persons through the crisis (Rogers & Soyka, 2004). Such intervention models are found to dehumanise suicidal persons due to their distancing and marginalising effects, as well as their potential to contribute to the stigma of suicidal persons (Rogers & Soyka, 2004). The pertinent question is, *after treatment what is next?* What does treatment of the underlying mental illness of suicide attempt does to a person who goes back to the same condition/context that originally triggered the mental illness and the subsequent attempt? These questions are asked against the background of concerns of hospitalisations of suicide attempts, with evidence showing that many persons who seek treatment for suicidal problems still go ahead to kill themselves (Pridmore, 2015). The overbearing focus on mental illness and its accompanying unitary and impersonal treatment options goes against the grain of Karl Jaspers (1959) decade-long admonition for a full human presence in people's phenomenological experience of suffering. A phenomenological approach promises to aid our understanding of suicide and suicidal behaviour, helping us to *understand* rather than to *explain* the behaviour (Pompili, 2010). From such a standpoint, we can better understand suicide in ways that can help sharpen the responsiveness of all sectors of the society, particularly, the mental health systems and the legal system, towards addressing the problem.

Fostering a Kinship between the Legal and Mental Health Systems in Suicide Prevention

The complementary role of the legal system in mental healthcare system has a long history. In Ghana, past legislations have provided the legal framework for how the mental health sector is organised, as well as the provision of the mental health care services. These legislations include the Criminal Offences Act, 1960 (29); Criminal Offences (Procedure) Act, 1960 (30); and the Mental Health Act, 1972, which is now replaced with the Mental Health Act, 2012 (Act 846). However, over the years, not much has been achieved in terms of enhancing the capacity of the legal sector towards the prevention of suicide. To address the problem, the Ghana Mental Health Authority, working in conjunction with the Judiciary, recently undertook a nationwide exercise to train judges and magistrates across the country on mental health, suicide and its prevention (Nyavi, 2017). The first author, being one of the facilitators for the training, noted situations where judges and magistrates narrated instances when they had to simply advise and discharge suicide attempters or refer them for further professional mental health help. These judges and magistrates took these discretionary measures rather than applying the full force of the law primarily because they considered the cases to be mostly socioeconomically and psychosocially driven. The training, thus, helped to strengthen the disposition of the judges and magistrates to help, as it equipped them with basic mental health and suicide literacy such as risk identification, warning signs, and prevention tips. The judges and magistrates, in turn, also shared their work conditions and the ramifications those conditions had on their own mental health, which prompted us to deliver training in stress-reducing therapies for their optimum wellbeing. Sustaining such partnerships is potentially good for the improvement in mental health and effective suicide prevention. Also, given that judges and magistrates are mainly law interpreters, the mental health sector can leverage on their unique experiences to push for law reforms as is currently being done in Ghana, where insights from the referenced (Nyavi, 2017) training has helped in the drafting of a petition to Ghana's parliament for the repeal of the anti-suicide laws. Basically, the petition seeks reforms at broader levels, including sharpening of the responsiveness of both the legislature and the judiciary to underlying psychological problems of defendants.

The attempt at "courting the courts' support" for helping persons experiencing suicidal crises can be well situated within the doctrine of therapeutic jurisprudence as advanced by Wexler and Winick (1992). Therapeutic jurisprudence recognises the law as a social force with consequences in the psychological domain. That is, the law does not operate in vacuum, there is always a spirit behind the letter of the law, a spirit that seeks to reflect the realities of the context and the person, and aims at advancing the social good and justice concerns. Therapeutic jurisprudence also examines the role of the law as a therapeutic agent and its enormous potential to "heal" (Wexler, 2008; Wexler & Winick, 1996). Thus, rather than advancing arguments on decriminalisation premised on pushing suicidal attempt completely away from the legal system to the mental health system, we can rather be promoting the responsiveness of the legal system towards (1) Diverting persons facing suicide attempt charges to the mental health system for help or (2) Helping in seeking social justice for the many in society who, for the lack of capacity to address the many social ills they are confronted with, opt for suicide attempt and suicide. Several cases of suicides in Ghana that follow abuses, social taunts, discrimination, and neglect of individuals could be well addressed particularly through the latter while not ignoring potential underlying psychiatric and psychosocial factors. Such approaches require effective collaboration among all the sectors, particularly the mental and legal systems.

Conclusion

Suicide is a complex phenomenon that is at the juncture of many disciplinary perspectives—biological, psychosocial, existential, law, economic and cultural. Effective prevention and intervention require a consideration of multiple approaches that focus on the population-level factors rather than on individuals-level factors only. Situating suicide as social suffering offers a perspective that fosters a kinship of all relevant sectors of society towards effective remediation. Efforts towards the decriminalisation of suicide attempt in Ghana and other countries, for instance, offer one such avenue where an effective collaboration between the mental health system and the legal system is needed not only to just expunge the anti-suicide laws but also to address the many social ills that give impetus for the choice of suicide among some persons.

References

Adinkrah, M. (2011). Epidemiologic characteristics of suicidal behavior in contemporary Ghana. *Crisis: The Journal of Crisis Intervention and Suicide Prevention, 32*(1), 31. https://doi.org/10.1027/0227-5910/a000056

Adinkrah, M. (2012). Better dead than dishonored: Masculinity and male suicidal behavior in contemporary Ghana. *Social Science & Medicine, 74*, 474–481. https://doi.org/10.1016/j.socscimed.2010.10.011

Adinkrah, M. (2015). Suicide and mortuary beliefs and practices of the Akan of Ghana. *OMEGA—Journal of Death and Dying, 74*(2), 138–163. https://doi.org/10.1177/0030222815598427

Adinkrah, M. (2018). Characteristics of elderly suicides in Ghana. *OMEGA—Journal of Death and Dying, 82*(1), 3–24. https://doi.org/10.1177/0030222818779527

Agyeman, N. K. (2019, November). *Don't decriminalise suicide—Haruna Iddrisu*. Graphic Online. Retrieved from https://www.graphic.com.gh/news/politics/ghana-news-don-t-decriminalise-suicide-haruna-iddrisu.html

Akotia, C. S., Knizek, B. L., Hjelmeland, H., Kinyanda, E., & Osafo, J. (2019). Reasons for attempting suicide: An exploratory study in Ghana. *Transcultural Psychiatry, 56*(1), 233–249. https://doi.org/10.1177/1363461518802966

Akotia, C. S., Knizek, B. L., Kinyanda, E., & Hjelmeland, H. (2014). "I have sinned": Understanding the role of religion in the experiences of suicide attempters in Ghana. *Mental Health, Religion & Culture, 17*(5), 437–448. https://doi.org/10.1080/13674676.2013.829426

Andoh-Arthur, J., Asante, K. O., & Osafo, J. (2015). Determinants of psychological help-seeking intentions of university students in Ghana. *International Journal for the Advancement of Counselling, 37*(4), 330–345. https://doi.org/10.1007/s10447-015-9247-2

Andoh-Arthur, J., Hjelmeland, H., Osafo, J., & Knizek, B. L. (2020). Substance use and suicide among men in Ghana: A qualitative study. *Current Psychology* 1–13. https://doi.org/10.1007/s12144-020-00644-0

Andoh-Arthur, J., Knizek, B. L., Osafo, J., & Hjelmeland, H. (2018). Suicide among men in Ghana: The burden of masculinity. *Death Studies, 42*(10), 658–666. https://doi.org/10.1080/07481187.2018.1426655

Andoh-Arthur, J., Knizek, B. L., Osafo, J., & Hjelmeland, H. (2019). Societal reactions to suicide in Ghana: A qualitative study of experiences of the bereaved. *Crisis: The Journal of Crisis Intervention and Suicide Prevention.* https://doi.org/10.1027/0227-5910/a000618

Asare-Doku, W. (2015). *Experiences and coping mechanisms of suicide attempters and their families in Ghana: A mixed method approach.* Unpublished Master's thesis, University of Ghana.

Badu, E., O'Brien, A. P., & Mitchell, R. (2018). An integrative review of potential enablers and barriers to accessing mental health services in Ghana. *Health Research Policy and Systems, 16*(1), 110. https://doi.org/10.1186/s12961-018-0382-1

Barke, A., Nyarko, S., & Klecha, D. (2011). The stigma of mental illness in southern Ghana: Attitudes of the urban population and patients' views. *Social Psychiatry and Psychiatric Epidemiology, 46*, 1191–1202. https://doi.org/10.1007/s00127-010-0290-3

Black, H. C., Garner, B. A., McDaniel, B. R., Schultz, D. W., & West Publishing Company. (1999). *Black's law dictionary* (Vol. 196). West Group.

Broz, L., & Münster, D. (Eds.). (2015). *Suicide and agency: Anthropological perspectives on self-destruction, personhood, and power.* Ashgate Publishing, Ltd.

Canetto, S. S., & Sakinofsky, I. (1998). The gender paradox in suicide. *Suicide and Life-Threatening Behavior, 28*(1), 1–23. Retrieved from https://www.researchgate.net/publication/13720598_The_Gender_Paradox_in_Suicide

Chisholm, D., Docrat, S., Abdulmalik, J., Alem, A., Gureje, O., Gurung, D., et al. (2019). Mental health financing challenges, opportunities and strategies in low- and middle-income countries: Findings from the Emerald project. *BJPsych Open, 5*(5). https://doi.org/10.1192/bjo.2019.24

De Witte, M. (2001). *Long live the dead! Changing funeral celebrations in Asante, Ghana.* Ghana Aksant Academic Publishers.

Der, E. M., Dakwah, I. A., Derkyi-Kwarteng, L., & Badu, A. A. (2016). Hanging as a method of suicide in Ghana: A 10 year autopsy study. *Pathology Discovery, 4*(1), 2. https://doi.org/10.7243/2052-7896-4-2

Durkheim, E. (1897/1966). *Suicide: A study in sociology.* Free Press.

Franklin, J. C., Ribeiro, J. D., Fox, K. R., Bentley, K. H., Kleiman, E. M., Huang, X., et al. (2017). Risk factors for suicidal thoughts and behaviors: A meta-analysis of 50 years of research. *Psychological Bulletin, 143*(2), 187–232. https://doi.org/10.1037/bul0000084

Glenn, C. R., Kleiman, E. M., Kellerman, J., Pollak, O., Cha, C. B., Esposito, E. C., et al. (2020). Annual research review: A meta-analytic review of world-wide suicide rates in adolescents. *Journal of Child Psychology and Psychiatry, 61*(3), 294–308. https://doi.org/10.1111/jcpp.13106

Hawton, K., Saunders, K. E., & O'Connor, R. C. (2012). Self-harm and suicide in adolescents. *The Lancet, 379*(9834), 2373–2382. https://doi.org/10.1016/S0140-6736(12)60322-5

Hjelmeland, H., Kinyanda, E., & Knizek, B. L. (2012). Mental health workers' views on the criminalization of suicidal behaviour in Uganda. *Medicine, Science and the Law, 52*(3), 148–151. https://doi.org/10.1258/msl.2012.011107

Hjelmeland, H., & Knizek, B. L. (2010). Why we need qualitative research in suicidology. *Suicide. and Life-Threatening Behavior, 40*(1), 74–80. https://doi.org/10.1521/suli.2010.40.1.74

Hjelmeland, H., Osafo, J., Akotia, C. S., & Knizek, B. L. (2014). The law criminalizing attempted suicide in Ghana. *Crisis, 35*(2), 132–136. https://doi.org/10.1027/0227-5910/a000235

Ikuenobe, P. (2017). African communal basis for autonomy and life choices. *Developing World Bioethics.* https://doi.org/10.1111/dewb.12161

Jack, H., Canavan, M., Ofori-Atta, A., Taylor, L., & Bradley, E. (2013). Recruitment and retention of mental health workers in Ghana. *PLOS One, 8*(2), e57940. https://doi.org/10.1371/journal.pone.0057940

Jacob, K. S. (2017). Suicide prevention in low-and middle-income countries: Part perceptions, partial solutions (Editorial). *British Journal of Psychology, 211*, 264–265.

Jaspers, K. (1959). *General psychopathology.* The John Hopkins University Press.

Kleinman, A., Das, V., & Lock, M. M. (Eds.). (1997). *Social suffering.* University of California Press.

Klonsky, E. D., May, A. M., & Saffer, B. Y. (2016). Suicide, suicide attempts, and suicidal ideation. *Annual Review of Clinical Psychology, 12*, 307–330. https://doi.org/10.1146/annurev-clinpsy-021815-093204

Korang, D. (2013, September). *In defence of the Law on suicide.* GhanaWeb Online. Retrieved from https://www.ghanaweb.com/GhanaHomePage/features/In-defence-of-the-law-of-suicide-287094

Kral, M. J. (1998). Suicide and the internalization of culture: Three questions. *Transcultural Psychiatry, 35*(2), 221–233. https://doi.org/10.1177/136346159803500203

Kuah-Pearce, K. E., Kleinman, A., & Harrison, E. (2014). Social suffering and the culture of compassion in a morally divided China. *Anthropology & Medicine, 21*(1), 1–7. https://doi.org/10.1080/13648470.2014.880873

Lubaale, E. C. (2017). The crime of attempted suicide in Uganda: the need for reforms to the law. *Journal of Law, Society and Development, 4*(1), 1–19. https://doi.org/10.25159/2520-9515/385

Mars, B., Burrows, S., Hjelmeland, H., & Gunnell, D. (2014). Suicidal behaviour across the African continent: A review of the literature. *BMC Public Health, 14*(1), 606. https://doi.org/10.1186/1471-2458-14-606

Mishara, B. L., & Weisstub, D. N. (2016). The legal status of suicide: A global review. *International Journal of Law and Psychiatry, 44*, 54–74. https://doi.org/10.1016/j.ijlp.2015.08.032

Moore, S. (2000). *The decriminalisation of suicide.* An unpublished doctoral dissertation, London School of Economics and Political Science, UK.

Naghavi, M., & Global Burden of Disease Self-Harm Collaborators. (2019). Global, regional, and national burden of suicide mortality 1990 to 2016: Systematic analysis for the Global Burden of Disease Study 2016. *BMJ, 364*, l94. https://doi.org/10.1136/bmj.l94

Neeleman, J. (1996). Suicide as a crime in the UK: Legal history, international comparisons and present implications. *Acta Psychiatrica Scandinavica, 94*(4), 252–257. https://doi.org/10.1111/j.1600-0447.1996.tb09857.x

Nyavi, G. A. (2017, June). *Judges trained on need to decriminalize attempted suicide.* Graphic Online. Retrieved from https://www.graphic.com.gh/news/general-news/judges-schooled-on-need-to-decriminalize-attempted-suicide.html

Osafo, J., Akotia, C. S., Andoh-Arthur, J., Boakye, K. E., & Quarshie, E. N.-B. (2018). "We now have a patient and not a criminal": An exploratory study of judges and lawyers' views on suicide attempters and the law in Ghana. *International Journal of Offender Therapy and Comparative Criminology, 62*(6), 1488–1508. https://doi.org/10.1177/0306624X17692059

Osafo, J., Akotia, C. S., Andoh-Arthur, J., & Quarshie, E. N.-B. (2015). Attempted suicide in Ghana: Motivation, stigma, and coping. *Death Studies, 39*(5), 274–280. https://doi.org/10.1080/07481187.2014.991955

Osafo, J., Akotia, C. S., Boakye, K. E., & Dickson, E. (2018). Between moral infraction and existential crisis: Exploring physicians and nurses' attitudes to suicide and the suicidal patient in Ghana. *International Journal of Nursing Studies, 85*, 118–125. https://doi.org/10.1016/j.ijnurstu.2018.05.017

Osafo, J., Akotia, C. S., Quarshie, E. N. B., Boakye, K. E., & Andoh-Arthur, J. (2017). Police views of suicidal persons and the law criminalizing attempted suicide in Ghana: A qualitative study with policy implications. *Sage Open*, *7*(3). https://doi.org/10.1177/2158244017731803

Pompili, M. (2010). Exploring the phenomenology of suicide. *Suicide and Life-Threatening Behavior*, *40*(3), 234–244. https://doi.org/10.1521/suli.2010.40.3.234

Pridmore, S. (2015). Mental disorder and suicide: A faulty connection. *Australian & New Zealand Journal of Psychiatry*, *49*(1), 18–20. https://doi.org/10.1177/0004867414548904

Quarshie, E. N. B., Asante, K. O., Andoh-Arthur, J., Asare-Doku, W., & Navelle, P. L. (2018). Suicide attempts and deaths in older persons in Ghana: A media surveillance approach. *Current Psychology*, 1–14. https://doi.org/10.1007/s12144-018-9932-5

Quarshie, E. N. B., Osafo, J., Akotia, C. S., & Peprah, J. (2015). Adolescent suicide in Ghana: A content analysis of media reports. *International Journal of Qualitative Studies on Health and Well-Being*, *10*(1), 27682. https://doi.org/10.3402/qhw.v10.27682

Quarshie, E. N.-B., Waterman, M. G., & House, A. O. (2020a). Adolescent self-harm in Ghana: A qualitative interview-based study of first-hand accounts. *BMC Psychiatry*, *20*(275). https://doi.org/10.1186/s12888-020-02599-9

Quarshie, E. N.-B., Waterman, M. G., & House, A. O. (2020b). Self-harm with suicidal and non-suicidal intent in young people in sub-Saharan Africa: A systematic review. *BMC Psychiatry*, *20*, 1–26. https://doi.org/10.1186/s12888-020-02587-z

Ranjan, R., Kumar, S., Pattanayak, R. D., Dhawan, A., & Sagar, R. (2014). (De-) criminalization of attempted suicide in India: A review. *Industrial Psychiatry Journal*, *23*(1), 4. https://doi.org/10.4103/0972-6748.144936

Roberts, M., Mogan, C., & Asare, J. B. (2014). An overview of Ghana's mental health system: Results from an assessment using the World Health Organization's Assessment Instrument for Mental Health Systems (WHO-AIMS). *International Journal of Mental Health Systems*, *8*(1), 16. https://doi.org/10.1186/1752-4458-8-16

Rogers, J. R., & Soyka, K. M. (2004). "One size fits all": An existential-constructivist perspective on the crisis intervention approach with suicidal individuals. *Journal of Contemporary Psychotherapy*, *34*(1), 7–22.

Sareen, H., & Trivedi, J. K. (2009). Legal implication of suicide problems specific to South Asia. *Delhi Psychiatry Journal*, *12*, 121–125. Retrieved from https://imsear.searo.who.int/handle/123456789/158934

Semrau, M., Evans-Lacko, S., Koschorke, M., Ashenafi, L., & Thornicroft, G. (2015). Stigma and discrimination related to mental illness in low- and middle-income countries. *Epidemiology and Psychiatric Sciences, 24*(5), 382–394. https://doi.org/10.1017/s2045796015000359

Shahtahmasebi, S. (2013). Examining the claim that 80–90% of suicide cases had depression. *Frontiers in Public Health, 1*, 62. https://doi.org/10.3389/fpubh.2013.00062

Shneidman, E. S. (1998). *The suicidal mind.* Oxford University Press.

Trivedi, J. K. (1997). Punishing attempted suicide: An anachronism of 20th century. *Indian Journal of Psychiatry, 39*, 87–89. Retrieved from https://pubmed.ncbi.nlm.nih.gov/21584053/

Uddin, R., Burton, N. W., Maple, M., Khan, S. R., & Khan, A. (2019). Suicidal ideation, suicide planning, and suicide attempts among adolescents in 59 low-income and middle-income countries: A population-based study. *The Lancet Child & Adolescent Health, 3*(4), 223–233. https://doi.org/10.1016/s2352-4642(18)30403-6

Wexler, D. B. (2008). Two decades of therapeutic jurisprudence. *Touro L. Rev., 24*, 17.

Wexler, D. B., & Winick, B. J. (1992). Therapeutic jurisprudence and criminal justice mental health issues. *Mental and Physical Disability Law Reporter, 16*(2), 225–231. Retrieved from https://www.jstor.org/stable/20783213?seq=1

Wexler, D. B., & Winick, B. J. (1996). *Law in a therapeutic key: Developments in therapeutic jurisprudence.* Carolina Academic Press.

White, J., Marsh, I., Kral, M. J., & Morris, J. (Eds.). (2015). *Critical suicidology: Transforming suicide research and prevention for the 21st century.* UBC Press.

World Health Organisation. (2014). *Preventing suicide: A global imperative.* WHO.

World Health Organisation. (2016). *Practice manual for establishing and maintaining surveillance systems for suicide attempts and self-harm.* WHO.

9

Issues of Competence, Experience and Psychological Awareness among Police who Prosecute Cases of Child Sexual Abuse in Ghana

Charlotte Omane Kwakye-Nuako

Introduction

An Executive Instrument (E.I. 4) gives prosecutorial powers to the police in Ghana to prosecute cases of summary jurisdiction. Thus, the penetrative sexual abuse of a child under 16 years (defilement), which is a second degree felony, falls under their ambit. When victims of crime engage with the police and other members of the criminal justice system, they want to be believed and they want the police to show competence in handling their cases (Antonsdóttir, 2018; Daly & Curtis-Fawley, 2006; Herman, 2005). In a context where the police service is under-resourced and the personnel lack the requisite training, their interaction with the police becomes even more difficult. An additional factor that affects police interaction with the populace is where they are perceived to have little training and are not friendly towards their clients. This does not augur

C. O. Kwakye-Nuako (✉)
Department of Forensic Science, University of Cape Coast,
Cape Coast, Ghana

© The Author(s), under exclusive license to Springer Nature Switzerland AG 2021   **191**
H. C. O. Chan, S. Adjorlolo (eds.), *Crime, Mental Health and the Criminal Justice System in Africa*, https://doi.org/10.1007/978-3-030-71024-8_9

well for victims who come into contact with them after a distressful experience.

This chapter looks at how the police who are clothed with prosecutorial powers function within the context where they are dealing with traumatised victims of child sexual abuse. The chapter uses the perspectives of the police prosecutors themselves and those of defense lawyers to understand the issues of competence and skill surrounding the function of policemen as prosecutors in this space. The chapter begins with a brief history and overview of the Police Service in Ghana, proceeds to discuss the theoretical basis for the chapter and continues with the methods, analysis and discussion sections.

History and Current Function of Policing in Ghana

Historically, policing as it exists now in Ghana, was a creation of the British colonial government (Pokoo-Aikins, 1998; Tankebe, 2008b). Before then, the traditional rulers had military and paramilitary groups and persons who kept the peace in various localities (Appiahene-Gyamfi, 2009; Boateng & Darko, 2016). Their current structure and operations thus bear vestiges of their colonial mandate. For instance, the colonial police force was to maintain law and order and to also protect the British economic interests along trade routes. All these were done in a way to protect the British against the indigenes. Post-independence governments assumed the use of the police as instruments by which they could subjugate the people for their own ends, thus perpetuating the colonial mandate (Atuguba, 2008; Tankebe, 2008a).

The police service in Ghana has evolved over the years with increase in personnel and a focus towards community policing (Pokoo-Aikins, 1998). This re-focus led to the inception of the Domestic Violence and Victim Support Unit (DOVVSU) with a mandate for all matters related to domestic violence, child rights, human trafficking and other gendered matters that border on criminality. Formerly called Women and Juvenile Unit (WAJU), the Unit has been in existence since 1998. Although the police at DOVVSU have been found to provide service to these vulnerable groups, there are still some challenges (Amoakohene, 2004; Darkwah & Prah, 2016). DOVVSU officers are a part of a community that is considerably patriarchal and thus underrate violence against women (Boakye, 2009). They have thus been found to provide insufficient help to their clients (Boateng & Lee, 2014). Added to this is the lack of logistics and human resource, which restrains them from providing support and follow-up services to the victims who report to their facility.

Police Prosecutors in Ghana

The police also work as prosecutors in Ghana. In 1976 an Executive Instrument (E.I. 4) entitled the "Appointment of Public Prosecutors Instrument", was promulgated by which the Attorney-General ceded a part of its prosecutorial powers to several bodies including the police. This means that any police officer from the rank of a Sergeant could be trained to function as a prosecutor irrespective of their former training. The prosecutorial powers of the police are however, limited to the lower courts—the District and Circuit Courts.[1]

The Legal and Prosecution Directorate of the Ghana Police Service is responsible for their training in collaboration with the regional prosecution units headed by senior police officers who are lawyers[2] (Ghana Police Service, 2018b). The JUPOL is a trained police officer who is a lawyer. Anecdotal reports suggest that the prosecutors are initially trained by the Legal and Prosecution Directorate and on quarterly basis they are expected to receive in-service training from the CID supported by lawyers from the Attorney General's Department.

In a 2018 Report by the EU's Accountability, Rule of Law and Anti-Corruption Programme (ARAP), it was found that although police prosecutors were an essential part of the justice delivery, they were poorly

---

[1] Ghana has two levels of court, namely the Superior courts (comprising of the Supreme Court, Court of Appeal and High Court) and Lower courts (comprising the Circuit and District Courts). The jurisdiction of the superior courts are set out in Ghana's 1992 Constitution and the Courts Act, 2003 (Act 459) (as amended) whereas the jurisdiction of the lower courts is set out in the latter.
[2] They are often referred to as Judicial Police Officers (JUPOL).

selected, poorly trained and not motivated. For instance, they had no job description (on rules and responsibilities of police prosecutors), no identifiable selection process, little or no previous experience of investigative work, and little pre-deployment training. The Police prosecutors are often not trained lawyers and there is no standing agreement between the Ghana School of Law and the Ghana Police Service to train the prosecutors. They are taken from among the police service, trained in minimum skills and deployed to the courts. Their competence and training is thus in question at the beginning of their duty. There are also internal issues that make the role of police prosecutors unattractive. They are not given incentives that other special units of the police are remunerated with and are also subject to arbitrary transfers (Accountability Rule of law and Anti-Corruption Programme, 2018). The interaction of this group of ill-trained and poorly motivated police officers with victims of child sexual abuse have not been investigated.

Theoretical Framework

The effectiveness of police work depends on the level of acceptance they receive from the community they serve. This has been discussed by Tyler in terms of procedural justice and legitimacy (Tyler, 2006). Studies conducted in Ghana have however, found that rather than procedural appropriateness, *police effectiveness* is a better predictor of community cooperation with the police (Pryce, 2018; Pryce, Johnson, & Maguire, 2016; Tankebe, 2009). The views of the general population in Ghana, and even Ghanaian immigrants, show a general distrust for the police and their activities (Pryce, 2018). This is mainly due to the inability of the citizenry to see the police as being effective in their work. For instance, victims of sexual abuse have consistently reported challenges in their interactions with the police during reporting (Darkwah & Prah, 2016) so that persons who have encountered the police in earlier victimisations are reluctant to report subsequent incidents to them due to their previous encounters with them (Boateng & Lee, 2014).

Therapeutic jurisprudence also suggests that the law as it is and how it is practiced has the ability to produce either therapeutic or anti-therapeutic consequences for the end user (Wexler, 1993, 2011). Thus, the extent to which the police are seen to be effective would enhance the therapeutic experience of victims of sexual abuse who have to work with the police in their double role as investigators and prosecutors. The term police is used here to refer to the Ghana Police Service as an institution.

Challenges of Victims and Caregivers Seeking Justice

Child sexual abuse is debilitating to both victims and their caregivers. In resource-poor environments, the absence of adequate resources coupled with the increased prevalence in urban poor areas (Wrigley-Asante, Owusu, Oteng-Ababio, & Owusu, 2016) makes it especially complicated and leads to a *triple victimisation* when they come into contact with the criminal justice system. Triple victimisation means that they are at once confronted with the debilitating effects of the abuse, they have to confront de-moralised criminal justice officers, and also have to deal with their own lack of economic resources to fully engage a system that offers no economic support (Mulambia, Miller, MacDonald, & Kennedy, 2018; Musiwa, 2018).

Studies conducted on victims of sexual crimes show that they require three things from the justice system: to have a voice (Daly & Curtis-Fawley, 2006; Herman, 2005), for their stories to be believed; an end to their victimisation; and finally, a speedy trial (Back, Gustafsson, Larsson, & Berterö, 2011; Eastwood, 2003). At the very least, they would like their cases to be treated with some seriousness and to obtain empathy from the persons they are dealing with (Daly & Bouhours, n.d.). Again, they look out for procedural justice in that, where the processes their cases are taken through are seen to be fair, they are likely to be satisfied even when they do not win (Antonsdóttir, 2018; Herman, 2005). Although in some countries, compensation is paid to them, studies in Western contexts have shown that the money paid for the offence has not been their focus—they rather preferred that the truth would be revealed in the trial and that they would have been treated with decency by the officers in the criminal justice system (Back et al., 2011).

One noticeable feature in most of these studies is that there are separate roles for the police and the prosecutors. The former serve as police personnel and the latter are usually lawyers. This is not the case in Ghana and in some African countries such as Malawi (Molyneux, Kennedy, Dano, & Mulambia, 2013; Mulambia et al., 2018). The police double as both investigators and prosecutors, meaning that victims and their caregivers are going to experience a more debilitating experience if they have a poor interaction with them.

This chapter argues that the dual position of the police in child sexual abuse cases in Ghana should be revisited. These are distressed people who encounter a harassing police service during initial intake and investigation (see Daly, 2014; Darkwah & Prah, 2016; Spohn & Holleran, 2001), and so this chapter makes the argument that after the initial investigation, the victims and their caregivers should not be made to continue dealing with the police as prosecutors. The aim of this chapter therefore was to explore the role of police prosecutors in their prosecution of child sexual abuse cases. It makes this exploration through the lenses of the police prosecutors themselves and defense lawyers who work with them in court.

Methods

Research Design

A qualitative method and specifically, a phenomenological research design was used to address the research question The data was analysed using thematic analysis because of its theoretical and epistemological flexibility (Braun & Clarke, 2006; Clarke & Braun, 2017). The data analysis employed an interpretative perspective and not merely a semantic approach.

Study Setting, Participants and Participant Recruitment

Ghana is a West African country that is made up 16 regions comprising people from different ethnic groups. Similar to other countries with common law jurisdictions, Ghana has a criminal justice system that encompasses the Police, Prisons and the Judiciary. The Ghana Police Service has among others, the mandate to apprehend offenders and ensure the safety of individuals within the country (Ghana Police Service Act, 1970, Act 350). Legal practice in Ghana is regulated by the Legal Professions Act, 1960 (Act 32 as amended) and is regulated by the General Legal Council (GBA, 2017). Prosecutorial duties are also carried out by lawyers in the Attorney General's Department. The Department has regional offices but not district offices.

A total of 14 participants were sampled using the purposive sampling technique (see Table 9.1). They comprised 6 defense lawyers (Mean$_{age}$ = 38.3; 83.3% male), 7 police prosecutors (Mean$_{age}$ = 46.1 years; 57% male) and 1 female legal prosecutor from the Attorney General's Department (see Table 9.1). About 77% of the participants had at least a first degree. In the process of gathering data, saturation was reached by the fourteenth participant (Fusch & Ness, 2015), hence the need to stop

Table 9.1 Demographic information of participants

Pseudonym	Sex	Age	Qualification	Occupation
DfnseL1K	M	45	First degree; BL	Defense lawyer
DfnseL2K	M	35	First degree; BL	Defense lawyer
DfnseL3K	M	45	First degree; BL	Defense lawyer
DfnseL4A	M	39	LLM; BL	Defense lawyer
DfnseL5A	F	32	First degree; BL	Defense lawyer
DfnseL6A	M	34	First degree; BL	Defense lawyer
Prosc1K	M	52	PhD (Div.), MBA, LLB	Police prosecutor
Prosc2K	F	47	First degree	Police prosecutor
Prosc3K	M	53	Diploma	Police prosecutor
Prosc4K	M	48	Post-secondary	Police prosecutor
Prosc5K	F	32	First degree; BL	A-G prosecutor
Prosc6A	M	42	First degree	Police prosecutor
Prosc7A	F	49	MBA	Police prosecutor

K = Kumasi; A = Accra; BL = Barrister at law

gathering more data at that point. Moreover, it was depth of information that was of essence rather than quantity (Smith & Osborn, 2008).

Ethics and Data Collection Procedure

Ethical approval for this study was obtained from the Ethical Committee for the Humanities at the University of Ghana, Legon (protocol: ECH 051/17-18). Institutional permission was also obtained from the Ghana Police Service and the Regional DOVVSU units in Accra and Kumasi to interview the police. Individual written and verbal consent was obtained from legal practitioners. Potential participants who were contacted had the objectives of the study explained to them. Their concerns were adequately addressed, and written consent obtained. Participants were given the opportunity to determine the place, date and time for the interviews, which they deemed would not pose any inconvenience. They were also at liberty to withdraw from the study at any time without penalty. Although psychological support was made available in case any of the participants needed one during or after the study, the study did not pose psychological harm to the participants beyond what they encounter in their daily lives. An interview guide was used in gathering information from participants. The interviews were tape-recorded, and later transcribed verbatim. The identity of participants was held anonymous and confidential through the use of pseudonyms.

Data Analysis and Validation

This was a qualitative study using thematic analysis (Braun & Clarke, 2006; Clarke & Braun, 2017) to understand the nuanced meanings of the role, training and other issues relating to the use of police prosecutors in defilement cases in Ghana. In terms of reflexivity, the researcher is a female who works both as a lawyer and a clinical psychologist. As a lawyer, she deals with mostly civil matters and thus came into the area of criminal law practice with a somewhat first-timer perspective. This helped her to approach the subject matter with some freshness as well as a practiced eye of legal knowledge.

The researcher ensured the trustworthiness of the study by following the guidelines of Lincoln and Guba (1985): credibility, transferability, confirmability, and dependability. Due process involved in conducting qualitative studies of this nature was adhered to—obtaining the right sample, how the data is was gathered and managed, analysed, and reported (Creswell, 2014; Levitt et al., 2018). Initially, the researcher selected individuals with adequate experience and knowledge of prosecution and defense of child sexual abuse cases. The researcher built rapport with the participants before the commencement of the interviews. This was to create an atmosphere that would enable them to freely give out relevant information. Sampling these specific participants made it possible for the transferability of findings to those with similar characteristics. Further, confirmability was ensured by allowing an independent researcher to also analyse the same data using the same procedures I followed. Some of the codes were merged with others and others were taken out. The overall process was made known to another researcher as a way of peer debriefing, to ensure the dependability of the study.

The transcripts were read and re-read for their latent meanings, codes were developed and these codes were grouped together into themes. The findings are discussed under these thematic areas.

Findings

Three themes with their respective sub-themes were found as follows: *inadequate legal training* (subordinate themes: police inexperienced, and training and re-training), *intimidating or friendly* (subordinate themes: intimidating to victims, and care for victims), and *cross fire of accusations* (subordinate themes: lack of technical competence, focus on incarceration, tripartite role of police should be broken and lawyers intimidate and delay process) (see Table 9.2).

Table 9.2 Themes and sub-themes

Themes	Sub-themes
Inadequate legal training	Police inexperienced
	Training and re-training
Intimidating or friendly	Intimidating to victims
	Care for victims
Cross fire of accusations	Lack of technical competence
	Focus on incarceration
	Tripartite role of police should be broken
	Lawyers intimidate and delay process

Inadequate Legal Training

Both the lawyers and the prosecutors agreed that there was much to be desired in the training of police prosecutors. Police are generally selected from the rank of Sergeant upwards. In practice, a police person with such a qualification and who has worked as an orderly/court officer in the court for a period of time may be trained in legal principles to become a prosecutor in the courts. This is in contrast with lawyers who are expected to go through a total of 4 to 5 years of training in order to qualify as lawyers:

> *As I was saying most of these police are not lawyers but with long-term policing they're prosecuting and so looking at the technical nature of it, the evidence to prove it is not easy. Sometimes ....you have to conduct thorough investigation ... how to interpret the evidence is sometimes difficult. E.g. what shows that the bruise that you found on her [victim] ... was by the man [perpetrator] or that the lady used her finger nails to scratch her vagina?* (DfnseL1, male defense lawyer, Kumasi)

The prosecution of sexual abuse cases is complex and this complexity is sometimes lost on the police since they lack the ability to properly evaluate the evidence. In a documentary review of court data of closed files of defilement cases in one gender-based court in Accra, it was observed that 12 of the 67 (17.9%) cases reviewed were withdrawn by the police because there was no proper due diligence of evidence required to prove the offence. For instance, the age of the victim had not been provided (Kwakye-Nuako, 2018). In other instances, the wrong charge had been assigned to the perpetrator, for example, indecent assault when there was penetration (and therefore warranting a charge of defilement).

The prosecutors at the Attorney General's department are therefore petitioned by caregivers of victims to take over cases.

> *And the police some of them lack training in this aspect, when it comes to sexual offences regarding children. So we decide to take it and do the prosecution ourselves … The police as I said, most of them lack training, ahaa, so then we decide to take it and do it.* (Prscctor5K, female legal prosecutor, Kumasi)

The police are given their initial training and subsequently re-trained by their Judicial Police or by other non-governmental organisations. The lack of in-depth training makes them inadequate in court, and This distinction in training is apparent. Thus the lawyers perceive most prosecutors to be incompetent while the police see themselves as doing their best.

The police on the other hand believe that although inadequate, they are indeed taken through some training and re-training. This is done at the initial stages when they are assigned prosecutorial duties. They are trained and re-trained by their superior officers or a non-governmental organisation:

> *But what we do is in-service training. We do in-service training for our prosecutors, refreshment courses, and so and so forth. Ahah that one, sometimes the IGP will assemble a team of lawyers from our legal directorate from Head Quarters to come and assist us and they do the in-service training for prosecutors.* (Prosc1K, male police prosecutor, Kumasi)

Under the social identity theory (Tajfel & Turner, 1979), individuals evaluate others by the categorisation of "them" and "us". Rutland and Brown (2001) argued that in a bid to increase one's self-esteem, individuals evaluate themselves in a positive light compared to out-group members. Hence, the lawyers perceived the police as incompetent to handle cases of sexual abuse, while the police saw themselves to be competent and well able to carry out their duties.

Intimidating or Friendly?

Their interactions with victims have been seen from two opposing sides; whereas to the prosecutors, they are acting as lawyers to the victims and providing them with the needed help and preparation for court, the lawyers on the other hand see them as sometimes intimidating the victims. Following from their inexperience in psychological issues, the police are seen to intimidate victims who come into contact with them. *"At times they're intimidated by the police officer in uniform—the victims"* (DfnseL1K, male defense lawyer, Kumasi). This is in consonance with the stereotypic belief that the police is persecutory and aggressive in their interventions (Oulmokhtar et al., 2011). On the other hand, the police believe that they take care of the victims. This is expected since their individual worth is tied to the image of the service. By portraying themselves as being experienced and competent, the image of the police service in general is enhanced. They prepare them for court, act as their lawyer in court, and so on:

> *Then after everything, then we tell them we are taking them to court and that when we go to court the accused will be there, they should not look at the accused person, look at the judge or "you look at me or your mother, you shouldn't be scared" then we tell them that, "there will be a judge, the judge is there for justice, the judge is your friend", like we try to make them feel comfortable, tell them things that will make them feel comfortable when they get to the court, so that one helps.* (Prosc 5K, female legal prosecutor, Kumasi)

Preparation is where the prosecutor has conference with the victim to know their story and what their testimonies will be in court. They shape the stories of the victims and also help them to understand what the process will be.

> *Before you go to court you should be able to know what your client will say. Here you take out all irrelevant facts so as not to waste the court's time. When there are discrepancies, you instruct the investigator to go back and sort them out. You instruct on the docket by writing with a red pen—you instruct the*

investigator to visit those places mentioned, interview people around. (Prosc7A female police prosecutor, Accra)

Thus depending on the profession of the person, the police were viewed in a different way. Although the policemen saw themselves as having adequate knowledge and experience in preparing victims for the court, the lawyers thought that they were rather ill-equipped to handle cases of that nature.

Cross Fire of Accusations

This theme expounds on the cross-accusations between the lawyers and the police prosecutors. The lawyers speak about the inability of the police prosecutors to understand and operationalise the nuances in criminal jurisprudence and an inordinate desire to incarcerate offenders. The police on the other hand see the lawyers as bullies who intimidate them with their legal jargons in court. They also see the lawyers as the ones who delay the court process by seeking for adjournments frequently, holding up cases, and putting other technical stumbling blocks in the way of the legal process.

> *They delay because when the ermm lawyers come, because the lawyer probably may have only some few cases to handle and that is his source of income, he will not always be coming, he will not always be regular at court. So they'll frustrate you with a lot of ... with a lot of erherhermm how do we call it ... errmm postponements ... adjournments, a lot of adjournments.* (Prosc1K, male police prosecutor, Kumasi)

Therapeutic jurisprudence suggests that the process and its actors concur to produce either therapeutic or non-therapeutic consequences for persons who seek retributive justice. A context in which two main actors within the court process seem to think badly of each other is bound to cause problems for the victims. They are likely to be caught within this cross fire and may be harmed by it. Such harm is not within the purview of this chapter but is imaginable in these circumstances.

Going forward, the lawyers believe that the three-fold work of the police involving the arrest, investigation and prosecution of cases, should be broken. They believe that due to the likelihood of corruption, the role of prosecuting cases should be stripped from them.

> *I am one person who is against the police prosecuting any case. Ghana is … I don't know about other jurisdictions but I think Ghana is probably going to be one of the few countries if there're other countries where one institution will arrest you, will prosecute you will investigate you … one institution. Clearly the end result will still benefit that institution. Their purpose is to fight crime they make a report and they arrest you. An investigator who wants you in jail will investigate you, then a prosecutor who wants to just finish the work started by the investigator and the police institution that arrested you will come forth and just do what they want to do. So you have three people form one. You know. They arrest you, they investigate you and they conclude on that investigation that you are guilty and the final one the prosecutor will just come in and … I think that It's only fair that they are given a specific role.* (DfnseL6A, male lawyer, Accra)

This lawyer believes that the multiple roles played by the police may create an avenue for corruption and overbearance.

Discussion

This study brings to the fore the role of the police as prosecutors in the adjudication of cases, specifically child sexual abuse cases from the perspectives of the police prosecutors themselves and defense lawyers. The findings from this study show that the training the police prosecutors receive is inadequate with regard to court practice and especially in contrast with what is received by the defense lawyers. This calls for an enhanced training procedure and process for the police prosecutors. It has been suggested therefore that the police should be trained by the various faculties of law and proceed to professional law training at the Ghana School of Law. Alternatively, it has also been suggested that the police recruit persons who have obtained their training in law from the various faculties, equip them with police training and use them as prosecutors (Accountability Rule of law and Anti-Corruption Programme (ARAP), 2018). The same organisation has recommended the delineation of the prosecutorial role of the Ghana Police Service from its investigative role. These are laudable recommendations and would go a long way to help improve the functions of the police as prosecutors.

The lawyers displayed a negative perception about the police prosecutors in general. This was mostly in relation to their training. Pryce (2018) has noted a general mistrust for the police and their activities. Such ingrained perceptions about the police could account for why lawyers displayed such negative perceptions about the police in this situation. It is explained that negative perceptions about the police stem from their view that the police is not competent enough to carry out their duties (Oulmokhtar et al., 2011; Pryce, 2018).

Their perception may also be explained using the Social Identity theory which evaluates others in a more negative light than the self (Tajfel & Turner, 1979). Stereotypes are considered to be overgeneralised standardised image, opinions or concepts about a group or members of that group (Moore, 2006). They serve to furnish us with information about social groups and justify the differences a person is likely to identify among social groups (Crandall et al., 2011). Tajfel and Turner (1979) put forward that people evaluate others on the basis of "us" and "them". It has been shown that people enhance their self-esteem by evaluating their in-group in favorable terms compared with an out-group (Ruthland & Brown, 2001). The police as a socio-professional category has a controversial outlook among other social groups (Oulmokhtar et al., 2011). They have been considered as incompetent, inefficient, aggressive in their interventions, persecutory, full of prejudices and poorly educated (Oulmokhtar et al., 2011).

The lawyers also viewed the police as intimidating to the victims although the prosecutors believed that they were doing their best for the victims. The views of the lawyers are supported by views of victims who come into contact with the police in Ghana following domestic violence (Darkwah & Prah, 2016). The challenges they encounter have (in some cases) led to the reluctance of those who have ever suffered victimisation to report subsequent cases to the police (Boateng & Lee, 2014). To an extent this confirms Wexler's (1993, 2011) assertion that the law and how it is implemented could become anti-therapeutic though it is expected to be therapeutic. Thus, perceived police incompetence and coldness carries with it the inability to provide a therapeutic atmosphere for victims of sexual abuse.

Again, the Ghana Police Service in their 2018–2020 policy document entitled Transformation Agenda, make room for victims and witnesses (Ghana Police Service, 2018a). The policy seeks to ensure that the police are responsive to victims, treat them with care and give them timely information. It is important to note that the current study was conducted between 2017 and 2019 while this transformation agenda was in place; however, the challenges advanced by the participants seem to be the same ones that the policy seeks to address. It thus suggests a possible disconnect between the policy and the behavior of the prosecutors. It may well be that the resources, tools and training required to implement those policies are yet to be presented to the police to ensure the full implementation of the policy directives.

Limitations and Suggestions for Future Research

This study focused on two main professionals in the criminal delivery space for child sexual abuse in Ghanaian courts. It would have been interesting to gather the views of the victims themselves. This would have helped to ascertain whether the negative perceptions of the lawyers about the police and vice versa were supported by the victims themselves. Other studies should endeavor to address this gap. Future studies may also benefit from the use of quantitative tools such as surveys to assess the views of the general populace about police prosecutors. Also, methods such as observational and ethnographic studies could be employed in future studies for a comprehensive understanding of this topic.

Conclusion and Recommendations

This chapter sought to explore the views of police prosecutors and lawyers on the issue of the use of police prosecutors in defilement cases in Ghana. Three main themes were generated from the interviews with police prosecutors and lawyers. The findings suggest that the police prosecutors are low on training, lack basic skills required to defend their cases in court (though they themselves think otherwise) and are easily bamboozled by lawyers. There also seems to be a turf war between the police prosecutors and the lawyers. The primary function of the police is to resolve conflicts. Their additional mandate as prosecutors therefore seems to be an "encroachment" on the domain of lawyers.

Again, the prosecution of sexual abuse cases, and especially those involving children, is very technical requiring expertise and skill. Studies conducted in other countries show that such cases are less likely to be prosecuted successfully due to child-related or evidence-related issues (see: Back, Gustafsson, & Berterö, 2013; Castelli & Goodman, 2014; Christensen, Sharman, & Powell, 2015). Thus for the successful prosecution of such cases, a certain level of skill is required. However, practical and economic exigencies and the people's right to justice, provide that where there is a harm there ought to be a remedy. The Attorney General's department is short-staffed and cannot go to all the villages and towns where the police are available, thus the practical solution of using police prosecutors. The suggestions of ARAP that the police establish some collaboration with the legal training institutions, is therefore a welcome call.

It is helpful that currently, some police officers and police prosecutors are training as lawyers and so should be better equipped to handle the technical aspects of the cases that they handle. This is a start in the general metamorphoses of the police service. It is, however, unclear whether their number will be sufficient to address the needs of persons who need help at the lower courts where cases of child sexual abuse are prosecuted. One other suggestion that might help is the de-coupling of the prosecutorial role of the police from their investigative role. It has been suggested that the police create a separate office which would be named the National Prosecutions Service (NPS) with a clear mandate, access to the

Attorney General's department and with full control of all criminal prosecutions from the District to the Regional levels (Accountability Rule of law and Anti-Corruption Programme, 2018).

Considering these practical exigencies, it is the view of this chapter that the selection and training of police prosecutors should be stringent and consistent. Their practical training in law should be further enhanced to help deal with the harm likely to be suffered by the victims and their caregivers as a result of their deficiencies in legal training and practice. It would be helpful for them to appreciate that seeking justice is a psychological need for victims and so to the extent that police prosecutors are seen to be helpful, would go a long way to enhance the therapeutic experience of justice seeking.

References

Accountability Rule of law and Anti-Corruption Programme. (2018). *Improving professional standards in criminal prosecutions: A Report on the work of Police Prosecutors* (Issue January). Retrieved from http://arapghana.eu/sia/web/uploads/documents/ARAP_Functional_Analysis_Report_-_Police_Prosecutors_250118.pdf

Amoakohene, M. I. (2004). Violence against women in Ghana: A look at women's perceptions and review of policy and social responses. *Social Science and Medicine, 59*(11), 2373–2385. https://doi.org/10.1016/j.socscimed.2004.04.001

Antonsdóttir, H. F. (2018). 'A witness in my own case': Victim–Survivors' views on the criminal justice process in Iceland. *Feminist Legal Studies, 26*(3), 307–330. https://doi.org/10.1007/s10691-018-9386-z

Appiahene-Gyamfi, J. (2009). Crime and punishment in the Republic of Ghana: A country profile. *International Journal of Comparative and Applied Criminal Justice, 33*(2), 309–324. https://doi.org/10.1080/01924036.2009.9678810

Atuguba, R. (2008). The colonial state lives on: Reflections on the colonial character of Ghana's police. *African Agenda, 11*(2), 14–16. Retrieved from http://ugspace.ug.edu.gh/handle/123456789/415

Back, C., Gustafsson, P. A., & Berterö, C. (2013). Sexually abused children – Prosecutors' experiences of their participation in the legal process in Sweden. *Psychiatry, Psychology and Law, 20*(2), 273–283. https://doi.org/10.1080/13218719.2012.666017

Back, C., Gustafsson, P. A., Larsson, I. B., & Berterö, C. (2011). Managing the legal proceedings: An interpretative phenomenological analysis of sexually abused children's experience with the legal process. *Child Abuse and Neglect, 35*(1), 50–57. https://doi.org/10.1016/j.chiabu.2010.08.004

Boakye, K. E. (2009). Culture and nondisclosure of child sexual abuse in Ghana: A theoretical and empirical exploration. *Law & Social Inquiry, 34*(4), 951–979. https://doi.org/10.1111/j.1747-4469.2009.01170.x

Boateng, F. D., & Darko, I. (2016). *Our past: The effect of colonialism on policing in Ghana. International Journal of Police Service and Management.* https://doi.org/10.1177/1461355716638114

Boateng, F. D., & Lee, H. D. (2014). Willingness to report sexual offenses to the police in Ghana. *Victims and Offenders, 9*(4), 436–454. https://doi.org/1 0.1080/15564886.2014.907848

Braun, V., & Clarke, V. (2006). Using thematic analysis in psychology. *Qualitative Research in Psychology, 3*(2), 77–101. https://doi.org/10.119 1/1478088706qp063oa

Castelli, P., & Goodman, G. S. (2014). Children's perceived emotional behavior at disclosure and prosecutors' evaluations. *Child Abuse and Neglect, 38*(9), 1521–1532. https://doi.org/10.1016/j.chiabu.2014.02.010

Christensen, L. S., Sharman, S., & Powell, M. (2015). Professionals' views on child sexual abuse attrition rates. *Psychiatry, Psychology and Law, 22*(4), 542–558. https://doi.org/10.1080/13218719.2014.960036

Clarke, V., & Braun, V. (2017). Thematic analysis. *The Journal of Positive Psychology, 9760*, 1–2. https://doi.org/10.1080/17439760.2016.1262613

Crandall, C. S., Bahns, A. J., Warner, R., & Schaller, M. (2011). Stereotypes as justifications of prejudice. *Personality and Social Psychology Bulletin, 37*(11), 1488–1498. https://doi.org/10.1177/0146167211411723

Creswell, J. W. (2014). *Research design: Qualitative, quantitative and mixed methods approaches* (4th ed.). SAGE Publications.

Daly, K. (2014). Reconceptualizing sexual victimization and justice. In A. P. Vanfraechem & F. Hdahinda (Eds.), *Routledge international handbook of victimology* (pp. 378–395). Routledge. https://doi.org/10.4324/9780203094532

Daly, K., & Bouhours, B. (n.d.). *Rape and attrition in the legal process: A comparative analysis of five countries.* March 2009.

Daly, K., & Curtis-Fawley, S. (2006). Justice for victims of sexual assault: Court or conference. In K. Heimer & C. Kruttschnitt (Eds.), *Gender, offending, and victimization* (pp. 1–65). New York University Press.

Darkwah, A. K., & Prah, M. (2016). *Beyond domestic violence laws: Women's experiences and perceptions of protection services in Ghana (Regional evidence papers)*. CEGENSA.

Eastwood, C. (2003). The experiences of child compainants of sexual abuse in the criminal justice system. In *Trends and issues in crime and criminal justice* (Vol. 250).

Fusch, P. I., & Ness, L. R. (2015). Are we there yet? Data saturation in qualitative research. *Qualitative Report, 20*(9), 1408–1416. https://doi.org/10.46743/2160-3715/2015.2281

Ghana Police Service. (2018a). *Communication and Public education strategy 2018–2020.*

Ghana Police Service. (2018b). *Service Manual.*

Herman, J. L. (2005). Justice from the victim's perspective. *Violence Against Women, 11*(5), 571–602. https://doi.org/10.1177/1077801205274450

Kwakye-Nuako, C. O. (2018). *The psychosocial context of withdrawals and discharges in court cases involving child sexual abuse in Accra: A documentary study.* University of Ghana School of Social Science Conference.

Levitt, H. M., Bamberg, M., Creswell, J. W., Frost, D. M., Josselson, R., & Suárez-Orozco, C. (2018). Journal article reporting standards for qualitative primary, qualitative meta-analytic, and mixed methods research in psychology: The APA publications and communications board task force report. *American Psychologist, 73*(1), 26–46. https://doi.org/10.1037/amp0000151

Molyneux, E. M., Kennedy, N., Dano, A., & Mulambia, Y. (2013). Sexual abuse of children in low-income settings: time for action. *Paediatrics and International Child Health, 33*(4), 239–246. https://doi.org/10.1179/2046905513Y.0000000087

Moore, J. R. (2006). Shattering stereotypes: A lesson plan for improving student attitudes and behavior toward minority groups. *The Social Studies, 97*(1), 35–39. https://doi.org/10.3200/TSSS.97.1.35-39

Mulambia, Y., Miller, A. J., MacDonald, G., & Kennedy, N. (2018). Are one-stop centres an appropriate model to deliver services to sexually abused children in urban Malawi? *BMC Pediatrics, 18*(1), 1–7. https://doi.org/10.1186/s12887-018-1121-z

Musiwa, A. S. (2018). How has the presence of Zimbabwe's victim-friendly court and relevant child protection policy and legal frameworks affected the management of intrafamilial child sexual abuse in Zimbabwe? The case of Marondera district. *Journal of Interpersonal Violence, 33*(11), 1748–1777. https://doi.org/10.1177/0886260517752154

Oulmokhtar, D., Krauth-Gruber, S., Alexopoulos, T., & Drozda-Senkowska, E. (2011). Police officers' stereotype content and its evolution over two decades: From "neither nice nor able" to "still not nice but able." *International Review of Social Psychology, 24*(3), 87–100. https://www.researchgate.net/publication/288388445_Police_officers'_stereotype_content_and_its_evolution_over_two_decades_From_neither_nice_nor_able_to_still_not_nice_but_able

Pokoo-Aikins, J. B. (1998). The Ghana police service: Changes after colonization. *The Police Journal: Theory, Practice and Principles, 71*(2), 176–178. https://doi.org/10.1177/0032258x9807100213

Pryce, D. K. (2018). Ghanaian immigrants' differential trust in and obligation to obey the US police and Ghana police: Findings from a qualitative study. *African Identities, 16*(4), 396–411. https://doi.org/10.1080/1472584 3.2018.1467751

Pryce, D. K., Johnson, D., & Maguire, E. R. (2016). Procedural justice, obligation to obey, and cooperation with procedural justice. *Criminal Justice and Behavior, 20*(10), 1–23. https://doi.org/10.1177/0093854816680225

Rutland, A., & Brown, R. (2001). Stereotypes as justifications for prior intergroup discrimination: Studies of Scottish national stereotyping. *European Journal of Social Psychology, 31*(2), 127–141. https://doi.org/10.1002/ejsp.25

Smith, J. A., & Osborn, M. (2008). Interpretative Phenomenological Analysis. In J. A. Smith (Ed.), *Qualitative Psychology: A practical guide to research methods* (pp. 53–80). SAGE Publications. http://med-fom-familymed-research.sites.olt.ubc.ca/files/2012/03/IPA_Smith_Osborne21632.pdf

Spohn, C. C., & Holleran, D. (2001). Prosecuting sexual assault: A comparison of charging decisions in sexual assault cases involving strangers, acquaintances, and intimate partners. *Justice Quarterly, 18*(3), 651–688. https://doi.org/10.1080/07418820100095051

Tajfel, H., & Turner, J. (1979). *An integrative theory of intergroup conflict. In The social psychology of intergroup relations* (pp. 33–47). Brooks Cole.

Tankebe, J. (2008a). Colonialism, legitimation, and policing in Ghana. *International Journal of Law, Crime and Justice, 36*, 67–84. https://doi.org/10.1016/j.ijlcj.2007.12.003

Tankebe, J. (2008b). Police effectiveness and police trustworthiness in Ghana: An empirical appraisal. *Criminology and Criminal Justice, 8*(2), 185–202. https://doi.org/10.1177/1748895808088994

Tankebe, J. (2009). Public cooperation with the police in ghana: Does procedural fairness matter? *Criminology, 47*(4), 1265–1293. https://doi.org/10.1111/j.1745-9125.2009.00175.x

Tyler, T. R. (2006). Psychological perspectives on legitimacy and legitimation. *Annual Review of Psychology, 57*(1), 375–400. https://doi.org/10.1146/annurev.psych.57.102904.190038

Wexler, D. B. (1993). Therapeutic jurisprudence and the criminal courts. *William & Mary Law Review, 35*(1), 279. Retrieved from https://www.researchgate.net/publication/248074727_Therapeutic_Jurisprudence_and_the_Criminal_Courts

Wexler, D. B. (2011). From theory to practice and back again in therapeutic jurisprudence: Now comes the hard part. *Monash University Law Review, 37*(1), 33–42. Retrieved from http://search.ebscohost.com/login.aspx?direct=true&db=a9h&AN=86195601&site=ehost-live&scope=site

Wrigley-Asante, C., Owusu, G., Oteng-Ababio, M., & Owusu, A. Y. (2016). Poverty and crime: Uncovering the hidden face of sexual crimes in urban low-income communities in Ghana. *Ghana Journal of Geography, 8*(81), 32–50.

Statutes Referred To

Ghana Police Service Act, 1970 (Act 350).
Legal Professions Act, 1960 (Act 32).

10

Mental Health of Prison Inmates in the Nigerian Criminal Justice System

Chiedu Eseadi

Introduction

The increase in prisoner populations worldwide and the call for the compassionate care of prisoners with mental illnesses necessitate an appraisal of correctional mental health services. Conducting such an assessment will help foster prisoners' rights, community reintegration and utilitarian safety and the development of correctional mental health legislation that is globally comparable (Olagunju et al., 2018). Several studies have shown that prison inmates have a high rate of mental illness (Assadi et al., 2006; Birmingham, Mason, & Grubin, 1996; Fatoye, Fatoye, Oyebanji, & Ogunro, 2006; Fazel & Danesh, 2002). Watson, Stimpson, and Hostick (2004) identified a range of health problems common among prisoners, including mental health concerns, substance abuse disorders and communicable diseases. Many of these health problems have been

C. Eseadi (✉)
Department of Educational Foundations, University of Nigeria,
Nsukka, Nigeria
e-mail: chiedu.eseadi@unn.edu.ng

© The Author(s), under exclusive license to Springer Nature Switzerland AG 2021
H. C. O. Chan, S. Adjorlolo (eds.), *Crime, Mental Health and the Criminal Justice System in Africa*, https://doi.org/10.1007/978-3-030-71024-8_10

213

confirmed in Nigerian prisons (Adesanya, Ohaeri, Ogunlesi, Adamson, & Odejide, 1997; Agbahowe, Ohaeri, Ogunlesi, & Osahon, 1998). Agbahowe et al. (1998) found a prevalence rate of 83.7% for psychiatric morbidity amongst prison inmates in Nigeria. Fatoye et al. (2006) found in their Nigerian prison study prevalence rates of 85.3% and 87.8% for depression and general psychiatric morbidity, respectively.

The high prevalence rates of psychiatric morbidity found in many prison studies indicate that prisoner populations are vulnerable to mental illness. This correlation could be attributed to many factors. Incarceration results in the loss of personal freedoms and opportunities for social support, interpersonal relationships, employment, social status and social roles (Butler & Allnutt, 2003). Adetula, Fatusin, and Adetula (2010) noted that life in Nigerian prisons is generally overly regimented, and all activities are stringently controlled. These circumstances regularly leave the prisoners mentally brutalised and with broken spirits.

The prison environment is often characterised by uncertainty, overcrowding, institutionalised regimens and a lack of recreational activities, all of which can be stressful. Prisoners are a marginalised population, and due to their incarceration, they may be denied privileges and benefits that others in society may enjoy. They are less likely to have their mental health needs recognised or treated (Birmingham et al., 1996). The assumed norm is that the majority of prison inmates are convicted offenders, and the minority are remanded inmates waiting to plead their cases. However, the past three decades in Nigeria have witnessed an inverted trend in the ratio of convicted prisoners to people awaiting trials (Abdulmalik, Adedokun, & Baiyewu, 2014). Inmates who are awaiting trial may feel hopeless and uncertain of their fate. Their circumstances can afflict them with severe psychological stress and result in deterioration of their mental health. The general condition of the health care delivery system in Nigeria further jeopardises prisoners' mental health.

Many inmates' mental health problems may be under-diagnosed in Nigeria. Several studies have confirmed the vulnerability and plausibility of prisoners with mental health problems becoming problematic for correctional staff and other inmates (Hilton & Simmons, 2001; Hoptman, Yates, Patalinjug, Wack, & Convit, 1999). However, empirical studies are lacking in the Nigerian context. According to Fazel and Danesh (2002), about 99% of available data from prison surveys are derived from Western populations. This rate highlights the need for more forensic psychiatric research in non-Western populations, especially Nigeria. Studies on mental health issues in Nigerian prisons can provide empirical evidence that can guide feasible prison reform.

An appraisal of the mental health policy in Nigeria by Odebiyi (1998) revealed the generally poor social attitude of the government and other stakeholders towards the mentally ill. Those in prisons are in an even worse situation as they are excluded from national policy. Mental health policies in Nigeria have not met the challenges of caring for the mentally ill in the populace, let alone the prison population.

Reports have shown that psychiatric morbidity in Nigerian prisons is more prevalent in the southern and western parts of Nigeria than in the north (Agbahowe et al., 1998; Aishatu, Armiya, Obembe, Moses, & Tolulope, 2013). The few studies of psychiatric morbidity among Nigerian prison inmates have mostly been conducted in the south and the west (Osasona & Koleoso, 2015). Several factors account for the mental health issues of the Nigerian prisoner population, including substance use disorders (Watson et al., 2004). The increasing use of substances by Nigeria prisoners may account for the high prevalence of mental health problems (Adesanya et al., 1997).

Incarceration patterns and prison facilities have been reported to handicap mental health services among inmates in Nigeria. Cases of maladjustment, mental disorder and post-release relapse among inmates have been traced to prison life and lock-up patterns. In most Nigerian remanded and convicted populations, the younger and older inmates are not separated into different cells, despite the standard minimum rules for imprisonment, which stipulate that prisoners should be locked up based on their demographics. Nonetheless, the observable synergistic efforts of multidisciplinary staff members and pre-existing intra-agency leaders towards collaboration in combating inmates' psychosocial and mental health needs are reducing barriers to providing mental health services (Atilola et al., 2017).

Current efforts to improve prisoners' mental health services and facilities in Nigerian prisons may prove superficial in the absence of a total overhaul of the criminal justice system. The current judicial psychological orientation relies on imprisonment as a disposal method for many offences. The strategic position of neuropsychiatric hospitals across the country offers an opportunity to effectively implement a task-shifting method for improving mental health service in prisons. These hospitals can help train, supervise and provide professional care along the referral pathway for mental health care. Several hospitals already run community outreach programmes that share human and material resources.

This book chapter discusses the mental health of prison inmates in the Nigerian criminal justice system. The subsequent sections give an overview of policies, studies and facilitators and barriers to addressing prisoner mental health in Nigeria. The chapter concludes with a discussion of practical implications.

Policies Addressing Prisoner Mental Health in Nigeria

Management of the Nigeria Correctional Service is based on the Nigeria Prison Act of 1972. Several researchers (Abdulmalik et al., 2019; Onyemelukwe, 2016; Sanni & Adebayo, 2014; Ugochukwu et al., 2020; Westbrook, 2011) have explored this body of principles to understand its strengths and weaknesses and offer recommendations. Several flaws in the Prison Act have led to a failure to address the antisocial behaviour of inmates. The Prison Act only addresses the surface issues of prisoners' psychological welfare. Section 8 discusses the removal and relocation of sick prisoners to the hospital. Regulation 22 refers to prisoners' diet, Regulation 25 refers to prisoners' bedding, and Regulation 28 addresses prisoners' cleanliness. No section of the Prison Act satisfactorily addresses the vital issues of reformation, rehabilitation and reorientation. The Prison Act is inadequate, as it neither serves the purpose of imprisonment nor fulfils the provision outlined in the 1999 constitution (Omaka, 2014).

The Nigerian prison system stresses the importance of custody over rehabilitation. It treats imprisonment as the implementation of retributive sanctions rather than complementing sentences with rehabilitation. To address this issue, the Sixth National Assembly amended the 1972

Prison Act to amend the errors; however, the amendment only peripherally focused on the rehabilitation, reformation and reorientation of inmates, and it did not acknowledge or incorporate the crucial role of mental health care (Onyekachi, 2016). This policy is not backed by the force of law. It is not statutory, which means it is subject to change.

The 2019 Nigerian Correctional Service Act revoked the Prison Act Cap. P29, Laws of the Federation of Nigeria, 2004, and addresses issues that were not considered under the revoked act. It presents clear rules and obligations for the Nigerian Correctional Service and outlines inmates' rights. Section 24 provides for inmates' mental health and related issues (Nigerian Correctional Service Act, 2019). If it appears to the superintendent that an inmate who is undergoing imprisonment or sentence of death is of unsound mind, she/he shall report the matter to the state controller of correctional services, who shall take further actions as stipulated in subsequent subsections of Sect. 24. The state controller may contact the Mental Health Review Board for a clinical assessment of the situation. The Mental Health Review Board is charged with reviewing and certifying conditions as clinically valid. The board must consist of a psychiatrist to act as the head of the board, a representative of federal or state psychiatric hospitals in the state or geopolitical zone, a clinical psychologist, a social worker and medical personnel from the custodial centre.

According to the Federal Ministry of Health (2013), people with severe mental disorders should be treated in a therapeutic rather than punitive environment. Prisoners with psychosis should be moved to the hospital. Less severe disorders are frequent among prisoners, and there should be synergy between health teams and prison staff to help correctional officers recognise mental disorders, conditions for referral to the hospital and the management of depression and suicidal risk in prison settings. The policy approach between the health sector and prisons staff in Nigeria seeks to maintain inter-sectoral liaisons to:

1. Construct joint plans to improve the conditions of people with mental health problems in prisons;
2. Develop good practices for the management of people with mental illness;
3. Ensure that prisons provide follow-up care;

4. Arrange training sessions for prison health care staff, ensure that mental health professionals (at least a psychiatric nurse) are available in each prison and maintain resources to attend to the medical care needs of the prison population;
5. Guarantee obedience to the policy concerning the transfer of people with mental illnesses to hospital facilities;
6. Ensure that psychiatrists are embedded in the prison health care system; and
7. Ensure that prison staff members recognise the human rights of mentally ill prisoners.

Research on Prisoner Mental Health in Nigeria

The issue of mental health deterioration in Nigerian prisons is not new. Several scholars have investigated the matter, using quantitative and qualitative methods to reveal prevalence rates, problems and prospects for change. Agboola, Babalola, and Udofia (2017) explored psychopathology among offenders in a Nigerian prison. The authors reported that most of the inmates were young offenders (62.8%), 57.4% scored 5 or above on the General Health Questionnaire, and 32.8% had depression. Their study found a high prevalence rate of psychopathology among prison inmates in Nigeria.

Abdulmalik et al. (2014) enquired into the prevalence and correlates of mental health problems among remanded inmates in a prison facility in Ibadan, Nigeria. Their study reported that 56.6% of this population had a mental illness. Depression was the most common condition (20.8%), followed by alcohol dependence (20.6%), substance dependence (20.1%), suicidality (19.8%) and antisocial personality disorder (18%).

Seeking to understand the effects of a group-focused cognitive-behavioural coaching programme on depressive symptoms, Eseadi, Obidoa, Ogbuabor, and Ikechukwu-Ilomuanya (2018) investigated a sample of 30 inmates from Nsukka prisons in Enugu, Nigeria, and found that the programme significantly reduced the depressive symptoms of inmates in the treatment group as against those in the control group.

Barkindo and Bryans (2016) reviewed the development of a basic prison-based de-radicalisation programme that took a cognitive restructuring approach to rehabilitate inmates in Nigeria. The study reported that the staff's basic awareness of the de-radicalisation programme content and participant management was minimal. Their risk assessment was rudimentary and focused only on the threat of escapes. There were no offending behaviour programmes, and specialist staff were in short supply and had no intervention training. Financial and physical resources were limited.

Olagunju et al. (2018) investigated mental health services in two urban Nigerian prisons to understand and prescribe intervention measures to meet inmates' psychological needs. The study was conducted among 179 inmates and revealed that schizophrenia (49.3%) was the most common clinical diagnosis, followed by mood disorders (29.6%). Approximately half of the participants (46.5%) used psychoactive substances. About one-fifth of the participants showed violent and/or dangerous tendencies. Most of the participants (88.4%) presented with an initial mental illness episode, and 14% had a previous correctional history.

Abiama and Etowa (2013) investigated 80 Calabar prison inmates, 70 of whom were male. They found that long-term imprisonment and solitary confinement negatively impacted the mental health of prison inmates.

Prisoner Mental Health Services in Nigeria: Opportunities and Hindrances

Opportunities

Implementation of Necessary Legislation

There are opportunities to strengthen prisoner mental health services in Nigeria. The revised National Mental Health Policy of 2013 has been officially adopted by the federal government. If this mental health bill is passed into law, it will provide another opportunity. The Federal Ministry of Health (FMOH) in 2008 established the National Mental Health Action Committee (NMHAC) to serve as a policy think tank and provide strategic guidance and supervision for the mental health agenda in prison and the general population. The NMHAC and the Mental Health Desk Officer should consider it a priority to guarantee the effective incorporation of mental health policies for inmates into successive revisions of the National Health Sector Strategic Development Plan.

Professional Training and Recruitment of Staff

Staffing opportunities require acknowledging the task-shifting method as effective in improving the mental health care services in Nigerian prisons. Mental health should be integrated into primary care, as advocated in the National Mental Health Policy. The Nigerian prison system should accept and apply the WHO's Mental Health Gap Action Programme-Intervention Guide (MHGAP-IG) to train non-specialist prison health care staff and wardens to spot mental health issues and intervene accordingly. The MHGAP-IG has been contextualised and modified for Nigeria according to Abdulmalik et al. (2013). The National Primary Health Care Development Agency (NPHCDA) is presently exploring the development of a curriculum for primary health care workers. Training programmes based on the MHGAP-IG have benefits, but facility managers tend to prefer a flexible training regimen and more staff recruitment. A Mental Health Desk Officer has been appointed at the level of the Federal Ministry of Health. However, the position has yet to be created at the regional and state levels, which would be required for grassroots implementation at prisons and satellite facilities. The revised Mental Health Policy advocates for a Mental Health Programme to be established and headed by a deputy director at a minimum.

Inter-Sectoral Collaboration

Many opportunities can be brought to fruition by national-level collaborations between the FMOH, relevant ministries, such as that of information, professional bodies, such as the Association of Psychiatrists in Nigeria and the Nigerian Medical Association, and governmental agencies, such as the NPHCDA. The revised Mental Health Policy outlines the role of relevant stakeholders and the necessity of inter-sectoral collaboration. Coordinated efforts could result in more productive inter-sectoral collaboration if well implemented.

Institution of Welfare Strategies

Community-based insurance schemes are meant to lessen the weight of chronic medical conditions, including some of the mental health issues of inmates, by improving financial access to care. Several states have social welfare intervention packages for prisoners. Advocacy and public health engagement activities in a few locations could be reinforced and enhanced to achieve better visibility and more impact. Finally, ethical protection protocols are available for the protection of the rights of individuals with mental illness, and they apply to inmates. Informed consent is required for participation in research, and ethical evaluation boards must review and approve research protocols.

Implementation of Monitoring and Evaluation Activities

There is no routine data collection for mental health conditions in the Nigerian health care system. However, the country has participated in major epidemiological studies, such as the WHO World Mental Health Surveys (Gureje, Lasebikan, Kola, & Makanjuola, 2006) and country reports based on the WHO Assessment Instrument for Mental Health Systems (WHO-AIMS, 2006). The revised Mental Health Policy recommends the formation of a monitoring and evaluation unit to be chaired by a deputy director.

Threats

Lack of Mental Health Professionals

The insufficient number of mental health professionals poses a significant threat to the effective delivery of services to the Nigerian prison population. For every 100,000 individuals in Nigeria, there are 0.19 nurses, 0.02 psychologists, 0.06 psychiatrists and 0.06 other health workers (WHO, 2011). The training of primary health care workers does not ensure the skill development necessary for recognising and assisting with mental health conditions.

Lack of Formal Collaborative Networks and Partnerships

The Nigerian Correctional Service relies on a centralised, hierarchical planning and management system. The lack of formal collaborative networks and partnerships with other sectors, such as health, social welfare, education and justice ministries, is a major concern. The involvement with mental health service users and caregivers is limited. Service users, such as prisoners, are not involved in mental health care service delivery. Their role is restricted to the clinical consultation process rather than offering input on the planning and execution of services. However, service user involvement is possible in the planning, execution and delivery of mental health services is possible and would benefit mental health services in the correctional service system.

Stigma, Discrimination and Poor Awareness

Pervasive stigma and discrimination against mentally unwell inmates pose significant threats and continue the low priority of addressing mental health issues in policymaking. Many people are aware of advocacy and public health crusades for health programmes addressing HIV and malaria, but few are aware of campaigns for prisoner mental health conditions.

Financial Constraints

The National Health Insurance Scheme reaches only 5% of the population and offers minimal coverage for mental health conditions. Most health care services, including those to address inmates' mental health, are only accessible via out-of-pocket payments. Interventions such as conditional cash transfer inducements, which exist for reproductive health programmes, are not available for mental health conditions. Poor funding is further reflected in the absence of a designated budget for prisoner mental health and the ad hoc basis for mental health spending from the general purse of non-communicable diseases. This lack of funding reduces the chances of employing enough health care personnel to manage mental health issues in prisons.

Poor Data Assessment and Inventory Systems

Inadequate data collection results in limited guidance for mental health service planning in Nigerian prisons. The lack of a robust, routine data collection paradigm for appraising the mental health conditions of inmates in the Nigerian health care system simply means that planning and decision-making for prisoner mental health services may not be evidence-based. Donor-funded programmes for communicable diseases, such as HIV/AIDS, malaria and tuberculosis, seem to be prioritised over mental health conditions in terms of the provision of regular reporting systems and data collection tools.

Implications for Practice

Comprehensive prison reform should involve all stakeholders, including prisoners. It should focus on considerable yet timely changes in promoting prison health and ensuring that Nigerian prisons are humane. The legal rights of the accused need to be reinterpreted. The undue delay and confinement of people awaiting trial is resulting in overcrowding in Nigerian prisons and must be curtailed. The employment of more judges, even on a part-time basis, could quicken the delivery of judgements. Prison can be made more humane without undercutting the public's interests. Reforms can help inmates and smooth their reintegration into society. The National Economic Empowerment and Development Strategy initiated by the Obasanjo administration could be extended to those in prisons, especially women and youths. The lives of many prisoners from low economic backgrounds may be better after exiting prison. However, introducing such a programme will entail a reorientation of the prison staff from the current modus operandi to new norms. More qualified employees will need to be recruited into the Nigerian Correctional Service health care units to maintain social order and professionalism. This step will impact the quality of staff members and inmates' outcomes. In the final evaluation, alternatives to prison, such as community service and parole systems, may be helpful than incarceration. These alternative measures, when properly designed and applied within the sociocultural context of Nigeria, may be more cost-effective, efficient and higher functioning than the present system.

Conclusion

Inmates' severe, persistent mental issues and psychoactive substance consumption are the main sources of mental health service utilisation in Nigerian prisons. In consonance with global best practices, there is a need for risk assessment involving the combined use of clinical and actuarial evaluation with validated tools. Multifaceted intervention strategies are needed to tackle the unmet mental needs of prisoners. The prison psychiatric unit needs to become more service friendly. The provision of long-term care facilities outside prison walls should be considered in addition to policies that are favourable to mentally ill offenders. The routine screening of prisoners is necessary for the early detection of mental illness and the development of prison health care services. Empirical evidence should guide indicators for evaluating the mental health system in Nigeria, the development of prison infrastructure, the delivery of capacity building exercises for policymakers, service users and researchers. Taking such steps will require expertise that may not be readily available or immediately become routine practice, but they should shape the goals of long-term health system planning in Nigeria.

References

Abdulmalik, J., Kola, L., Fadahunsi, W., Adebayo, K., Yasamy, M. T., Musa, E., et al. (2013). Country contextualization of the mental health gap action programme intervention guide: A case study from Nigeria. *PLoS Medicine, 10*(8), e1001501. https://doi.org/10.1371/journal.pmed.1001501

Abdulmalik, J., Olayiwola, S., Docrat, S., Lund, C., Chisholm, D., & Gureje, O. (2019). Sustainable financing mechanisms for strengthening mental health systems in Nigeria. *International Journal of Mental Health Systems, 13*(1), 38. https://doi.org/10.1186/s13033-019-0293-8

Abdulmalik, J. O., Adedokun, B. O., & Baiyewu, O. O. (2014). Prevalence and correlates of mental health problems among awaiting trial inmates in a Prison facility in Ibadan, Nigeria. *African Journal of Medicine and Medical Sciences, 43*(Suppl 1), 193. Retrieved from https://pubmed.ncbi.nlm.nih.gov/26689928/

Abiama, E. E., & Etowa, P. E. (2013). The impact of long-term incarceration and solitary confinement on the mental health of prison inmates in Nigeria. *Nigerian Journal of Psychological Research, 9.* Retrieved from https://www.semanticscholar.org/paper/THE-IMPACT-OF-LONG-TERM-INCARCERATION-AND-SOLITARY-Abiama-Etowa/ae86dd55601c8c612a244b7ad781f7d2aa1e7d2b

Adesanya, A., Ohaeri, J. U., Ogunlesi, A. O., Adamson, T. A., & Odejide, O. A. (1997). Psychoactive substance abuse among inmates of a Nigerian prison population. *Drug and Alcohol Dependence, 47*(1), 39–44. https://doi.org/10.1016/s0376-8716(97)00067-7

Adetula, A., Fatusin, A. F., & Adetula, G. A. (2010). The prison subsystem culture: Its attitudinal effects on operatives, convicts and the free society. *IFE PsychologIA: An International Journal, 18*(1), 189–205. https://doi.org/10.4314/ifep.v18i1.51662

Agbahowe, S. A., Ohaeri, J. U., Ogunlesi, A. O., & Osahon, R. (1998). Prevalence of psychiatric morbidity among convicted inmates in a Nigerian prison community. *East African Medical Journal, 75*(1), 19–26. Retrieved from https://pubmed.ncbi.nlm.nih.gov/9604530/

Agboola, A., Babalola, E., & Udofia, O. (2017). Psychopathology among offenders in a Nigeria prison. *International Journal of Clinical Psychiatry, 5*(1), 10–15. https://doi.org/10.5923/j.ijcp.20170501.02

Aishatu, Y., Armiya, U., Obembe, A., Moses, D. A., & Tolulope, O. A. (2013). Prevalence of psychiatric morbidity among inmates in Jos maximum security prison. *Open Journal of Psychiatry, 3*(1), 12–17. https://doi.org/10.4236/ojpsych.2013.31003

Assadi, S. M., Noroozian, M., Pakravannejad, M., Yahyazadeh, O., Aghayan, S., Shariat, S. V., et al. (2006). Psychiatric morbidity among sentenced prisoners: Prevalence study in Iran. *The British Journal of Psychiatry, 188*(2), 159–164. https://doi.org/10.1192/bjp.188.2.159

Atilola, O., Ola, B., Abiri, G., Sahid-Adebambo, M., Odukoya, O., Adewuya, A., et al. (2017). Status of mental-health services for adolescents with psychiatric morbidity in youth correctional institutions in Lagos. *Journal of Child & Adolescent Mental Health, 29*(1), 63–83. https://doi.org/10.2989/17280583.2017.1321550

Barkindo, A., & Bryans, S. (2016). De-radicalising prisoners in Nigeria: Developing a basic prison based de-radicalisation programme. *Journal for Deradiclization, 7.* Retrieved from https://journals.sfu.ca/jd/index.php/jd/article/view/56

Birmingham, L., Mason, D., & Grubin, D. (1996). Prevalence of mental disorder in remand prisoners: Consecutive case study. *BMJ, 313*(7071), 1521–1524. https://doi.org/10.1136/bmj.313.7071.1521

Butler, T., & Allnutt, S. (2003). *Mental illness among New South Wales prisoners.* Sydney, NSW: Corrections Health Service.

Eseadi, C., Obidoa, M. A., Ogbuabor, S. E., & Ikechukwu-Ilomuanya, A. B. (2018). Effects of group-focused cognitive-behavioral coaching program on depressive symptoms in a sample of inmates in a Nigerian prison. *International Journal of Offender Therapy and Comparative Criminology, 62*(6), 1589–1602. https://doi.org/10.1177/0306624x16687046

Fatoye, F. O., Fatoye, G. K., Oyebanji, A. O., & Ogunro, A. S. (2006). Psychological characteristics as correlates of emotional burden in incarcerated offenders in Nigeria. *East African Medical Journal, 83*(10), 545–552. https://doi.org/10.4314/eamj.v83i10.9467

Fazel, S., & Danesh, J. (2002). Serious mental disorder in 23 000 prisoners: A systematic review of 62 surveys. *The Lancet, 359*(9306), 545–550. https://doi.org/10.1016/s0140-6736(02)07740-1

Federal Ministry of Health. (2013). *National Policy for Mental Health Services Delivery Nigeria*. Abuja, Nigeria: Federal Ministry of Health. Retrieved from http://cheld.org/wp-content/uploads/2015/02/national_policy_for_mental_health_service_delivery__2013_.pdf

Gureje, O., Lasebikan, V. O., Kola, L., & Makanjuola, V. A. (2006). Lifetime and 12-month prevalence of mental disorders in the Nigerian Survey of Mental Health and Well-Being. *The British Journal of Psychiatry, 188*(5), 465–471. https://doi.org/10.1192/bjp.188.5.465

Hilton, N. Z., & Simmons, J. L. (2001). The influence of actuarial risk assessment in clinical judgments and tribunal decisions about mentally disordered offenders in maximum security. *Law and Human Behavior, 25*(4), 393–408. https://doi.org/10.1023/a:1010607719239

Hoptman, M. J., Yates, K. F., Patalinjug, M. B., Wack, R. C., & Convit, A. (1999). Clinical prediction of assaultive behavior among male psychiatric patients at a maximum-security forensic facility. *Psychiatric Services, 50*(11), 1461–1466. https://doi.org/10.1176/ps.50.11.1461

Nigerian Correctional Service Act, § 24. (2019). Retrieved from https://placng.org/wp/wpcontent/uploads/2019/08/Nigerian-Correctional-Service-Act-2019.pdf

Odebiyi, A. (1998). *Appraisal of the mental health care policy in Nigeria* (Vol. 4). Development Policy Centre.

Olagunju, A. T., Oluwaniyi, S. O., Fadipe, B., Ogunnubi, O. P., Oni, O. D., Aina, O. F., et al. (2018). Mental health services in Nigerian prisons: Lessons from a four-year review and the literature. *International Journal of Law and Psychiatry, 58*, 79–86. https://doi.org/10.1016/j.ijlp.2018.03.004

Omaka, A. C. (2014). Decongesting prisons in Nigeria: The EBSU Law Clinic model. *International Journal of Clinical Legal Education, 20*(2), 533. https://doi.org/10.19164/ijcle.v20i2.21

Onyekachi, J. (2016). Problems and prospects of administration of Nigerian prison: Need for proper rehabilitation of the inmates in Nigeria prisons. *Journal of Tourism & Hospitality, 5*(4), 1–14. https://doi.org/10.4172/2167-0269.1000228

Onyemelukwe, C. (2016). Stigma and mental health in Nigeria: Some suggestions for law reform. *Journal of Law, Policy and Globalization, 55*, 63–68. Retrieved from https://core.ac.uk/download/pdf/234650863.pdf

Osasona, S. O., & Koleoso, O. N. (2015). Prevalence and correlates of depression and anxiety disorder in a sample of inmates in a Nigerian prison. *The*

International Journal of Psychiatry in Medicine, 50(2), 203–218. https://doi.org/10.1177/0091217415605038

Sanni, A. A., & Adebayo, F. O. (2014). Nigerian Mental Health Act 2013 assessment: A policy towards modern international standards. *American Academic & Scholarly Research Journal, 6*(1), 27. Retrieved from https://www.semanticscholar.org/paper/Nigerian-Mental-Health-Act-2013-Assessment%3A-A-Sanni-Adebayo/0c1003435722808207caad738 06097dbb5f16b2b

Ugochukwu, O., Mbaezue, N., Lawal, S. A., Azubogu, C., Sheikh, T. L., & Vallières, F. (2020). The time is now: Reforming Nigeria's outdated mental health laws. *The Lancet Global Health, 8*(8), e989–e990. https://doi.org/10.1016/s2214-109x(20)30302-8

Watson, R., Stimpson, A., & Hostick, T. (2004). Prison health care: A review of the literature. *International Journal of Nursing Studies, 41*(2), 119–128. https://doi.org/10.1016/s0020-7489(03)00128-7

Westbrook, A. H. (2011). Mental health legislation and involuntary commitment in Nigeria: A call for reform. *Washington University Global Studies Law Review, 10*, 397. Retrieved from https://openscholarship.wustl.edu/cgi/viewcontent.cgi?article=1022&context=law_globalstudies

WHO. (2011). Country profile of Nigeria. In *Mental health atlas of the WHO* (pp. 348–351). WHO.

WHO-AIMS. (2006). *World Health Organization assessment instrument for mental health systems-WHO-AIMS version 2.2*. World Health Organization.

Part II

The Police, Correctional and Legal System

11

The Experiences of People Who Use Drugs and Their Encounters with the Police in Ghana

Feikoab Parimah, Charlotte Omane Kwakye-Nuako, Maria-Goretti Ane, Timothy Pritchard Debrah, Mary Eyram Ashinyo, and Samuel Cudjoe Hanu

Introduction

Drug use is prevalent in most societies around the world. Problematic drug use refers to pharmacologically related self-destructive behaviour (United Nations Office on Drugs and Crime, 2010). The world drug

F. Parimah (✉)
Basic Research, Advocacy and Initiative Networks, Kwabenya, Accra, Ghana

Department of Psychology, University of Western Cape, Cape Town, South Africa

C. O. Kwakye-Nuako
Department of Forensic Science, University of Cape Coast, Cape Coast, Ghana

M.-G. Ane
International Drug Policy Consortium, Accra, Ghana

report indicated that in 2014, 250 million people between 15 and 54 years of age used at least one drug (UNODC, 2016), of whom 29 million were problematic drug users who required treatment. In 2013, 37,800 illicit drug-related deaths were recorded in Africa (UNODC, 2015).

Studies on problematic drug use have been conducted in several African countries, including Ghana. Onifade et al. (2011) showed the types, spread and characteristics of drug treatment centres in Nigeria and noted that 50% of such centres in Southwestern Nigeria perform internal and external assessments of treatment processes and outcomes. In Ghana, marijuana, cocaine and heroin are the most abused drugs (Affinnih, 1999). Agbakpe, Kwakye-Nuako, Bruce, and Bekoe (2011) added that although the rate of alcohol dependence is unknown, alcohol is considered the most abused substance in the Ghanaian population. Some drug users become problematic drug users and patronise the services of drug rehabilitation centres in Ghana. In exploring the factors that account for relapse among problematic drug users at some drug rehabilitation centres in Ghana, Appiah, Danquah, Nyarko, Ofori-Atta, and Aziato (2017) found that religio-cultural and familial factors, a sense of loss, peer influence and treatment-based issues initiated and maintained the cycle of relapse.

Psychosocial Effects of Drug Use

Drug use affects users' lives in different ways. Apart from the development of a criminal lifestyle, which brings individuals into conflict with

T. P. Debrah
School of Nursing and Midwifery, University of Cape Coast, Cape Coast, Ghana

M. E. Ashinyo
Department of Quality Assurance, Ghana Health Service Headquarters Ministries, Accra, Ghana

S. C. Hanu
Accra Psychiatric Hospital, Accra, Ghana

the law, several ripple effects can result from problematic drug use. Teesson et al. (2015) noted that people who use drugs (PWUDs) face challenges such as unemployment, familial and social problems and legal issues. Drug use hinders the realisation of accomplishments and personal health and worsens the quality of life of the family members of abusers (Choate, 2015; Wu, 2010). The negative effects inhibit the proper functioning of society.

The use of psychoactive substances produces psychological effects that can be 'positive' to the drug user or detrimental to their mental health. Drug users are often enticed to continue using drugs due to the euphoria that comes with use (Marlatt & VandenBos, 1997). However, drug use can result in mental health problems. The association between marijuana use and the psychosis spectrum operates on a continuum including threshold delusions, hallucinations, odd or unusual thoughts, and perceptual illusions (Gage, Hickman, & Zammit, 2016; Moore et al., 2007; Van Os, Linscott, Myin-Germeys, Delespaul, & Krabbendam, 2009). Moss, Chen, and Yi (2014) showed that some marijuana users also use other drugs, and poly-drug use is strongly related to psychotic-like experiences (Gage et al., 2014; Van Dam, Earleywine, & DiGiacomo, 2008).

The use of psychoactive substances may increase the risk of suicidal ideation, attempts and behaviours (Brent, Baugher, Bridge, Chen, & Chiappetta, 1999; Gould et al., 1998; Shaffer et al., 1996). Young people who use marijuana, tobacco, cocaine and other illicit drugs are more likely to report suicidal ideation (Brener, Hassan, & Barrios, 1999; Thompson, Moody, & Eggert, 1994). The number of drugs used appears to be more relevant in predicting suicidal behaviour than the types of drugs used (Borges, Walter, & Kessler, 2000; Kwon, Yang, Park, & Kim, 2013; Wilcox, Conner, & Caine, 2004). Thus, poly-drug use is a stronger predictor of suicidal ideation than mono-drug use. The ripple effects of problematic drug use provide a basis for exploring the experiences of PWUDs in Ghana and the extent of the effects of drug use on their lives. This study will extend the research of Appiah et al. (2017), who focused on the factors that accounted for relapse among PWUDs in Ghana. In this study, we sought to answer the question, 'How does drug use impact the lives of PWUDs in Ghana?'

Drug Use and the Development of Criminal Behaviour

Several models have drawn links between crime and drug use (Bennett, Holloway, & Farrington, 2008; Bowser, Word, & Seddon, 2014; Colman & Vandam, 2009; Martin, Macdonalds, & Ishiguro, 2013; Walters, 2014). Some scholars have emphasised the significance of reaching a broader understanding of the association to advance social policy (Hammersley, 2011; Seddon, 2000). In explaining the association between drug use and crime, Goldstein (1985) provided a tripartite model that described the links from economic-compulsive, systemic and psychopharmacological perspectives. The economic-compulsive view-point holds that expensive drug use leads to criminal behaviour because the user needs money to purchase drugs. The systemic viewpoint holds that violent crimes, such as assault and armed robbery, are associated with illegal drug markets (Bennett et al., 2008; Colman & Vandam, 2009; Seddon, 2000). The psychopharmacological perspective proposes that the psychoactive effects of drug use may lead to criminal behaviour (Boles & Miotto, 2003; Prichard & Payne, 2005) as well as violence (Macdonald, Erickson, Wells, Hathaway, & Pakula, 2008). Seddon (2000) argued that the deterministic view of a direct causal association between drug use and crime is inadequate and proposed that the association involves a multi-faceted, multilevel interaction process. Scholars have found supporting evidence for each of these perspectives (Facchin & Margola, 2016).

It has been shown that problematic drug users in Ghana engage in illegal activities, such as stealing, to finance drug use (Affinnih, 1999). However, the extent of the influence of drug use on the development of criminal behaviour is unknown. To answer this question, we conducted an exploratory study to investigate the experiences of PWUDs in Ghana.

Drug Policy, the Police and Interactions with PWUDs

Countries have taken various approaches to manage their populations' drug use (Belackova, Ritter, Shanahan, & Hughes, 2017; Chapman, Spetz, Lin, Chan, & Schmidt, 2016; Klieger et al., 2017). Klantschnig (2016) revealed that Nigeria's drug policy is highly repressive, coercive and unpopular. Ghana's laws on drug possession and use are equally repressive. Under Ghana's Narcotics (Enforcement and Sanctions) Act, 1994, Act 236, the possession, use, manufacture, supply or trade of psychoactive substances is criminal if the activity is not backed by legal authority. Such offences can result in a range of jail sentences from 5 to 25 years of imprisonment. The government's repressive attitudes influence how the police enforce the law. Several studies have suggested that the decriminalisation of drug use and possession may significantly reduce imprisonment and improve access to health and social benefits (Belackova et al., 2017; Massin, Carrieri, & Roux, 2017; Stevens & Hughes, 2016).

National laws can shape police operations in various ways (Hughes, Barratt, Ferris, Maier, & Winstock, 2018), which can result in cross-national differences in police encounters. Hughes et al. (2018) showed that police encounters in Norway, Sweden and Finland often lead to arrest. They also found differences between countries regarding the types and locations of encounter; for instance, stop-and-search was the most reported activity in Columbia and Greece (Hughes et al., 2018). Hughes et al. (2018) and Friedman et al. (2006) indicated that the street-level enforcement of drug laws has mostly failed in deterring drug supply and use. Abadie et al. (2018) demonstrated that repressive policing has failed in preventing drug use and distribution among people who inject drugs (PWIDs) in central Puerto Rico. The shift in emphasis from repression to rehabilitation and treatment is projected to have a positive effect on the quality of life and health of PWIDs.

There is a legal distinction between PWUDs who consume and the people who use drugs as a commodity for trade in Ghana.[1] The former group is usually arrested for use, possession and supply, whereas the latter group is arrested for import, export or manufacturing. Some people report to psychiatric facilities with substance-related psychiatric problems (Appiah et al., 2017). Although Hughes et al. (2018) and Friedman et al. (2006) have indicated that the street-level enforcement of drug laws has a minimal impact on deterrence, it is unclear how police encounters in

---

[1] See the 2020 Narcotics Control Commission Act, which the president confirmed in May 2020. It replaces the now-repealed Narcotic Drugs (Control, Enforcement and Sanctions) Law of 1990 (PNDCL 236). The new law allows for monetary payment for drug possession for use instead of incarceration.

Ghana impact the lives of PWUDs. This issue deserves attention because in Ghana, policing is characterised by unethical practices and corruption, and little is known about how police treat PWUDs.

Police corruption bedevils most transitional societies (Gerber & Mendelson, 2008). As in other countries, the police in Ghana have been saddled with perceptions of being corrupt and unfriendly with victims (Boateng & Darko, 2016; Tankebe, 2008). These two factors contribute to decreased confidence in the police and their legitimacy. Oulmokhtar, Krauth-Gruber, Alexopoulos, and Drozda-Senkowska (2011) asserted that the public views the police as controversial, prejudiced, persecutory and aggressive. Such perceptions and people's personal experiences with the police impact the operations and effectiveness of the institution. The Centre for Democratic Development found that in a 2000 nationwide survey of 1500 households in Ghana, more than half of the respondents indicated that they paid some form of bribe to police officers (CDD-Ghana, 2000). Tankebe (2010) found that assessments of police corruption reforms predicted Ghanaians' confidence in police effectiveness. An increase in police efforts in tackling corruption increased public perceptions of police effectiveness in providing security, and vicarious experiences of police corruption diminished confidence in police effectiveness (Tankebe, 2010).

Provisions have been made in the law for police officers in Ghana to screen people who might have a mental illness, including problematic drug use, when they encounter the criminal justice system (Act 846, Section 76 (1)). However, people with mental illnesses in Ghana may not receive the proper attention they deserve and may not be diverted from the criminal justice system (Adjorlolo, 2016). The repressive nature of Ghana's drug laws suggests that PWUDs may not be rehabilitated. We sought to answer the question, 'What are the experiences of PWUDs when they encounter the police in Ghana?'

This study had three objectives. We explored how drug use influences the lives of PWUDs, how drug use leads to the development of criminal behaviour among PWUDs and how PWUDS describe their experiences with the police in Ghana.

Methods

Research Design

A phenomenological research design with semi-structured interviews was adopted to gather data from PWUDs at several drug rehabilitation centres in Ghana. Interpretative Phenomenological Analysis (IPA) helps explain complex, emotionally laden topics (Smith & Osborn, 2015) and helps capture the details of individuals' lived experiences (Smith, Flowers, & Larkin, 2009). IPA has three philosophical underpinnings. The phenomenological aspect refers to the idea of producing an account of a lived experience regarding a specific phenomenon (in this case, problematic drug use). The interpretative aspect refers to the recognition that humans are sense-making organisms and that researchers must make sense of the phenomenon of which the participants are trying to make sense. The idiographic aspect entails a commitment to making sense of a specific case before making general claims (Smith & Osborn, 2015). We used this research design to explore the phenomenon of drug use and its effects on PWUDs based on what they shared about their experiences. We sought to make sense of how PWUDs' drug use shaped their lives, including their experiences with the police. We analysed the experiences of the PWUDs on an individual level and then assessed the descriptions collectively.

Study Setting

We recruited PWUDs undergoing drug rehabilitation in three regions in Ghana, namely Volta, Greater Accra and Ashanti. Most drug rehabilitation centres are located in these regions. Anecdotal evidence suggests that there are one, two and eleven rehabilitation centres in Volta, Ashanti and Greater Accra, respectively. These numbers were verified by the centres that served as the study settings, which are part of an association that meets on occasion. We visited ten centres, but four are privately owned, and we could not obtain institutional permission from some of them.

Ultimately, we used four private residential centres and two government-owned centres, one of which was outpatient and the other residential.

The government-owned centres used the 12-step approach to treatment (see Narcotics Anonymous World Services, 2008). This approach requires drug users to (1) admit that they had become powerless over the substance they used and that their lives had become unmanageable; (2) believe that a power greater than them could restore them to sanity; (3) decide to turn their will and lives over to the care of God; (4) make a searching, fearless moral inventory of themselves; (5) admit to God, themselves and another human being the exact nature of their wrongs; (6) be ready for God to remove all these defects of character; (7) humbly ask God to remove the shortcomings; (8) make a list of everyone that they had harmed and make amends to them; (9) make amends directly to the listed people wherever possible, except when doing so may injure them or others; (10) continue to take a personal inventory and promptly admit errors; (11) pray and meditate to improve conscious contact with God and pray for knowledge of God's will and the power to execute it; and (12) carry this message to other substance users and practice these principles in all affairs.

An undisclosed token fee is charged at the centres before a person is admitted to the centre. Upon admission, the clients go through detoxification if an assessment shows there is a need for it. Medication may also be given based on the clients' needs. The private rehabilitation centres are owned by either private individuals or non-governmental organisations. They are often operated by faith-based organisations and offer free services based on the financial state of clients. Sometimes, they charge an undisclosed token fee if they perceive that the client is capable of paying. Some of them combine faith and the 12-step treatment programme. Some rely solely on faith (prayers) and clients' willingness to change. Those that use the 12-step treatment programme encourage their clients to detoxify.

Participants and Sample Selection

We adopted a purposive sampling strategy to select PWUDs so that we could adequately cover the problematic drug users at each of the rehabilitation centres. None of the participants dropped out of the study. This project was part of a larger study that looked at the experiences of PWUDs in rehabilitation centres in Ghana. We recruited 38 male PWUDs (age range = 19–59; mean age = 38, SD = 10.40). This sample was adequate, as the study sought to achieve depth of information rather than extensive analysis (Smith & Osborn, 2008). Twenty-nine of the participants were single, and nine were married. Eight of the participants had attained university-level education (Table 11.1), and the majority of them were Christian (n = 34). One participant did not indicate his religious affiliation. The inclusion criteria were that the participant had been at the facility for at least one month and did not experience psychotic or withdrawal symptoms at the time of the study. No prospective female recruits met the criteria for inclusion. The participants needed to be 18 years or older and had used cocaine, heroin, marijuana, alcohol or a combination of these drugs. The inclusion criteria were achieved with the help of the

Table 11.1 Demographic characteristics of sample (N = 38)

Variable		N
Age (M = 38, SD = 10.40)		
Religious affiliation:	Christianity	34
	Islam	3
Marital status:	Married	9
	Single	29
Level of education:	Primary education	5
	High school	16
	College of education	2
	Diploma—Information Technology	2
	Diploma—Accounting	2
	Diploma—Nurse	1
	Higher National Diploma	1
	Diploma	1
	Degree	8

counsellors at the various centres, who were well acquainted with the clients and their mental health status and records.

Ethical Issues and Data Collection Procedure

The study obtained ethical clearance from the institutional review board of the Noguchi Memorial Institute for Medical Research (protocol: NMIMR-IRB 075/17-18). Institutional permission was also obtained from the various rehabilitation centres that were visited. The participants signed informed consent forms, and they were given the option to withdraw from the study at any time. We assured them of the confidentiality and anonymity of their responses through the use of pseudonyms. Psychological services in the form of counselling were made available for any participant who required it. The participants were not exposed to any conditions other than what they usually encounter in their ordinary daily lives. To help the participants express themselves more freely, we sought to establish rapport, reduce the participants' tension and gain their trust. The interviews were conducted in a quiet, calm place to reduce interference.

An interview schedule was used to gather data. According to Smith (1995), a schedule is not intended to be prescriptive and does not dictate the exact course of the interview. We asked the participants, 'please can you give me a brief history about yourself?'; 'what led to your current state?'; 'give a detailed description of your experiences with the drug(s) you were using'; 'how do you personally feel about your state (i.e., problematic drug use)?'; 'what was the experience like when you first came into contact with the police?'; and 'concerning your condition, how has your relationship with your family been?'. The questions were piloted with one PWUD to ensure that they would elicit responses that could help answer our research questions. During the interviews, we adapted the questions based on the context when intriguing issues arose, and used probing questions when appropriate (Smith, 1995). Semi-structured interviews can take an hour or more depending on the topic (Smith & Osborn, 2003). However, interviews in Mole, Kent, Hickson, and Abbott (2019) lasted between 20 and 39 minutes. In this study, the interviews lasted between 30 and 40 minutes. Only one interview session was conducted with each participant; there were no follow-up interviews. Each interview was completed on the day it was conducted. However, we contacted the participants for clarification when necessary. We stopped gathering data when no new information emerged from the interviews.

Data Analysis

We performed a thematic analysis of the data (Braun & Clarke, 2006). Braun and Clarke (2006) suggested the use of a six-stage approach to thematic analysis. The steps include reading and rereading the transcript to learn about the data, generating initial codes using semantic and latent meanings, searching for themes, reviewing the themes, defining and naming the themes and finally writing about them. The first author read through the data several times. The first two authors performed manual coding of the responses that appeared to address the research questions. We independently generated and grouped the codes according to common underlying ideas or themes (Creswell & Poth, 2018). Then, we sorted the codes into themes and sub-themes. Finally, we gathered the findings and selected quotations to support them.

Trustworthiness

We sought to ensure the credibility, dependability, confirmability and transferability of our findings (Lincoln & Guba, 1985). Following Creswell's (2014) recommendation, we paid careful attention to how the data were gathered, stored, analysed and reported to ensure credibility. We verified that the participants were PWUDs who could provide responses about their experiences, including with the police. We built a rapport with the participants to encourage them to be honest. The interviews were conducted by two male researchers with degrees in psychology and experience in gathering qualitative data. The study and the processes involved in conducting the research were made known to an independent research team to ensure dependability. After generating the initial themes, the second author followed the steps outlined by Braun and Clarke (2006) to further elaborate on themes based on the data. To ensure confirmability, the first two authors met to compare the congruence of the themes they had generated. Differences in themes were discussed and resolved so that the final themes reflected the participants' responses. These measures reduced the chance of possible biases. By recruiting appropriate participants and following the due process involved in conducting a qualitative study of this nature, we sought to ensure the transferability of the findings to individuals with similar characteristics and in a similar context.

Findings

Three themes were extracted from the responses. (1) The participants discussed the feeling of ecstasy. (2) They described the psychosocial consequences of drug use, which included the sub-themes of psychological effects, the development of criminality, the disruption of lifestyles and breakdowns in familial relationships. (3) Finally, they discussed aspects of their encounters with the police. This topic included the sub-themes of sudden, unannounced sweeps, ghettos, bribery and the non-deterrence of arrest (Table 11.2).

Table 11.2 Superordinate and subordinate themes

Superordinate themes	Subordinate themes	N
Ecstasy		26
Psychosocial consequences of drug use	• Psychological effect	34
	• Development of criminality	20
	• Disruption of life	21
	• Breakdown in familial relationship	19
Police encounter		
	• Ghetto	23
	• Sudden and unannounced swoops	16
	• Bribery	13
	• Non-deterrence of arrest	22

Ecstasy

Nearly 70% of the participants (*n* = 26) described an intense pleasure that comes with taking drugs. This theme encompasses depictions of the feelings that problematic drug users derive from using drugs. The pleasure sustains their drug use. Caleb explained:

> I feel differently…and it makes my brain and my head…feel happy. Yeah, I feel happy, and I feel sweet. In my head, there is nothing, there is no enjoyment apart from this particular enjoyment that I feel right now. (Caleb, 35)

Caleb is a poly-drug user, and he described the feeling as incomparable, which suggests that he could not give up this enjoyment. The statement 'I feel differently' presupposes that he was previously having certain feelings which could no longer be compared to his new state. How will he be able to forgo the euphoria if 'there is no enjoyment apart from this particular enjoyment that I feel right now'? He could not dissociate himself from the ecstatic feelings that he derived from using drugs. To sustain the new heightened feeling, he had to continue using drugs.

Psychosocial Consequences of Drug Use

Drugs can have different effects on users. The participants reported some of the effects that drugs had on them, which we clustered into psychological effects, the disruption of one's lifestyle, breakdowns in familial relationships and the development of criminality.

Psychological effects. Thirty-four participants indicated that after using drugs they sometimes experience distorted perceptions. One participant recounted how he saw himself as bigger than everyone else after consuming drugs, which is a case of hallucination. He also felt that something was deceiving him, but he did not know what it was. He now sees that it was the drug that thwarted his perception and made him see himself as bigger than everyone else. He ascribed a spiritual connotation to the influence of the drugs, saying, 'the feeling and the spirit entered me'.

But one day, I went to get some in the ghetto. I don't know what it was. After taking it, I felt bigger than everybody on earth…The feeling and the spirit entered me. I saw everybody as smaller than me. So, when I came back to my senses, I asked myself, 'how come yesterday I wasn't so, but today I feel bigger than everybody else?' That means something is deceiving me. (Boahen, 35)

The psychological effects of drugs can also manifest in attempted suicide. One respondent became depressed after nursing thoughts that he was destined to become a PWUD. Suicide presented a way to end his misery. His state of misery was a compound effect of the unsuccessful attempt by him and his family to stop his substance abuse. He felt that he was a nuisance to his family.

So, I woke up one day and decided maybe that is my destiny. I decided to end it all. I wanted to commit suicide [because] that was how depressed I was. You know, life didn't make sense to me, but God works in mysterious ways. I hanged myself. I woke up one morning and took my sponge. Everybody was celebrating that 'today he is going to bathe'…So, they were celebrating throughout the house. Little did they know I had ill intentions…I entered my room, removed my fan, tied it to the hook and hanged myself, but it wasn't easy. I didn't die. It broke off, and I fell down. I was lying unconscious [when] my brother chanced upon me and told my mum what I had done. You know, at that point, the pity my family had left…they were like, 'once he is trying to kill himself, go and report him'. Let's go and report him. This is a fine opportunity to send him to jail. But, my mum was like, maybe the guy really means change. (Mike, 26)

Mike felt that his family showed a lack of empathy for him. Following the failed suicide attempt, they handed him over to the police to keep him away from the family and drugs. This case of family alienation due to attempted suicide offers a vivid description of how Ghanaians stigmatise those who attempt suicide. The law stipulating that 'whoever attempts to commit suicide shall be guilty of misdemeanour' (1960 Criminal Code, Act 29, Section 57) probably informed the family's decision to contact the police. Instead of seeing a need for psychological help, they acted as if he had committed a punishable deed.

Development of criminality. Twenty participants discussed how drug use caused them to engage in criminal behaviour. This theme encompasses the connection between drug use and committing crimes. After they spend their life earnings on drugs, PWUDs typically have to decide whether they will engage in some form of criminal activity to raise money to finance their drug use. Maxwell explained:

> The use of cocaine will definitely make one go into stealing, especially when one is suffering from going 'cold turkey'. You might even cut your finger off for money to get cocaine. If you have nobody to help you, it is not easy. I was not a thief, but I turned into one because of drugs. (Maxwell, 44)

The statement that 'You might even cut your finger off for money to get cocaine' shows the extent to which PWUDs will go to finance their drug use. The comment that 'I was not a thief, but I turned into one because of drugs' suggests that it was not his intention to become a thief and that drug use compelled him to do so. If stealing was the only way to finance his drug use, he had to resort to it. In this case, stealing was not an end but a means to an end (i.e., funding his drug use).

Disruption of one's lifestyle. The disruption of one's lifestyle refers to how drug use interrupts a person's endeavours. Twenty-one participants said that using drugs had stopped their education.

> Some jokes are expensive, and it's an expensive one that ended me here. Because of that, I had to pause my education. Right now, I have deferred my semester to come and be here. (Bright, 20)

Bright temporarily stopped his university education to spend time at the rehabilitation centre. He described the use of drugs as an expensive joke, which had the side effect of derailing his academic trajectory.

Drug use also interrupts one's work life. Alfred described his state as

> Yes, of course, personally, I'm okay. But it looks like after having left the office for a couple of weeks, now there are certain things that I'm supposed to handle. Personal business, communication-wise, is something. I'm not

on my cell to make calls to check whether the business is on track. A whole lot is going on, so it looks like I am finding myself in an awkward position. (Alfred, 42)

While Alfred was spending time at the rehabilitation centre, he had to put aspects of his productive life on hold until he recovered. He indicated that his admission into the facility had cut him off from his business, leaving him in an 'awkward position'.

Breakdowns in familial relationships. Some participants (*n* = 19) revealed how drug use affected their relationships with their significant others. This theme describes how drug use damages the relationships between substance abusers and their family members.

> My conduct has caused all my relations to live abroad. I have children, and I have successfully learnt a trade—spraying. My mother told me that because I have sold all of her clothing, she cannot return to Ghana, and that's very true. I had a good relationship with my children, but because I was into cocaine…I had no time for the children. This made all of the mothers travel with the children. That leaves only my elder daughter, who is a nurse in Accra. Because I use drugs, when I call her, she does not respond. (Yaw, 44)

Yaw's situation led his family members to leave him alone in the country. He indicated that initially, he had a good relationship with his children. However, due to his condition, their mothers took them away from him. His elder daughter also avoids him because of his condition. Other participants mentioned that their families disregarded or reported them to the police when they attempted suicide.

Police Encounters

Poly-drug users often clash with the law because of their illicit drug use. The participants explained that they are often accosted in ghettos through police sweeps. After accosting the drug users, the police often required a bribe in exchange for their release.

Ghettos. Many participants (*n* = 23) revealed that they were often accosted in ghettos. 'Ghetto' is the term that the PWUDs used to refer to the shelters where they congregated for drug supply and use. They are converging points for substance abusers. Drug peddlers can easily locate drug abusers in such places, and they serve as a 'home' for drug users.

> One day, we were in the ghetto, smoking, and I think that time it was a general operation. The police came into the ghetto, went and started chasing people and things all over…By then I was so high that I was asleep. (Mensah, 19)

Mensah, a poly-drug user, states that it was in the ghetto that the police accosted him. Although drug users are generally aware that ghettos are a police target, PWUDs continue to frequent them because they can most easily acquire drugs there. To satisfy his craving for drugs, Mensah was in a ghetto, and the police accosted him even though he was high.

Unannounced sweeps. Some of the participants (*n* = 16) described in detail how the police accosted them. This theme describes the police's modus operandi for arresting PWUDs. James set the scene, saying, 'I was in the ghetto, smoking, thinking everything was alright, thinking I was free from my family'. James had fled his home to a ghetto to find solace. Although family can be a haven for some drug users, the disagreements that some PWUDs have with their families lead them to search for another home in a ghetto to have some peace of mind. James found a place where he felt that he belonged and could obtain a level of intimacy. Then, suddenly, he was arrested as part of a police sweep. The suddenness of the sweep disrupted an otherwise peaceful state of affairs.

> As I was in the ghetto, we were chatting, and we were talking about musicians and footballers who have prospered…Eh?! Before I could say 'jack', I was in the grip of the police! (James, 29)

Bribery. Thirteen participants indicated that they had to bribe the police to be released. Sunday described the series of events as follows:

On a Monday, we were supposed to go and have a blood test. On the way there, I made a few calls, got some money, settled everything, and they let us go. (Sunday, 28)

Sunday suggests that some kind of transaction happened between him, his colleagues and the police before a blood test could be taken. The release of these PWUDs depended on their ability to pay money.

Non-deterrence of arrests. More than half of the poly-drug users (*n* = 22) indicated that being arrested and confined at the police station did not deter them from using drugs. One of the participants thought it worsened his addiction. The police accost PWUDs to deter them or potential substance abusers. However, with substance abuse, such actions do not dissuade PWUDs. Bossman said that after his arrest he began devising other ways of using drugs to outwit the police. A friend convinced him that the probability of being caught when consuming cocaine is low. He accepted this logic, which led him to socialise 'with the junkies', and he 'eventually became a junky also'.

That experience [with the police] made my addiction even worse. It was that experience in the police station that made me involve myself in cocaine and rock...I was told by my friends that when you are smoking cocaine, eh, you will not be caught, but when you smoke marijuana, you will be caught. So, I listened to them and engaged with the junkies. So, I eventually became a junkie also. (Bossman, 29)

Stephen corroborated the limited preventive nature of police arrests, stating,

Oooh, no, no. That one does nothing. That one alone, I just feel that now I have to change where I smoke...But it doesn't tell me that I have to stop or something like that, no. (Stephen, 35)

Upon his release, Stephen sought ways to use drugs without being arrested, which led him to change his location for smoking marijuana. The arrest did not convince him to stop taking drugs. In such a state, the only objective that he understood was to feed his craving for drugs without being caught.

Discussion

In our interviews, we explored how drug use has influenced the lives of PWUDs in Ghana, how drug use can lead to the development of criminal behaviour and drug users' encounters with the police. The findings clustered around three themes: ecstasy; the psychosocial consequences of drug use, with the sub-theme of psychological effects, the development of criminality, the disruption of one's lifestyle and breakdowns in familial relationships; and police encounters, with the sub-themes of ghettos, sudden and unannounced police sweeps, bribery and the non-deterrence of arrests.

How Drug Use Influence the Lives of PWUDs

Consistent with Marlatt and VandenBos (1997), the euphoria associated with the use of drugs sustained the participants' drug use. Marlatt and VandenBos (1997) explained that people with substance use disorders desire immediate gratification without thinking about the remote effects of drugs on their lives.

Psychological effects, such as hallucinations and attempted suicide, were some of the effects that drugs had on the lives of the PWUDs in this study. These findings align with other studies (see Gage et al., 2014; Van Dam et al., 2008) that have observed that PWUDs report psychotic-like experiences, such as perceptual illusions. They confirm the findings of Brent et al. (1999) and Shaffer et al. (1996), who found that drug use is a risk factor for attempted suicide. Borges et al. (2000) and Wilcox et al. (2004) demonstrated that the number rather than the type of drugs used is strongly associated with suicidal behaviour. Poly-drug use is a strong predictor of suicide attempts (Kwon et al., 2013). In the study, we found that several of the poly-drug users had contemplated suicide.

How Drug Use Leads to the Development of Criminal Behaviour

The PWUDs in our study developed criminal behaviours due to their drug use, confirming the economic-compulsive perspective of the drug–crime relationship. The economic-compulsive view proposes that expensive drug use culminates in criminal behaviour because users have to devise every means possible to finance their drug use (Goldstein, 1985). Bennett et al. (2008) supported this perspective by suggesting that PWUDs commit crimes, such as stealing property, to fund their drug use. In the same vein, Colman and Vandam (2009) conceptualised the drug–crime relationship as a linear cause-and-effect association, where the individual commits a crime as a means to an end (i.e., acquiring money to feed an addiction).

Further, our study confirmed that the use of drugs leads to disruptions in the lifestyles of PWUDS and breaks down familial relationships, as has been established in the literature (Teesson et al., 2015). Our findings align with Choate (2015), who observed that drug use impacts the proper operation of the family system. The participants' drug use affected their relationships with family members and disrupted their careers in part because they had to stay in the rehabilitation centres to complete their treatment programmes. This finding supports Teesson et al. (2015), who indicated that drug use leads to social challenges, such as unemployment.

The Police Encounters of PWUDs

We observed that officers often accosted PWUDs through sweeps, which appeared to be the police's modus operandi. Ghana's laws criminalise the possession and use of drugs such as heroin, cocaine and marijuana (Criminal Procedure Code 1960, Act 29), mandating the police to arrest anyone found culpable. Several studies have established differences in the legal approaches that countries adopt to tackle drugs (Belackova et al., 2017; Chapman et al., 2016; Klieger et al., 2017). Hughes et al. (2018) indicated that police encounters in some Nordic countries (e.g., Norway) were likely to lead to arrest and that there are differences in the types and locations of law enforcement encounters. They observed that the police in Greece and Columbia rely on a stop-and-search mode (Hughes et al., 2018), which is contrary to the sweep mode adopted by Ghana's police. Our study established that police sweeps, which were the primary type of police contact among our participants, are generally sudden and disruptive for PWUDs.

Though the police frequently conduct sweeps, PWUDs continue to converge in ghettos. They serve as meeting places for PWUDs and drug suppliers. The participants also talked about the need for PWUDs to bribe the police for their release. PWUDs go to ghettos knowing that they can buy their way out by bribing the police. The police and the drug users ensure that the cycle of sweep-bribery-ghetto continues. The police's attitude seems to reinforce drug users' continued meeting in ghettos, raising the issue of police legitimacy and trust (Boateng & Darko, 2016; Tankebe, 2008). This study confirms Boateng and Darko (2016) and Tankebe (2008), who demonstrated why the Ghana Police Service continues to be saddled with corruption.

The participants' encounters with the police through sweeps did not deter them from drug use. This finding supports Friedman et al. (2006) and Hughes et al. (2018), who asserted that the street-level enforcement of drug laws is ineffective. Abadie et al. (2018) showed that repressive policing in Puerto Rico also failed to prevent drug use. In Ghana, the lack of efficacy could be attributed to addiction or the ability of PWUDS to bribe the police to release them when arrested. The decriminalisation of possession and use of drugs may help reduce imprisonments and lead to increased health and social benefits (Belackova et al., 2017; Massin et al., 2017; Stevens & Hughes, 2016).

Limitations and Recommendations

This study shares several important findings regarding the experiences of PWUDs, including their encounters with the police. However, these findings can only be transferred to male problematic drug users. Our inability to gain institutional permission to access four of the drug rehabilitation centres made it impossible to learn about the experiences of PWUDs at those centres. We recommend that future studies seek to gather data from those centres. Scholars could also extend the scope to cover other actors in the criminal justice system, such as lawyers and judges. Similarly, drug users' experiences with their counsellors and colleagues in the rehabilitation centres could be explored. Recently, a new drug law was implemented, and future studies could observe how law enforcement agencies are enforcing it.

Conclusion

The study has brought to light the detrimental effects of problematic drug use in Ghana. We observed the disruption of lifestyles and the development of criminal behaviour. Problematic drug users need to be identified so that they can receive rehabilitation. Their unchecked drug use may negatively impact the economy and society. The government or private stakeholders should provide more rehabilitation centres, and admission should be affordable to encourage people to undergo rehabilitation. The police's corrupt practices are not helping reduce problematic drug use; they seem to reinforce it. Proper checks and balances should be implemented to tackle corruption within the Ghana Police Service. The police should also be educated on the nature of drug use and addiction to help them better appreciate the plight of PWUDs. They should learn to empathise with PWUDs rather than extort money from them. People who come into contact with the criminal justice system should undergo mental health and drug use screenings so that they can be redirected when it is appropriate.

References

Abadie, R., Gelpi-Acosta, C., Davila, C., Rivera, A., Welch-Lazoritz, M., & Dombrowski, K. (2018). "It ruined my life": The effects of the war on drugs on people who inject drugs (PWID) in rural Puerto Rico. *International*

Journal of Drug Policy, 51, 121–127. https://doi.org/10.1016/j. drugpo.2017.06.011

Adjorlolo, S. (2016). Diversion of individuals with mental illness in the criminal justice system in Ghana. *International Journal of Forensic Mental Health,* 15(4), 382–392. https://doi.org/10.1080/14999013.2016.1209597

Affinnih, Y. H. (1999). A preliminary study of drug abuse and its mental health and health consequences among addicts in Greater Accra, Ghana. *Journal of Psychoactive Drugs,* 31(4), 395–403. https://doi.org/10.1080/0279107 2.1999.10471769

Agbakpe, G. F. K., Kwakye-Nuako, C. O., Bruce, D., & Bekoe, A. A. (2011). Relationship between substance abuse, study behavior and academic performance: A case study of senior high students of some selected schools in the Accra Metropolis. *Ghana International Journal of Mental Health,* 3(1), 1–7. Retrieved from http://apps.ug.edu.gh/ghana-ijmh/images/vol_3_2011.pdf

Appiah, R., Danquah, S. A., Nyarko, K., Ofori-Atta, A. L., & Aziato, L. (2017). Precipitants of substance abuse relapse in Ghana: A qualitative exploration. *Journal of Drug Issues,* 47(1), 104–115. https://doi.org/10.1177/0022042616678612

Belackova, V., Ritter, A., Shanahan, M., & Hughes, C. E. (2017). Assessing the concordance between illicit drug laws on the books and drug law enforcement: Comparison of three states on the continuum from decriminalised to punitive. *International Journal of Drug Policy,* 41, 148–157. https://doi.org/10.1016/j.drugpo.2016.12.013

Bennett, T., Holloway, K., & Farrington, D. P. (2008). The statistical association between drug misuse and crime: A meta-analysis. *Aggression and Violent Behavior,* 13, 107–118. https://doi.org/10.1016/j.avb.2008.02.001

Boateng, F. D., & Darko, I. N. (2016). Our past The effect of colonialism on policing in Ghana. *International Journal of Police Science and Management,* 18(1), 13–20. https://doi.org/10.1177/1461355716638114

Boles, S. M., & Miotto, K. (2003). Substance abuse and violence: A review of the literature. *Aggression and Violent Behavior,* 8, 155–174. https://doi.org/10.1016/S1359-1789(01)00057-X

Borges, G., Walter, E. E., & Kessler, R. C. (2000). Associations of substance use, abuse and dependence with subsequent suicidal behavior. *American Journal of Epidemiology,* 151(8), 781–789. https://doi.org/10.1093/oxfordjournals.aje.a010278

Bowser, B. P., Word, C. O., & Seddon, T. (2014). *Understanding drug use and abuse: A global perspective*. Palgrave Macmillan.

Braun, V., & Clarke, V. (2006). Using thematic analysis in psychology. *Qualitative Research in Psychology, 3*(2), 77–101. https://doi.org/10.119 1/1478088706qp063oa

Brener, N., Hassan, S., & Barrios, L. (1999). Suicidal ideation among college students in the United States. *Journal of Consulting and Clinical Psychology, 67*, 1004–1008. https://doi.org/10.1037//0022-006x.67.6.1004

Brent, D. A., Baugher, M., Bridge, J., Chen, T., & Chiappetta, L. (1999). Age- and sex-related risk factors for adolescent suicide. *Journal of the American Academy of Child and Adolescent Psychiatry, 38*, 1497–1505. https://doi.org/10.1097/00004583-199912000-00010

CDD-Ghana. (2000). *The Ghana Governance and Corruption Survey: Evidence from Households, Enterprises and Public Officials*. Ghana Anti-Corruption Coalition.

Chapman, S. A., Spetz, J., Lin, J., Chan, K., & Schmidt, L. A. (2016). Capturing heterogeneity in medical marijuana policies: A taxonomy of regulatory regimes across the United States. *Substance Use & Misuse, 51*(9), 1174–1184. https://doi.org/10.3109/10826084.2016.1160932

Choate, P. W. (2015). Adolescent alcoholism and drug addiction: The experience of parents. *Behavioral Science, 5*, 461–476. https://doi.org/10.3390/bs5040461

Colman, C., & Vandam, L. (2009). Drugs and crime: Are they hand in glove? A review of the literature. In *Contemporary issues in the empirical study of crime* (pp. 21–48). Maklu.

Creswell, J. W. (2014). *Research design: Qualitative, quantitative and mixed methods approaches* (4th ed.). Sage Publications.

Creswell, J. W., & Poth, C. N. (2018). *Qualitative inquiry and research design: Choosing among five approaches* (4th ed.). Sage Publications.

Facchin, F., & Margola, D. (2016). Researching lived experience of drugs and crime: A phenomenological study of drug-dependent inmates. *Qualitative Health Research, 26*(12), 1627–1637. https://doi.org/10.1177/1049732315617443

Friedman, S. R., Cooper, H. L. F., Tempalski, B., Keem, M., Friedman, R., Floma, P. L., et al. (2006). Relationships of deterrence and law enforcement to drug related harms among drug injectors in US metropolitan areas. *AIDS, 20*(1), 93–99. https://doi.org/10.1097/01.aids.0000196176.65551.a3

Gage, S., Hickman, M., & Zammit, S. (2016). Association between cannabis and psychosis: Epidemiologic evidence. *Biological Psychiatry, 79*, 549–556. https://doi.org/10.1016/j.biopsych.2015.08.001

Gage, S. H., Hickman, M., Heron, J., Munafò, M. R., Lewis, G., Macleod, J., et al. (2014). Associations of cannabis and cigarette use with psychotic experiences at age 18: Findings from the Avon Longitudinal Study of Parents and Children. *Psychological Medicine, 44*(16), 3435–3444. https://doi.org/10.1017/s0033291714000531

Gerber, P. T., & Mendelson, E. S. (2008). Public experiences of police violence and corruption in contemporary Russia: A case of predatory policing? *Law and Society Review, 42*, 1–44. https://doi.org/10.1111/j.1540-5893.2008.00333.x

Goldstein, P. J. (1985). The drug/violence Nexus: A tripartite conceptual framework. *Journal of Drug Issues, 39*, 143–174. https://doi.org/10.1177/002204268501500406

Gould, M. S., King, R., Greenwald, S., Fisher, R., Schwab-Stone, M., Kramer, R., et al. (1998). Psychopathology associated with suicidal ideation and attempts among children and adolescents. *Journal of the American Academy of Child and Adolescent Psychiatry, 37*(9), 915–923.

Hammersley, R. (2011). Pathways through drugs and crime: Desistance, trauma and resilience. *Journal of Criminal Justice, 39*, 268–272. https://doi.org/10.1016/j.jcrimjus.2011.02.006

Hughes, C. E., Barratt, M., Ferris, J. A., Maier, L. J., & Winstock, A. R. (2018). Drug-related police encounters across the globe: How do they compare? *International Journal of Drug Policy, 56*, 197–207. https://doi.org/10.1016/j.drugpo.2018.03.005

Klantschnig, G. (2016). The politics of drug control in Nigeria: Exclusion, repression and obstacles to policy change. *International Journal of Drug Policy, 30*, 132–139. https://doi.org/10.1016/j.drugpo.2015.10.012

Klieger, S. B., Gutman, A., Allen, L., Pacula, R. L., Ibrahim, J. K., & Burris, S. (2017). Mapping medical marijuana: State laws regulating patients, product safety, supply chains and dispensaries. *Addiction, 112*(12), 2206–2216. https://doi.org/10.1111/add.13910

Kwon, M., Yang, S., Park, K., & Kim, D. (2013). Factors that affect substance users suicidal behavior: A view from the Addiction Severity Index in Korea. *Annals of General Psychiatry, 12*(1), 35. https://doi.org/10.1186/1744-859x-12-35

Lincoln, Y. S., & Guba, E. G. (1985). *Naturalistic inquiry*. Sage Publications.

Macdonald, S., Erickson, P. G., Wells, S., Hathaway, A., & Pakula, B. (2008). Predicting violence among cocaine, cannabis, and alcohol treatment clients. *Addictive Behaviors, 33,* 201–205. https://doi.org/10.1016/j.addbeh.2007.07.002

Marlatt, G. A., & VandenBos, G. R. (Eds.). (1997). *Addictive behaviors: Readings on etiology, prevention, and treatment.* American Psychological Association. https://doi.org/10.1037/10248-000

Martin, G., Macdonalds, S., & Ishiguro, S. (2013). The role of psychosocial characteristics in criminal convictions among cocaine and gambling clients in treatment. *International Journal of Mental Health and Addiction, 11,* 162–171. https://doi.org/10.1007/s11469-012-9406-1

Massin, S., Carrieri, M. P., & Roux, P. (2017). De jure decriminalisation of cannabis use matters: Some recent trends from France. *International Journal of Drug Policy, 24*(6), 634–635. https://doi.org/10.1016/j.drugpo.2013.04.008

Mole, L., Kent, B., Hickson, M., & Abbott, R. (2019). 'It's what you do that makes a difference': An interpretative phenomenological analysis of health care professionals and home care workers experiences of nutritional care for people living with dementia at home. *BMC Geriatrics, 19*(1), 250. https://doi.org/10.1186/s12877-019-1270-4

Moore, T., Zammit, S., Lingford-Hughes, A., Barnes, T. R. E., Jones, P. B., Burke, M., et al. (2007). Cannabis use and risk of psychotic or affective mental health outcomes: A systematic review. *Lancet, 370*(9584), 319–328. https://doi.org/10.1016/s0140-6736(07)61162-3

Moss, H., Chen, C., & Yi, H. (2014). Early adolescent patterns of alcohol, cigarettes, and marijuana polysubstance use and young adult substance use outcomes in a nationally representative sample. *Drug and Alcohol Dependence, 136,* 51–62. https://doi.org/10.1016/j.drugalcdep.2013.12.011

Narcotics Anonymous World Services. (2008). *Narcotics anonymous* (6th ed.). Narcotics Anonymous World Services Inc.

Onifade, P. O., Somoye, E. B., Ogunwobi, O. O., Ogunwale, A., Akinhanmi, A. O., & Adamson, T. A. (2011). A descriptive survey of types, spread and characteristics of substance abuse treatment centers in Nigeria. *Substance Abuse Treatment, Prevention, and Policy, 6*(25). https://doi.org/10.1186/1747-597X-6-25

Oulmokhtar, D., Krauth-Gruber, S., Alexopoulos, T., & Drozda-Senkowska, E. (2011). Police officers' stereotype content and its evolution over two decades: from "neither nice nor able" to "still not nice but able". *Revue*

Internationale de Psychologie Sociale, 3(24), 87–100. https://www.cairn.info/revue-internationale-de-psychologie-sociale-2011-3-page-87.htm

Prichard, J., & Payne, J. (2005). *Alcohol, drugs and crime: A study of juveniles in detention*. Australian Institute of Criminology. https://doi.org/10.1037/e583062012-001

Seddon, T. (2000). Explaining the drug-crime link: Theoretical, policy and research issues. *Journal of Social Policy, 29*, 95–107. https://doi.org/10.1017/s0047279400005833

Shaffer, D., Gould, M. S., Fisher, P., Trautman, P., Moreau, D., Kleinman, M., et al. (1996). Psychiatric diagnosis in child and adolescent suicide. *Archives of General Psychiatry, 53*, 339–348. https://doi.org/10.1001/archpsyc.1996.01830040075012

Smith, J., & Osborn, M. (2008). Interpretative phenomenological analysis. In J. Smith (Ed.), *Qualitative psychology: A practical guide to research methods* (pp. 53–80). Sage Publications.

Smith, J. A. (1995). Semi-structured interviewing and qualitative analysis. In *Rethinking methods in psychology*. Sage.

Smith, J. A., Flowers, P., & Larkin, M. (2009). *Interpretative phenomenological analysis: Theory, method and research*. Sage.

Smith, J. A., & Osborn, M. (2003). Interpretative Phenomenological Analysis. In *A practical guide to research methods*. Sage.

Smith, J. A., & Osborn, M. (2015). Interpretative phenomenological analysis as a useful methodology for research on the lived experience of pain. *British Journal of Pain, 9*(1), 41–42. https://doi.org/10.1177/2049463714541642

Stevens, A., & Hughes, C. (2016). Dépénalisation et santé publique: politiques des drogues et toxicomanies au Portugal. *Mouvements, 2*(86), 22–33. https://doi.org/10.3917/mouv.086.0022

Tankebe, J. (2008). Colonialism, legitimation and policing in Ghana. *International Journal of Law, Crime and Justice, 36*(1), 67–84. https://doi.org/10.1016/j.ijlcj.2007.12.003

Tankebe, J. (2010). Public confidence in the police: Testing the effects of public experiences of police corruption in Ghana. *British Journal of Criminology, 50*, 296–319. https://doi.org/10.1093/bjc/azq001

Teesson, M., Marel, C., Darke, S., Ross, J., Slade, T., Burns, L., et al. (2015). Long term mortality, remission, criminality and psychiatric comorbidity of heroin dependence: 11-year findings from the Australian Treatment Outcome Study. *Addiction, 110*(6), 986–993. https://doi.org/10.1111/add.12860

Thompson, E. A., Moody, K. A., & Eggert, L. L. (1994). Discriminating suicide ideation among high-risk youth. *Journal of School Health, 64,* 361–367. https://doi.org/10.1111/j.1746-1561.1994.tb06205.x

UNODC. (2010). *World Drug Report 2010.* United Nations.

UNODC. (2015). *World drug report 2015.* United Nations.

UNODC. (2016). *World Drug Report 2016.* United Nations.

Van Dam, N. T., Earleywine, M., & DiGiacomo, G. (2008). Polydrug use, cannabis, and psychosis-like symptoms. *Human Psychopharmacology, 23*(6), 475–485. https://doi.org/10.1002/hup.950

Van Os, J., Linscott, R., Myin-Germeys, I., Delespaul, P., & Krabbendam, L. (2009). A systematic review and meta-analysis of the psychosis continuum: Evidence for a psychosis proneness–persistence–impairment model of psychotic disorder. *Psychological Medicine, 39*(2), 179–195. https://doi.org/10.1017/s0033291708003814

Walters, G. D. (2014). Crime and substance misuse in adjudicated delinquent youth: The worst of both worlds. *Law and Human Behavior, 38,* 139–150. https://doi.org/10.1037/lhb0000050

Wilcox, H. C., Conner, K. R., & Caine, E. D. (2004). Association of alcohol and drug use disorders and completed suicide: An empirical review of cohort studies. *Drug and Alcohol Dependence, 76,* S11–S19. https://doi.org/10.1016/j.drugalcdep.2004.08.003

Wu, L. T. (2010). Substance abuse and rehabilitation: Responding to the global burden of diseases attributable to substance abuse. *Substance Abuse and Rehabilitation, 1,* 5–11. https://doi.org/10.2147/sar.s14898

12

Evaluating the Predictors of Stress among Police Officers: A Current Psychosocial Analysis from Nigeria

Oluwagbenga Michael Akinlabi

Introduction

Policing is one of the most stressful and physically demanding occupations in the world (Anshel, 2000; Anshel, Robertson, & Caputi, 1997; Dempsey & Forst, 2019). The American Institute of Stress classified police work has highly stressful and that it is among the top ten stress-producing jobs (The American Institute of Stress, 2020). Police officers are more likely to report and be diagnosed with psychological problems and stress-related physical complaints than workers in other professions (Can, Hendy, & Karagoz, 2015; Dempsey & Forst, 2019; The American Institute of Stress, 2020). They are often exposed to situations and events at work that may be beyond the threshold of normal human experiences (Anderson, Litzenberger, & Plecas, 2002; Anshel et al., 1997). This could range from critical incidents such as situations in which they face threats

O. M. Akinlabi (✉)
Department of Social Sciences, Northumbria University,
Newcastle upon Tyne, UK
e-mail: Oluwagbenga.akinlabi@northumbria.ac.uk

© The Author(s), under exclusive license to Springer Nature Switzerland AG 2021
H. C. O. Chan, S. Adjorlolo (eds.), *Crime, Mental Health and the Criminal Justice System in Africa*, https://doi.org/10.1007/978-3-030-71024-8_12

to their physical well-being, or that of a fellow police officer, or a victim within the community, and it can also include a dispatch to road traffic fatality. It is evident that when stress becomes chronic, it can lead to a plethora of other problems affecting officers at work and in other socio-personal aspect of their lives (Anderson et al., 2002; Anshel, 2000).

Research has shown that stressors occur at different and multiple stages across life, and that they can also present different levels of severity and chronicity (Keyes, Hatzenbuehler, & Hasin, 2011). Other studies have also confirmed that there are different sources of stress in the police (see Can et al., 2015; Cullen, Lemming, Link, & Wozniak, 1985; Keyes et al., 2011); however, four specific classifications are identified as prominent among others—organisational stressors, operational stressors, external stressors and personal stressors (see Dempsey & Forst, 2019; Violanti & Aron, 1994). According to Dempsey and his colleague, external stress is produced by real physical threats and a heightened sense of imminent dangers which can include dangerous assignments in which there are physical confrontations, shoot-outs and involvement in auto pursuits (Anderson et al., 2002; Collins & Gibbs, 2003). Organisational stress often results from the quasi-military structure of the police in which officers work at odd hours with little or no weekend or holidays, the strict regimental discipline placed on officers, lack of control over workload, workplace bullying and bias, and the general condition and atmosphere at work (Collins & Gibbs, 2003; Dempsey & Forst, 2019; Guile, Tredoux, & Foster, 1998).

Personal stress is often caused by officer's socio-personal interactions with others within their organisation. Personal stressors also involve events or conditions that occur in an individual's life that may have adverse effect on them or their family's well-being. *Operational stress* comes from the daily need to confront criminals and to deal with derelicts, mentally disturbed offenders and drug addicts, and the constant awareness and need to engage in dangerous activity to protect the public. Also, police officers are consistently cautious about their actions and inactions in a bid to avoid legal liability (Chapin, Brannen, Singer, & Walker, 2008; Dempsey & Forst, 2019; Violanti & Aron, 1994).

There have been significant results associated with these classifications in extant literature. For example, in a study conducted by Anderson et al.

(2002) using samples of police officers from 12 municipal police departments in British Columbia, the results indicate that police officers experience both physical and psychosocial stress and that officers anticipate stress as they go about their duty. The research further established that police officers suffer anticipatory stress at the start of their shifts and that the highest level of stress is experienced prior to and during critical incidents. Other research on police stress and stressors have suggested that overexposure of officers to stress may lead to a greater likelihood of job dissatisfaction, sleep disorder, absenteeism, weak immune system, short and long-term illness, divorce, burnout, early retirement, PTSD, diminished awakening cortisol response pattern, poor performance, low morale and premature death (see Alexopoulos, Palatsidi, Tigani, & Darviri, 2014; Anderson et al., 2002; Anshel, 2000; Anshel et al., 1997; Barnes, Brown, Krusemark, Campbell, & Rogge, 2007; Gerber, Hartmann, Brand, Holsboer-Trachsler, & Pühse, 2010; Ma et al., 2015; Renden et al., 2017; Violanti et al., 2017).

Similarly, in a 2007 study of 'the role of mindfulness in romantic relationship satisfaction and responses to relationship stress', Barnes and his colleagues asserted that individuals whose careers frequently exposed them to challenging and stressful situations often reports significant reduction in communication skills, and this outcome is also associated with divorce and break-up in relationships (Barnes et al., 2007). In a study conducted to examine how specific shift system is associated with stress, sleep and health among 460 Swiss Police, Gerber et al. (2010) found that shift work is associated with increased social stress, work discontent and sleep complaints among Swiss Police. Gerber and his colleagues also found that stress was associated with increased sleep complaints and lower scores in perceived health (see also Cannizzaro et al., 2020).

Broadly speaking, increased work-related stress has also been linked with a few other health challenges such as high blood pressure and coronary heart disease. Violanti et al. (2017) utilising the Spielberger Police Stress Survey examined the association between the top five highly rated and bottom five least-rated work stressors among police officers. In their analysis, Violanti and his colleagues found that there was a significant negative linear association between total stress index of the top five rated work stressors and slope of the awakening cortisol regression line. The result suggests that police events considered to be highly stressful by the officers may likely be associated with disturbances similar to awakening cortisol pattern. In their Danish study, Jensen et al. (2019) assessed the impact of organisational change at work on cardiovascular disease (CVD), and they found that there was an excess risk of CVD in the year following change in management and employee layoff. The study also confirmed that exposure to any organisational change has strong link to an increased risk of CVD (see also Bunker et al., 2003; de Rijk, 2020; Hanson et al., 2020).

Policing and Sources of Stress in Nigeria: Towards an Empirical Analysis

Work-related stress among police is a global issue, and police officers in Nigeria are no exception. Though police officers in Nigeria have considerable power to use force (see Akinlabi, 2018), they are often confronted with the arduous operational demand that may be detrimental to their psychological and physiological well-being (Idubor, Aihie, & Igiebor, 2015). They are routinely exposed to traumatic and disturbing situations such as intimate partner violence, abused of children, fatal motor vehicle accidents, ritualised killings and homicide (Idubor et al., 2015; John-Akinola, Ajayi, & Oluwasanu, 2020; Lateef, 2019). Significantly adding to these operational stresses are the everyday challenges in their socio-personal lives and the public expectations of police effectiveness in solving crimes in their community (Akinlabi, 2018). Officers are under strain to put their lives on the line to maintain law and orders in their communities. The fact that police officers are recruited with excellent physical and psychological health assessment but retire early on medical advice or die from job-related stress disorders demonstrates that the cost of stress is enormous.

In Nigeria, police officers are often confronted with various job stressors that are significantly different, both in quality and quantity, in comparison to their counterparts in the developed West. Also, while police officers in the developed West have pre- and post-exposure strategies in place to mitigate the effect of stress, officers in Nigeria receive little or no support in the management of stress at work and in their personal lives (Lateef, 2019). Like most developing countries, working in Nigeria can be incredibly challenging. The only dichotomy between Nigeria and other contexts is the way and manner in which Nigeria operates as a complex sociopolitical and ethnically divided society. Policing a socially and politically divided society like Nigeria presents an enormous stress for police officers in Nigeria (Adebayo, Sunmola, & Udegbe, 2008). During their day-to-day activities, police officers are frequently exposed to violence from criminals, and often engage in rescue operations of civilians from armed robbers and other gunmen they deal directly with the hardest criminals and the worst of the society. Sometimes, they watched their colleagues killed or maimed in the course of their legitimate duties (Lateef, 2019).

Every year more police officers commit suicide than are murdered by criminals (Adediran, 2020; Chopko, Palmieri, & Facemire, 2014; Miller, 2005). However, the media often deploy most of their resources to report police corruption than the everyday challenges police officers confront in the line of duty. Due to public and media backlash, officers are also under tremendous pressure to perform their duties effectively. While doing this, they are also susceptible to losing their jobs for committing the slightest blunder. This is how risky and challenging it is to be a police officer in Nigeria. These occupational stressors can have significant effect on officers' mental health morbidity. Studies have shown that officers' poor mental health well-being can be harmful at a professional level, on organisational effectiveness and for public safety (John-Akinola et al., 2020; Purba & Demou, 2019; Wakil, 2015).

A number of studies conducted in Nigeria have confirmed a significant connection between police work and job-related stress (Adegoke, 2014; Idubor et al., 2015; John-Akinola et al., 2020; Lateef, 2019; Odedokun, 2015; Ogungbamila & Fajemirokun, 2016; Omolayo, 2012). For example, in a recent study conducted in Edo State Nigeria, Idubor et al. (2015) investigated the effect of work-related stress on the health status of 1000 police officers and found a significant relationship between stress and health status of the sampled police officers. Specifically, they found that officers who reported a significant high score on both organisational and operational stressors also reported poor health and low quality of life.

In a study conducted by Ogungbamila and Fajemirokun (2016), they investigated the extent to which gender and marital status moderated the relationship between job stress and occupational burnout, and they found that job stress significantly predicted occupational burnout among the police in such a way that a heightened level of job stress also resulted to an increased level of occupational burnout. The study also confirmed that gender moderated the effects of job stress on occupational burnout. That is, female officers reported a higher level of occupational burnout that their male counterparts. Similarly, marital status moderated the relationship between job stress and occupational burnout. In other words, those who were married reported a higher level of occupational burnout than those who were unmarried.

Similarly, in a study conducted among 153 police officers in Ekiti State, Omolayo (2012) found effect for gender and rank. The study revealed that female police officers and those who are of low cadre (i.e. junior rank) are more likely to experience higher stress at work than others not in these categories. While gender is confirmed in many studies, there are other studies that reported that men are more susceptible to stress than their female counterparts (Morash, Kwak, & Haarr, 2006; Violanti et al., 2016), some reported similar effects between male and female (Spielberger & Reheiser, 1994) and some supported Omolayo (2012)'s findings that females are more prone to work-related stress and other associated factors such as PTSD than males (Bowler et al., 2010).

In assessing the coping strategy for stress among the police, Wakil (2015) confirmed that police officers who experienced stress adopt unconventional coping strategies such as the use of alcohol, smoking and religiosity rather than seek professional help to cope with stress. A similar study examining the experiences of stress and coping mechanism among police officers in Ibadan confirmed that a high proportion of the sample (80 percent) reported experiences of stress. The study also revealed that only a few (37 percent) of the officers had good coping mechanism and that knowledge about workplace stressors is scant among the police (John-Akinola et al., 2020).

Looking critically at current evidence, research has demonstrated that there is a huge psychological, economical and health cost of stress; and that there are multidimensional predictors of stress. Studies have also established that there are variegated outcomes of stress in individual's lives. In this current study, therefore, I empirically assessed the pattern, occurrence and prevalence, as well as the global effects of stress among police officers in Nigeria. To do this: (i) I assessed the pattern and prevalence stress among the police; (ii) I examined the psychosocial variables that predict organisational and operational police stress; and (iii) using relevant argument in literature, I also assessed whether there is a significant relationship between stress and a self-reported effect of stress in the police. While causality cannot be established in a study like this, it would be interesting, however, to assess whether one can establish a significant relationship between some of the independent variables and stress, and how stress would in turn interact with self-reported 'effect of stress' among the police.

Method

Data

The data for this study were collected through a cross-sectional survey of 706 police officers in southwest geopolitical zone in Nigeria. The sample for this study was predominantly police officers within the ranks of constable, corporal, sergeant and inspector, and they were randomly selected from Zone 2 and Zone 11 of the Nigeria Police Zone Commands. The Zone 2 and Zone 11 include Lagos, Ogun, Osun, Ondo and Oyo State. To draw sample for this study, five police commands in each of the five states were selected at random. A total of 750 questionnaires were administered through convenience sampling technique. After four weeks of administering pen-and-paper questionnaires, with support from two research assistants, the research team was able to retrieve 717 questionnaires (i.e. 95.6 percent response rate); however, only 706 questionnaires (i.e. 94.1 percent) were found useful and relevant for the current analysis. Accordingly, the socio-demographic characteristics of the research participants are presented in Table 12.1.

Table 12.1 Demographic and control variables

Demographics	(%)	Demographics	(%)
Gender		*Marital status*	
Male	56.8	Never married	13.6
Female	43.2	Married	83.1
		Separated/divorced	3.3
Age		*Ethnicity*	
18–30	41.6	Hausa	4.1
31–40	30.7	Igbo	13.3
41–50	15.0	Yoruba	66.0
51–60	12.6	Others	16.6
Rank		*During the past 12 months, how would you rate your health?*	
Constable	54.4	Poor	14.3
Corporal	26.3	Fair	31.0
Sergeant	14.7	Good	15.2
Inspector	4.5	Very good	29.9
		Excellent	9.6
During the past 12 months, how would you rank experiences of stress in your personal life?		*During the past 12 months, how much effect has stress had on your health?*	
No stress	6.1	None	6.1
Almost no stress	16.3	Hardly any	17.6
Relatively little stress	19.4	Some	28.8
Moderate amount of stress	23.8	A lot	47.6
A lot of stress	34.4		
During the past 12 months, have you taken any steps to control or reduce stress in your life?		*If you were stress, what type of help would you seek?*	
No	94.1	Spiritual	38.8
Yes	5.9	Medical/psychological	29.2
		Combination of both	32.0

As an important limitation in this study, it is important to note that because the data were collected through a convenience sampling technique, caution must be taken not to assume that the results in this study are analogous to the entire population of the police in Nigeria. It is also important to emphasise that cross-sectional surveys are generally not suitable to establish causality; as such, this current study will not be establishing causality but to systematically assess statistical relationships between the variables in this study.

Measures

A range of questionnaires were utilised to address the research questions in this study. These instruments and their relevance to this study are described below.

Police Stress Questionnaire

The police stress questionnaire was developed by McCreary and Thompson (2006) to assess the relationship between stress and health status of police officers. McCleary and Thompson have argued that the more stress people experience, the poorer their physical and mental health. In fact, studies have shown that people with higher stress level tend to report lower overall health and well-being, and a more adverse health symptoms such as sleep disturbances and high blood pressure are at a greater risk of coronary heart disease, hypertension, diabetes and auto-immune disorders. The police stress questionnaire is in two levels—measuring both organisational and operational levels of stress, that is, Operational Police Stress Questionnaire (PSQ-Op) and Organisational Police Stress Questionnaire (PSQ-Org). Each of the two levels of instruments contained 20 items/questions, and they are measured on a seven-point scale that ranges from 1 (No stress at all) to 7 (A lot of stress). For this current study, the reliability coefficient of the combined instrument yielded a Cronbach alpha $\alpha = 0.74$; *Mean* = 5.12; *SD* = 0.49 and individually, Operational Police Stress Questionnaire (PSQ-Op) has $\alpha = 0.83$; *Mean* = 5.14; *SD* = 0.79 and Organisational Police Stress Questionnaire (PSQ-Org) yielded $\alpha = 0.67$; *Mean* = 5.10; *SD* = 0.60, respectively. In both instruments, a high score indicates higher levels of stress.

Effect of Stress on General Well-being

The Effect of Stress on General Well-being in this study is a one-item variable that was tested using the question, 'During the past 12 months, how much effect has stress had on your general well-being?' The question was developed by the researcher to assess the global effect of stress on the general well-being of the research participants. In this study, the variable is included in the analysis as a dependent variable, and it is measured in terms of 'None' (1) to 'A lot' (4).

Demographic and Control Variables

Demographic variables for this study included age, gender, ethnicity, marital status and ranks. Other five questions/variables were added as control variables, and they included the following: (1) During the past 12 months, how would you rate your health? (2) During the past 12 months, how would you rank experiences of stress in your personal life? (3) During the past 12 months, have you taken any steps to control or reduce stress in your life? (4) If you were stressed, what type of help would you seek?

Results

The central focus of this study is to assess the pattern, occurrence and prevalence, as well as the global effects of stress among police officers in Nigeria. Tables 12.2 and 12.3 present the mean scores, standard deviations and the full wordings of the organisational and operational police stress questionnaires. Looking at the analyses in Tables 12.2 and 12.3, it is evident that the measures of organisational and operational stresses are positively skewed. This indicates that the mean of each item in the two questionnaires are higher than the median score. That is, response on each item indicates that there is a high occurrence and prevalence of organisational and operational stresses among the police.

Bivariate Correlation

In Table 12.4, a Pearson product-moment correlation was conducted to assess the relationship between the variables in this study. A significant bivariate correlation was established for some of the variables, and they

Table 12.2 Means and standard deviation of organisational police stress questionnaire

Variable items	Mean	SD
Dealing with co-workers	5.25	1.78
The feeling that different rules apply to different people (e.g. favouritism)	5.81	1.64
Feeling like you always have to prove yourself to the organisation	5.99	1.26
Excessive administrative duties	5.76	1.38
Constant changes in policy/legislation	4.69	2.07
Staff shortages	5.87	1.70
Bureaucratic red tape	5.58	1.52
Too much computer work	5.47	1.39
Lack of training on new equipment	5.86	1.47
Perceived pressure to volunteer free time	5.64	1.55
Dealing with supervisors	5.15	1.78
Inconsistent leadership style	5.38	1.74
Lack of resources	5.93	1.89
Unequal sharing of work responsibilities	5.45	1.82
If you are sick or injured your co-workers seem to look down on you	2.63	1.38
Leaders overemphasise the negatives (e.g. supervisor evaluations, public complaints)	4.74	1.56
Internal investigations	3.61	1.52
Dealing the court system	2.47	1.29
The need to be accountable for doing your job	4.90	1.64
Inadequate equipment	5.90	1.70

Note: Responses ranges from "No stress at all" (1) to "A lot of stress" (7)

were mostly in the expected directions. Specifically, operational police stress ($r = .832$, $p < .01$) has the highest bivariate correlation with organisational police stress. Though the high correlation coefficient should violate collinearity assumption, however, further analysis will be conducted using Variance Inflation Factors and Tolerance to establish if this assumption was violated. Other correlations were within the expected limits (see Table 12.4).

Multiple Regression

Tables 12.5 and 12.6 present the findings for three multiple regression analyses. Preliminary analysis confirmed that no assumptions were

Table 12.3 Means and standard deviation of operational police stress questionnaire

Variable items	Mean	SD
Shift work	5.20	1.77
Working alone at night	5.50	1.71
Overtime demands	5.90	1.47
Risk of being injured on the job	5.65	1.53
Work-related activities on days off (e.g. court, community events)	3.59	1.95
Traumatic events (e.g. MVA, domestics, death, injury)	3.27	1.95
Managing your social life outside of work	4.62	1.57
Not enough time available to spend with friends and family	5.40	1.55
Paperwork	5.10	1.59
Eating healthy at work	5.54	1.58
Finding time to stay in good physical condition (e.g. regular exercise)	5.04	1.80
Fatigue (e.g. shift work, overtime)	5.38	1.72
Occupation-related health issues (e.g. back pain)	5.81	1.48
Lack of understanding from family and friends about your work	5.53	1.55
Making friends outside the job	4.60	2.12
Upholding a 'higher image' in public	4.84	1.44
Negative comments from the public	5.91	1.46
Limitations to your social life (e.g. who your friends are, where you socialise)	5.29	1.58
Feeling like you are always on the job	5.03	1.56
Friends/family feel the effects of the stigma associated with your job	5.59	1.54

Note: Responses ranges from "No stress at all" (1) to "A lot of stress" (7)

Table 12.4 Descriptive statistics and correlations

	1	2	3	4	5	6	7
(1) Operational police stress	1	.832**	.118**	.331**	-.096*	.023	-.003
(2) Organisational police stress		1	.106**	.345**	-.045	.007	.006
(3) Type of help			1	.070	-.022	-.003	.153**
(4) Stress reduction				1	-.077*	-.072*	.061
(5) Effect of stress on wellbeing					1	-.061	-.056
(6) Stress in personal life						1	-.043
(7) Death of a loved one							1

$N = 706$

Note: Statistically significant at $*p < .05$; $**p < .005$; $***p < .001$

Table 12.5 Predicting organisational and operational stress

Variable	Organisational police stress		Operational police stress	
	β	t	β	t
Age	.055	1.334	−.003	−.062
Gender	−.095*	−2.294	.059	1.428
Ethnicity	−.017	−.458	.047	1.248
Marital tatus	−.015	−.397	.029	.775
Ranks	−.058	−1.477	.022	.555
Health status	−.153***	−1.408	−.129***	−1.763
Stress in personal life	.170***	2.484	.161***	1.890
Stress reduction	−.007	−.174	−.004	−.097
Types of help	−.085*	−2.060	−.083*	−1.756
R	.37***		.12***	
R2	.13***		.05***	
F	2.112***		2.048***	

Note: Statistically significant at *$p < .05$; **$p < .005$; ***$p < .001$

Table 12.6 Predicting effect of stress on general well-being

Variable	β	t	R	R²	F
Age	−.068**	−2.980	.84***	.705***	150.704***
Gender	.044*	1.951			
Ethnicity	.029	1.392			
Marital tatus	−.035	−1.698			
Ranks	.016	.742			
Health status	−.018	−.853			
Stress in personal life	.799***	35.225			
Stress reduction	.005	.253			
Types of help	.089**	3.949			
Operational police stress	.005	.217			
Organisational police stress	.044*	2.099			

Note: Statistically significant at *$p < .05$; **$p < .005$; ***$p < .001$

violated. Collinearity diagnostic using Tolerance and Variance Inflation Factor were performed to avoid problems of multicollinearity. The collinearity diagnostic revealed that Tolerance values were above .10 and Variance Inflation Factors were below 10 for all the items in the analysis (see Field, 2018; Pallant, 2010; Tabachnick & Fidell, 2013). In Table 12.5, a multiple regression analyses were conducted to investigate the predictors of organisational and operational police stress. The two dependent variables were tested separately using nine demographic control and independent variables (i.e. age, gender, ethnicity, marital status, ranks, health status, stress in personal life, stress reduction and types of help). In Table 12.6, the effect of stress on general well-being was tested using 11 demographic control and independent variables (i.e. age, gender, ethnicity, marital status, ranks, health status, stress in personal life, stress reduction, types of help, operational police stress and organisational police stress).

In Table 12.5, the analysis indicated that nine variables in the model jointly accounted for 13 percent [$F(9, 697) = 2.112$; $p < .001$] total variance in organisational police stress, and four variables were statistically significant as follows: stress in personal- life ($\beta = 0.170$; $p < .001$), health status ($\beta = -0.153$; $p < .001$), gender ($\beta = -0.095$; $p < .05$) and types of help ($\beta = -0.085$; $p < .05$). The result shows that policemen who reported stress in their personal life had health-related challenges and sought unorthodox or alternative treatment for stress are more likely to experience organisational police stress.

Likewise, nine variables in the analysis jointly accounted for 5 percent [$F(9, 697) = 2.048$; $p < .001$] total variance in operational police stress. Individually, three variables predicted operational police stress as follows: stress in personal life ($\beta = 0.161$; $p < .001$), health status ($\beta = -0.129$; $p < .001$) and types of help ($\beta = -0.083$; $p < .05$). The result shows that police officers who reported stress in their personal life, had health-related challenges and sought alternative or unorthodox help for stress are more likely to experience operational police stress. Interestingly, this shows that there is a similar response patterns among police officers in Nigeria when they are assessed on organisational and operational police stress.

In Table 12.6, the result indicated that the eleven variables in this analysis jointly accounted for 70 percent [$F(11, 695) = 150.704$; $p < .001$] total variance in the effect of stress on general well-being. Individually, five variables predicted effects of stress on general well-being as follows: stress in personal life ($\beta = 0.799$; $p < .001$), types of help ($\beta = 0.089$; $p < .005$), age ($\beta = -0.068$; $p < .005$), gender ($\beta = 0.044$; $p < .05$) and organisational police stress ($\beta = -0.044$; $p < .05$). The result indicates that being female and young, having experiences of stress in personal life, seeking an orthodox help for stress and reporting organisational police stress may likely heightened the effect of stress on the general well-being of the police officers.

Discussion

This current study advances prior research and understanding on stress and stressors in the police. The study empirically assessed the occurrence and prevalence, as well as the effects of stress among police officers. This chapter also considers what current research could contribute to police practice, and the general implication for research and policymaking in Nigeria. As Newman and Beehr (1979) suggested, one of the first steps in handling job stress is to identify the factors which may likely predict or be related to stress. The current study confirmed this assertion. Using McCleary and Thompson's police stress questionnaires, this study demonstrated that there are existing factors that are related to the two categories of stress in the police. The first category being the nature of police work and how it often exposes police officers to stress, and the second category being the nature of police organisation.

Looking the occurrence and prevalence of stress in the police, the means and the standard deviation of the operational and organisational police stress questionnaires showed that stress is prevalent among the police. The analyses also showed that the individual items in the questionnaires were positively skewed. That is, the mean of each item in the two questionnaires are higher than the median score. This indicates that there are high occurrences and prevalence of organisational and operational stresses among the police. It makes sense, therefore, to argue that the police experiences both organisational and operational stress in Nigeria. Studies have shown that the police in Nigeria is faced with both organisational and operational challenges such as inadequate equipment, poor conditions of service, nepotism, corruption, insufficient education and training and a poor public image (Akinlabi & Murphy, 2018; Alemika, 1988; Idubor et al., 2015)

In the regression analyses, the results indicated that the current health status, stress in individual officer's life and the types of help being sought have significant effect on both organisational and operational police stress. The result confirmed that those who reported poor health status also reported high level of both organisational and operational police stress. Since this is an existing self-reported poor health condition, it is difficult to establish whether stress was responsible for the poor health status. Nevertheless, the result established a negative relationship between the two variables, indicating that self-reported poor health status can have a significant effect on self-reported stress in the police. The result also demonstrated that gender is a significant predictor of organisational police stress but not for operational police stress.

In this study, female police officers reported a relatively low organisational police stress than their male counterparts. Though, gender in this case corroborates previous studies, it however, contradicts previous studies that reported similar or a higher stress level in female officers than their male colleagues (see Idubor et al., 2015; Ogungbamila & Fajemirokun, 2016; Omolayo, 2012; Verma, Balhara, & Gupta, 2011; Wakil, 2015). While it is difficult to provide a simplistic explanation for this contradiction, it is important to point out that Nigeria is a complex society in which men are expected to be the breadwinner and the sole provider for both nuclear and extended families. The sociocultural expectations coupled with the challenges at work may likely be responsible for the higher stress level in policemen.

Overall, the current analysis confirms the divergent views in gender and stress research. For example, some studies indicated men are more susceptible to stress than their female counterparts (Morash et al., 2006; Violanti et al., 2016), some reported similar effects between male and female (Spielberger & Reheiser, 1994) and some supported Omolayo (2012)'s findings that females are more prone to work-related stress and other associated factors such as PTSD than males (Bowler et al., 2010). This study also established that police officers who sought unorthodox or alternative treatment for stress are more likely to experience both organisational and operational police stress. Invariably, this indicates that those who sought medical and psychological support will likely experience less stress or have better coping strategies.

The second part of the regression analyses assessed the effect of stress on the general well-being of police officers in Nigeria. In this analysis, age, gender, stress in the personal life of the police officers, types of help sought, and organisational police stress have significant effect on the general well-being of police officers. Specifically, the result revealed that younger policewomen, who had experienced stress in their personal lives, who had sought orthodox help for stress, as well as reported organisational police stress may likely report that stress has a lot of effect on their general well-being than their male counterparts. Among the variables and constructs in this analysis, 'stress in personal life' stands out with the highest beta value. This finding supports existing studies by confirming that prolonged personal experiences of stress could have a strong negative effect on general well-being (see Denovan & Macaskill, 2017; Wersebe, Lieb, Meyer, Hofer, & Gloster, 2018). Similarly, studies have shown that prolonged stress is associated with poor health and adverse health outcomes (Fawzy & Hamed, 2017), and that when challenges of personal stress exceed person's ability to cope effectively, it may likely have adverse effect on general well-being (Denovan & Macaskill, 2017; Fawzy & Hamed, 2017; Räsänen, Lappalainen, Muotka, Tolvanen, & Lappalainen, 2016). It is important to note that, though some of these studies are not primarily focused on policing, they are, however, relevant for comparative purposes.

Conclusion

This study provided an empirical understanding of the occurrence and prevalence of stress in the police as well as the effects of stress among police officers. The findings in this study, particularly, confirmed that the nature of police work and the stifling environment in which they work have significant effect on how police do their job. It also offered new insights on how stress associated with working for (and in) the police may impair their general well-being. To enhance the effectiveness of the police, police agencies must establish intervention programmes that are aimed at reducing stress and promoting coping strategies among the police. Such programmes should be designed to deal with and to address organisational and operational stressors. Also, it is important that specific stress management programmes be implemented for police officers in Nigeria.

Nigeria Police Force should initiate and adopt training programmes that would help 'supervisors' to identify signs of stress and to implement a stress reduction strategies and policies within and outside the police. In addition, officers should be encouraged to track their stressors by keeping journals of situations that create stress in their lives and their coping strategies or what they do to respond to them. Generally, officers should be exposed to stress management techniques such as developing healthy relationships at work, establishing boundaries, taking time off to recharge, keeping positive attitude, being assertive instead of aggressive at work and towards the positive, exercising regularly, eating healthy and well-balanced diets, and, finally, accepting that there are events that they cannot control but they can choose how to respond.

Lastly, since this study is among the few empirical pieces of research to address the issues of police stress in Nigeria, more work is clearly needed, especially in experimental or quasi-experimental research, to flesh out a finely nuanced questions that are not addressed in the current study. This will generate a body of work or evidence that can help guide future policies on police mental health and general well-being.

Appendix

Table 12.7 Percentages of each item in organisational police stress questionnaire

Variable items	1	2	3	4	5	6	7
Dealing with co-workers	6.7	4.1	6.5	7.9	19.5	25.8	29.5
The feeling that different rules apply to different people (e.g. favouritism)	5.7	1.7	1.3	7.5	13.5	22.1	48.3
Feeling like you always have to prove yourself to the organisation	0.8	0.6	3.5	7.4	18.4	20.3	49.0
Excessive administrative duties	1.0	2.5	3.3	10.1	19.5	22.5	41.1
Constant changes in policy/legislation	7.5	16.0	8.2	9.6	14.7	15.2	28.8
Staff shortages	6.7	1.7	1.3	3.7	16.0	16.9	53.8
Bureaucratic red tape	3.8	1.1	0.8	16.6	22.5	15.6	39.5
Too much computer work (or too much paperwork where there is no computer)	1.3	1.6	5.9	13.0	27.5	19.7	31.0
Lack of training on new equipment	4.7	1.1	0.8	0.3	27.5	20.7	44.9
Perceived pressure to volunteer free time	3.4	3.1	2.5	10.1	17.1	25.8	38.0
Dealing with supervisors	5.4	6.8	6.9	8.8	21.2	22.4	28.5
Inconsistent leadership style	3.0	7.4	6.7	8.8	16.3	21.8	36.1
Lack of resources	9.3	2.3	1.7	1.7	8.2	16.0	62.5
Unequal sharing of work responsibilities	7.5	3.8	2.8	6.7	19.0	21.2	39.0
If you are sick or injured, your co-workers seem to look down on you	21.5	23.9	42.4	3.7	2.4	2.5	3.5
Leaders overemphasise the negatives (e.g. supervisor evaluations, public complaints)	4.7	6.2	5.8	22.2	29.0	18.7	13.3

(continued)

Table 12.7 (continued)

Variable items	1	2	3	4	5	6	7
Internal investigations	11.9	14.9	16.7	22.9	28.2	2.8	2.8
Dealing the court system	23.1	31.2	35.6	3.7	0.7	4.2	1.6
The need to be accountable for doing your job	3.8	8.6	4.7	16.4	29.3	17.3	19.8
Inadequate equipment	6.7	2.5	1.4	1.7	11.2	24.6	51.8

Note: Responses ranged from No stress at all (1) to A lot of stress (7) and are expressed in percentages

Table 12.8 Percentages of each item in operational police stress questionnaire

Variable items	1	2	3	4	5	6	7
Shift work	6.2	5.4	4.5	10.8	21.8	21.7	29.6
Working alone at night	3.8	6.5	3.4	7.5	18.1	22.4	38.2
Overtime demands	2.5	1.4	3.7	6.9	17.4	17.0	51.0
Risk of being injured on the job	2.8	3.0	3.1	9.6	20.0	21.8	39.7
Work-related activities on days off (e.g. court, community events)	10.9	29.5	12.6	19.7	7.1	4.1	16.1
Traumatic events (e.g. MVA, domestics, death, injury)	19.7	20.1	29.7	5.8	5.1	7.4	12.2
Managing your social life outside of work	6.2	5.8	5.1	25.2	28.3	18.6	10.8
Not enough time available to spend with friends and family	3.4	2.5	5.7	10.1	26.8	20.1	31.4
Paperwork	4.0	5.5	4.0	14.7	28.3	21.7	21.8
Eating healthy at work	2.5	3.8	3.7	14.4	16.1	21.2	38.1
Finding time to stay in good physical condition (e.g. regular exercise)	7.1	5.9	5.0	12.0	22.8	21.8	25.4
Fatigue (e.g. shift work, overtime)	4.1	6.9	3.7	8.5	20.1	22.7	34.0
Occupation-related health issues (e.g. back pain)	2.4	1.6	4.5	8.1	17.6	19.1	46.7
Lack of understanding from family and friends about your work	3.3	3.0	3.8	10.1	22.2	22.7	35.0
Making friends outside the job	7.4	15.4	13.3	10.9	14.3	4.2	34.4
Upholding a 'higher image' in public	3.7	3.8	5.2	24.6	29.9	20.0	12.7
Negative comments from the public	1.8	2.7	3.4	3.4	26.9	7.4	54.4
Limitations to your social life (e.g. who your friends are, where you socialise)	3.8	3.3	5.9	10.5	27.6	21.4	27.5
Feeling like you are always on the job	3.5	6.2	4.2	16.0	28.6	22.2	19.1
Friends/family feel the effects of the stigma associated with your job	1.6	3.8	3.8	15.0	17.1	18.0	40.7

Note: Responses ranged from No stress at all (1) to A lot of stress (7) and are expressed in percentages

References

Adebayo, D., Sunmola, A., & Udegbe, I. (2008). Workplace fairness and emotional exhaustion in Nigeria police: The moderating role of gender. *Anxiety, Stress, and Coping, 21*(4), 405–416. https://doi.org/10.1080/10615800701415456

Adediran, I. (2020, 6 February). Police Inspector 'commits suicide' over murder charge. *Premium Times Nigeria*. Retrieved from https://www.premiumtimesng.com/news/top-news/375979-police-inspector-commits-suicide-over-murder-charge.html

Adegoke, T. (2014). Effects of occupational stress on psychological well-being of police employees in Ibadan Metropolis, Nigeria. *African Research Review, 8*(1), 302–320. https://doi.org/10.4314/afrrev.v8i1.19

Akinlabi, O. M. (2018). Why do Nigerians cooperate with the police? Legitimacy, procedural justice, and other contextual factors in Nigeria. In D. Oberwittler & S. Roche (Eds.), *Police-citizen relations across the world: Comparing sources and contexts of trust and legitimacy* (pp. 127–149). Routledge.

Akinlabi, O. M., & Murphy, K. (2018). Dull compulsion or perceived legitimacy? Assessing why people comply with the law in Nigeria. *Police Practice and Research, 19*(2), 186–201. https://doi.org/10.1080/15614263.2018.1418170

Alemika, E. O. (1988). Policing and perceptions of police in Nigeria. *Police Studies, 11*(4), 161–176. Retrieved from https://heinonline.org/HOL/LandingPage?handle=hein.journals/polic11&div=35&id=&page

Alexopoulos, E. C., Palatsidi, V., Tigani, X., & Darviri, C. (2014). Exploring stress levels, job satisfaction, and quality of life in a sample of police officers in Greece. *Safety and Health at Work, 5*(4), 210–215. https://doi.org/10.1016/j.shaw.2014.07.004

Anderson, G. S., Litzenberger, R., & Plecas, D. (2002). Physical evidence of police officer stress. *Policing: An International Journal of Police Strategies & Management, 25*(2), 399–420. https://doi.org/10.1108/13639510210429437

Anshel, M. H. (2000). A conceptual model and implications for coping with stressful events in police work. *Criminal Justice and Behavior, 27*(3), 375–400. https://doi.org/10.1177/0093854800027003006

Anshel, M. H., Robertson, M., & Caputi, P. (1997). Sources of acute stress and their appraisals and reappraisals among Australian police as a function of previous experience. *Journal of Occupational and Organizational Psychology, 70*(4), 337–356. https://doi.org/10.1111/j.2044-8325.1997.tb00653.x

Barnes, S., Brown, K. W., Krusemark, E., Campbell, W. K., & Rogge, R. D. (2007). The role of mindfulness in romantic relationship satisfaction and responses to relationship stress. *Journal of Marital and Family Therapy,* *33*(4), 482–500. https://doi.org/10.1111/j.1752-0606.2007.00033.x

Bowler, R. M., Han, H., Gocheva, V., Nakagawa, S., Alper, H., DiGrande, L., et al. (2010). Gender differences in probable posttraumatic stress disorder among police responders to the 2001 World Trade Center terrorist attack. *American Journal of Industrial Medicine, 53*(12), 1186–1196. https://doi.org/10.1002/ajim.20876

Bunker, S. J., Colquhoun, D. M., Esler, M. D., Hickie, I. B., Hunt, D., Jelinek, V. M., et al. (2003). "Stress" and coronary heart disease: psychosocial risk factors. *Medical Journal of Australia, 178*(6), 272–276. https://doi.org/10.5694/j.1326-5377.2003.tb05193.x

Can, S. H., Hendy, H. M., & Karagoz, T. (2015). LEOSS-R: four types of police stressors and negative psychosocial outcomes associated with them. *Policing: A Journal of Policy and Practice, 9*(4), 340–351. https://doi.org/10.1093/police/pav011

Cannizzaro, E., Cirrincione, L., Mazzucco, W., Scorciapino, A., Catalano, C., Ramaci, T., et al. (2020). Night-time shift work and related stress responses: A study on security guards. *International Journal of Environmental Research and Public Health, 17*(2), 562. https://doi.org/10.3390/ijerph17020562

Chapin, M., Brannen, S. J., Singer, M. I., & Walker, M. (2008). Training police leadership to recognize and address operational stress. *Police Quarterly, 11*(3), 338–352. https://doi.org/10.1177/1098611107307736

Chopko, B. A., Palmieri, P. A., & Facemire, V. C. (2014). Prevalence and predictors of suicidal ideation among US law enforcement officers. *Journal of Police and Criminal Psychology, 29*(1), 1–9. https://doi.org/10.1007/s11896-013-9116-z

Collins, P., & Gibbs, A. (2003). Stress in police officers: A study of the origins, prevalence and severity of stress-related symptoms within a county police force. *Occupational Medicine, 53*(4), 256–264. https://doi.org/10.1093/occmed/kqg061

Cullen, F. T., Lemming, T., Link, B. G., & Wozniak, J. F. (1985). The impact of social supports on police stress. *Criminology, 23*(3), 503–522. https://doi.org/10.1111/j.1745-9125.1985.tb00351.x

de Rijk, A. (2020). Coronary heart disease and return to work. *Handbook of Disability, Work and Health,* 1–20. https://doi.org/10.1007/978-3-319-75381-2_24-1

Dempsey, J. S., & Forst, L. S. (2019). *An introduction to policing* (9th ed.). Cengage Learning.

Denovan, A., & Macaskill, A. (2017). Stress and subjective well-being among first year UK undergraduate students. *Journal of Happiness Studies, 18*(2), 505–525. https://doi.org/10.1007/s10902-016-9736-y

Fawzy, M., & Hamed, S. A. (2017). Prevalence of psychological stress, depression and anxiety among medical students in Egypt. *Psychiatry Research, 255*, 186–194. https://doi.org/10.1016/j.psychres.2017.05.027

Field, A. (2018). *Discovering statistics using IBM SPSS statistics* (5th ed.). Sage.

Gerber, M., Hartmann, T., Brand, S., Holsboer-Trachsler, E., & Pühse, U. (2010). The relationship between shift work, perceived stress, sleep and health in Swiss police officers. *Journal of Criminal Justice, 38*(6), 1167–1175. https://doi.org/10.1016/j.jcrimjus.2010.09.005

Guile, G., Tredoux, C., & Foster, D. (1998). Inherent and organisational stress in the SAPS: An empirical survey in the Western Cape. *South Africa Journal of Psychology, 28*(3), 129–134. https://doi.org/10.1177/008124639802800302

Hanson, L. L. M., Rod, N. H., Vahtera, J., Virtanen, M., Ferrie, J., Shipley, M., et al. (2020). Job insecurity and risk of coronary heart disease: Mediation analyses of health behaviors, sleep problems, physiological and psychological factors. *Psychoneuroendocrinology, 118*, 104706. https://doi.org/10.1016/j.psyneuen.2020.104706

Idubor, E., Aihie, J. O., & Igiebor, G. O. (2015). The effect of occupational stress on health status of public officers: The case of Nigeria police. *International Journal of Development and Sustainability, 4*(4), 398–414. https://www.semanticscholar.org/paper/The-effect-of-occupational-stress-on-health-status-Idubor-Aihie/182bc5ecf2900063a8588377 19707bb 0eb4f398b

Jensen, J. H., Flachs, E. M., Skakon, J., Rod, N. H., Bonde, J. P., & Kawachi, I. (2019). Work-unit organizational changes and risk of cardiovascular disease: A prospective study of public healthcare employees in Denmark. *International Archives of Occupational and Environmental Health, 93*(4), 409–419. https://doi.org/10.1007/s00420-019-01493-6

John-Akinola, Y. O., Ajayi, A. O., & Oluwasanu, M. M. (2020). Experience of stress and coping mechanism among police officers in south western Nigeria. *International Quarterly of Community Health Education, 41*(1), 7–14. https://doi.org/10.1177/0272684x19900878

Keyes, K. M., Hatzenbuehler, M. L., & Hasin, D. S. (2011). Stressful life experiences, alcohol consumption, and alcohol use disorders: The epidemiologic evidence for four main types of stressors. *Psychopharmacology, 218*(1), 1–17. https://doi.org/10.1007/s00213-011-2236-1

Lateef, A. (2019). *Exploring the factors responsible for occupational stress among police officers in Nigeria.* Minnesota: Walden University.

Ma, C. C., Andrew, M. E., Fekedulegn, D., Gu, J. K., Hartley, T. A., Charles, L. E., et al. (2015). Shift work and occupational stress in police officers. *Safety and Health at Work, 6*(1), 25–29. https://doi.org/10.1016/j.shaw.2014.10.001

McCreary, D. R., & Thompson, M. M. (2006). Development of two reliable and valid measures of stressors in policing: The operational and organizational police stress questionnaires. *International Journal of Stress Management, 13*(4), 494–518. https://doi.org/10.1037/1072-5245.13.4.494

Miller, L. (2005). Police officer suicide: Causes, prevention, and practical intervention strategies. *International Journal of Emergency Mental Health, 7*(2), 101. https://pubmed.ncbi.nlm.nih.gov/16107042/

Morash, M., Kwak, D. H., & Haarr, R. (2006). Gender differences in the predictors of police stress. *Policing: An International Journal of Police Strategies & Management.* https://doi.org/10.1108/13639510610684755

Newman, J. E., & Beehr, T. A. (1979). Personal and organizational strategies for handling job stress: A review of research and opinion. *Personnel Psychology, 32*(1), 1–43. https://doi.org/10.1111/j.1744-6570.1979.tb00467.x

Odedokun, S. A. (2015). Differential influence of demographic factors on job burnout among police officers in Ibadan, Oyo state. *Mediterranean Journal of Social Sciences, 6*(3 S1), 520. https://doi.org/10.5901/mjss.2015.v6n3s1p520

Ogungbamila, B., & Fajemirokun, I. (2016). Job stress and police burnout: Moderating roles of gender and marital status. *IAFOR Journal of Psychology and the Behavioural Sciences, 2*(3), 17–32. https://doi.org/10.22492/ijpbs.2.3.02

Omolayo, B. (2012). Effect of gender and status on job stress among police officers in Ekti State of Nigeria. *Bangladesh e-Journal of Sociology, 9*(1), 38–42. Retrieved from https://www.researchgate.net/publication/329281893_Effect_of_Gender_and_Status_on_Job_Stress_among_Police_Officers_in_Ekti_State_of_Nigeria

Pallant, J. (2010). *SPSS survival manual: A step by step guide to data analysis using SPSS.* McGraw-Hill.

Purba, A., & Demou, E. (2019). The relationship between organisational stressors and mental wellbeing within police officers: A systematic review. *BMC Public Health, 19*(1), 1286. https://doi.org/10.1186/s12889-019-7609-0

Räsänen, P., Lappalainen, P., Muotka, J., Tolvanen, A., & Lappalainen, R. (2016). An online guided ACT intervention for enhancing the psychological wellbeing of university students: A randomized controlled clinical trial. *Behaviour Research and Therapy, 78*, 30–42. https://doi.org/10.1016/j.brat.2016.01.001

Renden, P. G., Landman, A., Daalder, N. R., de Cock, H. P., Savelsbergh, G. J., & Oudejans, R. R. (2017). Effects of threat, trait anxiety and state anxiety on police officers' actions during an arrest. *Legal and Criminological Psychology, 22*(1), 116–129. https://doi.org/10.1111/lcrp.12077

Spielberger, C. D., & Reheiser, E. C. (1994). The job stress survey: Measuring gender differences in occupational stress. *Journal of Social Behavior and Personality, 9*(2), 199. Retrieved from https://psycnet.apa.org/record/1995-03735-001

Tabachnick, B. G., & Fidell, L. S. (2013). *Using multivariate statistics* (6th ed.). Pearson.

The American Institute of Stress. (2020). *Workplace Stress.* The American Institute of Stress. Retrieved 20 June from https://www.stress.org/workplace-stress

Verma, R., Balhara, Y. P. S., & Gupta, C. S. (2011). Gender differences in stress response: Role of developmental and biological determinants. *Industrial Psychiatry Journal, 20*(1), 4. https://doi.org/10.4103/0972-6748.98407

Violanti, J. M., & Aron, F. (1994). Ranking police stressors. *Psychological Reports, 75*(2), 824–826. https://doi.org/10.2466/pr0.1994.75.2.824

Violanti, J. M., Fekedulegn, D., Andrew, M. E., Hartley, T. A., Charles, L. E., Miller, D. B., et al. (2017). The impact of perceived intensity and frequency of police work occupational stressors on the cortisol awakening response (CAR): Findings from the BCOPS study. *Psychoneuroendocrinology, 75*, 124–131. https://doi.org/10.1016/j.psyneuen.2016.10.017

Violanti, J. M., Fekedulegn, D., Hartley, T. A., Charles, L. E., Andrew, M. E., Ma, C. C., et al. (2016). Highly rated and most frequent stressors among police officers: Gender differences. *American Journal of Criminal Justice, 41*(4), 645–662. https://doi.org/10.1007/s12103-016-9342-x

Wakil, A. A. (2015). Occupational stress among Nigerian police officers: An examination of the coping strategies and the consequences. *African Research Review, 9*(4), 16–26. https://doi.org/10.4314/afrrev.v9i4.2

Wersebe, H., Lieb, R., Meyer, A. H., Hofer, P., & Gloster, A. T. (2018). The link between stress, well-being, and psychological flexibility during an Acceptance and Commitment Therapy self-help intervention. *International Journal of Clinical and Health Psychology, 18*(1), 60–68. https://doi.org/10.1016/j.ijchp.2017.09.002

13

A Study of Drug Use and Socio-Demographic Characteristics of Male Prisoners in Ghana

Feikoab Parimah, Jonathan Osei Owusu, and Sylvester Anthony Appiah-Honny

Introduction

Over the years, nations around the world have battled drug use and its attendant problems. Aning and Pokoo (2014) and Klantschnig (2016) indicated that the problem of narcotics is prevalent in African countries, especially in West Africa. Kumah-Abiwu (2019) supported this assertion. The West Africa Commission on Drugs (2014) declared that the increasing use of narcotic drugs within West Africa is a serious public health issue. Drug use has led to thousands of deaths in Africa (United Nations Office on Drugs and Crime, 2015).

F. Parimah (✉)
Basic Research, Advocacy and Initiative Networks, Accra, Ghana

Department of Psychology, University of Western Cape, Cape Town, South Africa

J. O. Owusu • S. A. Appiah-Honny
POS Foundation, Accra, Ghana

© The Author(s), under exclusive license to Springer Nature Switzerland AG 2021
H. C. O. Chan, S. Adjorlolo (eds.), *Crime, Mental Health and the Criminal Justice System in Africa*, https://doi.org/10.1007/978-3-030-71024-8_13

The prevalence of crimes such as robbery and narcotics trafficking in Ghana has been documented (Oteng-Ababio, Owusu, Wrigley-Asante, & Owusu, 2016). Affinnih (1999a) indicated that the most frequently abused drugs in Accra, Ghana, are marijuana, cocaine and heroin. Most drug users (about 79%) in that study were addicted to drugs, and 33% funded their use through illegal means such as stealing. Although it is not indigenous to Africa, marijuana is the drug most commonly abused in Ghana (Affinnih, 1999b), and it is considered a problem that permeates the social strata in Ghana (Adu-Gyamfi & Brenya, 2015).

Drug Use in Prison

Drug use among prisoners has been established in the literature. Kolind and Duke (2016) noted that many prisoners use drugs, and that most people who use drugs have probably been in prison. Prisons are a high-risk environment for drug initiation and use (Kolind & Duke, 2016), and marijuana is the most commonly used drug in such institutions (Ritter, Broers, & Elger, 2013). Prisoners' 'concern for time seems to be an almost constant and painful state of mind' (Galtung, 1961, p. 113), and they therefore use marijuana and other illicit drugs to help them cope with their sentences. Drug use in prison is not only a coping strategy for prisoners (Bengtsson, 2012), it is also a part of prisoner social networks, culture and economics (Wheatley, 2007). O'Hagan and Hardwick (2017) asserted that the use of drugs in prison is enabled by the social relationships that are more easily established among drug users.

Demand for drugs has encouraged the growth of drug supply, distribution and trade in prison. The supply of drugs in prison can come from an external source, such as visitors, or an internal source, such as among prisoners (Turnbull, Stimson, & Stillwell, 1994). The use of marijuana and heroin among prisoners depends on their prison's establishment of control strategies (Bullock, 2003). Tompkins (2015) noted that the use of drugs in prisons is linked to prison policy and the availability of drugs.

Several studies have suggested that drug supply is irregular in prison, leading prisoners to use drugs occasionally (Mjåland, 2016) or change their drug use pattern (Bullock, 2003). Bullock (2003) posited that the unavailability of desirable drugs hinders prisoners' maintenance of problematic drug use levels. There is a high probability that recently incarcerated heroin users will switch to other opiates depending on availability (Kolind & Duke, 2016).

Drug Use in Prisons in Africa

Drug use among prisoners has been observed in some African countries (e.g., Kinyanjui & Atwoli, 2013; Uganda Prisons Service, 2009). The use of marijuana, heroin, cocaine, amphetamine, tranquilisers and sedatives has been recorded among inmates in a prison in Kenya (Kinyanjui & Atwoli, 2013). Uganda Prisons Service (2009) reported that lifetime drug use (e.g., marijuana, cigarettes/tobacco and alcohol) among the prison population is high in Uganda. The use of marijuana is a problem that cuts across the social strata in Ghana (Adu-Gyamfi & Brenya, 2015). However, little is known about marijuana use in prisons in Ghana.

Age and Drug Use in Prison

Several studies have found an association between age and drug use in prison (Cope, 2000; Edgar & O'Donnell, 1998). Edgar and O'Donnell (1998) showed that adult prisoners reported more drug use in prison than young prisoners. Similarly, Arndt, Turvey, and Flaum (2002) observed that older prisoners were more likely to use alcohol than younger prisoners. Nevertheless, Davoren et al. (2015) reported that younger prisoners used more illicit drugs than older prisoners, and this finding was confirmed by Fazel, Hayes, Bartellas, Clerici, and Trestman (2016). Cope (2000) found that among prisoners aged between 16 and 21 years, marijuana was the most commonly used drug. Cope (2000) added that many of the study participants had used the drug prior to incarceration. The prison environment forced them to modify their drug use, but marijuana remained the drug that they most commonly abused.

Parker, Aldridge, and Measham (1998) explained that normalisation accounts for why young people use drugs. Normalisation refers to the process through which 'stigmatized or deviant individuals or groups become included in many features of everyday life as their identities or behaviour become increasingly accommodated and perhaps eventually valued' (Parker, 2005, p. 205). Many scholars have used normalisation to understand drug use among adolescents and young adults, and Erickson and Hathaway (2010) called for the theory to be extended to adults. Extending the theory of normalisation to adults requires considering contextual and cultural factors associated with illicit drug use rather than narrowly focusing on peer influence and the individual (Duff et al., 2012). Pennay and Moore (2010) stressed the importance of examining specific contexts and settings within which drugs are used and argued that normalisation works differently in diverse settings. Duff et al. (2012) demonstrated that normalisation theory could be extended to adults and other contexts. Normalisation may help explain the prevalence of drug use among older adults (Edgar & O'Donnell, 1998) and younger adults in prison (Cope, 2000).

Younger prisoners may be more organised, ensuring the effective distribution of drugs in prison (Cope, 2000). Moreover, older prisoners are likely to experience the loss of friends, loved ones and their social networks (Majekodunmi, Obadeji, Oluwole, & Oyelami, 2017). This factor may affect the rate at which people outside prison can give drugs to adult prisoners. Young prisoners are more likely than adults to have more extensive social networks and more contacts outside prison, which may facilitate their drug use by regularly providing supply.

Being an older adult prisoner does not necessarily mean that one is nearing the end of a sentence. Cope (2000) showed that prisoners often modified their drug use for particular gains, such as parole. Those who have served long periods in prison and are nearing the end of their sentences may change their behaviour (Cope, 2000). This dynamic may account for the variation in drug use between older and younger prisoners. Based on this premise, in this study, we asked, 'what is the association between age and the use of marijuana and other drugs among prisoners in Ghana?' We sought to reveal the association between age and drug use among prisoners, which has yet to be established in the Ghanaian context.

Robbery, Recidivism and Drug Use

The type of offense committed has been shown to be associated with specific types of drug use. Offenders who test positive for the use of drugs such as marijuana at the time of arrest (Zhang, 2004) may continue to use drugs in prison (Tompkins, 2015). Brochu et al. (2001) documented that among prisoners in Canada (from within the past six months to time of incarceration), 33.7% and 24.5% had used drugs and marijuana, respectively, at least once a week. Further, they showed that 25% indicated using illicit drugs on the day of the robbery. The association between psychoactive drug use and criminality is the onset of addiction and the funds needed to finance addiction (Brochu et al., 2001). Pernanen, Cousineau, Brochu, and Sun (2002) documented that 25% of prisoners in a federal prison in Canada reported that they had committed robbery to buy drugs, and 12% had committed robbery to buy alcohol and other illicit drugs.

Drug abuse has been associated with criminal recidivism (Mannerfelt & Håkansson, 2018). Belenko (2006) indicated that there is a high probability that prisoners who use drugs often in prison will reoffend. Prisoners with drug use problems who are not rehabilitated in prison are likely to reoffend when released into society to raise funds to finance their drug use. Although there have been reports of recidivism rates in Ghana, they have been unreliable due to a lack of proper mechanisms to distinguish between first-time offenders and reoffenders (Antwi, 2015). The extent of the association between reoffending and drug use in Ghana is unknown.

We sought to answer the following questions: (1) What is the relationship between a first-time robbery conviction and the use of marijuana or other drugs among prisoners in Ghana? (2) What is the relationship between a reoffending robbery conviction and the use of marijuana or other drugs among prisoners in Ghana?

Mental Health and the Criminal Justice System

There is empirical evidence that child abuse survivors may engage in drug abuse later in life (Kendler et al., 2000). Swogger, Conner, Walsh, and Maisto (2011) showed a significant association between surviving child abuse and drug use among prisoners. This finding is consistent with the finding of Sergentanis et al. (2014) that childhood maltreatment is associated with illicit drug use among male prisoners in Greece. People may use addictive drugs to cope with the stress associated with traumatic childhood experiences (Teixeira, Lasiuk, Barton, Fernandes, & Gherardi-Donato, 2017). Offenders who are not screened for possible therapy before or during incarceration, may end up using drugs and compounding their problems.

Mental Health and the Criminal Justice System in Ghana

A relatively large proportion of people in Ghana have mental illnesses (Read & Doku, 2012), and individuals in the Ghanaian criminal justice system may have mental health issues (Adjorlolo, 2016). Two possible contributing factors include the non-existence of systematic routine mental illness screenings at court and in prison and criminal justice officers' bias against offenders with mental illness (Adjorlolo, 2016). People in conflict with the law who have mental illnesses may be processed through the criminal justice system (Edgely, 2009). Ibrahim, Esena, Aikins, O'Keefe, and McKay (2015) found that more than half of the inmate population at a prison in Ghana showed signs of severe mental distress. Prisoners' mental distress and subsequent drug use may result from child abuse, as suggested by Teixeira et al. (2017). This type of offender should be identified through proper screening channels and receive some form of therapy in prison. Unfortunately, the prison system in Ghana does not perform screenings (Adjorlolo, 2016).

Part of the diversion legislation in Ghana, Act 846, states that 'a person arrested for a criminal act and in police custody shall be assessed by a mental health practitioner within forty-eight hours if there is suspicion of mental disorder' (Section 76 (1), p. 34). This mandate requires police officers to legally divert offenders with mental illness from the criminal justice system. However, offenders who have survived child abuse are probably being processed through Ghana's criminal justice system. The lack of routine systematic mental illness screening of offenders in Ghana (Adjorlolo, 2016) means that it is probable that this category of offender is not receiving appropriate attention. We argue that this category of offender is likely to use drugs in prison to help them cope (Teixeira et al., 2017) and that they should be identified for possible therapy. In this study, we asked, 'what is the association between child abuse and marijuana or other drug use among prisoners in Ghana?'

Materials and Methods

Study Setting, Population and Sample

Ghana has 44 prisons, which are generally classified as juvenile, special, open and agriculture settlement camp, local, female, maximum security, medium security or central (Ghana Prisons Service, 2019). The current prison population in Ghana is 15,463 (World Prison Brief, 2019). The Ghana Prisons Service (2019) stated that 98.8% of the total prison population is male and 1.2% is female. In 2015, 234 inmates were convicted of narcotic drug possession, whereas 3267 and 501 were convicted of stealing and robbery, respectively (Ghana Prisons Service, 2019). Using a cross-sectional survey, we purposively sampled 253 male prisoners (average age = 31.26, SD = 10.19) from the Nsawam Medium Security Prison and the Kumasi and Takoradi Central Prisons. These facilities host some of the largest inmate populations in Ghana and include different types of offenders. In this study, we only included prisoners who had been convicted of offenses that were property related or against an individual or public order. The participants also needed to be literate in English. Inmates who were convicted of murder and were serving life sentences were excluded from the study. Most of the participants were Christian (n = 200), and many had attained secondary education (n = 118; Table 13.1). Eighty-four (36.5%) of the participants had been convicted of robbery for the first time, whereas 33 (14.0%) were robbery reoffenders (Table 13.1). Less than half of the participants indicated that they had suffered child abuse (44.9%).

Table 13.1 Demographic characteristics of participants

Variable	Total (%)
Ever suffered childhood abuse (Yes = 110, No = 135)	110 (44.9)
Age: Mean = 31.26 (*SD* = 10.19)	
First time of being convicted for robbery (Yes = 84, No = 146)	84 (36.5)
Re-offender—robbery (Yes = 33, No = 203)	33 (14.0)
Educational level:	
Primary	13 (5.2)
Junior high school	73 (29.1)
Senior high school	118 (47.0)
Tertiary	47 (18.7)
Religious affiliation:	
Christian	200 (80.3)
Muslim	31 (12.4)
Traditional	9 (3.6)
Other	9 (3.6)

Data Collection Procedure

We obtained ethics approval (protocol: NMIMR-IRB 087/17-18) from the Noguchi Memorial Institute for Medical Research, an institutional review board (IRB) at the University of Ghana. The Ghana Prisons Service granted us access to male prisoners at the Nsawam Medium Security Prison and the Takoradi and Kumasi Central Prisons. First, a prison officer informed the prefects (i.e., representatives of cells who are mandated to maintain order) and asked them to announce the study and invite inmates to participate. The exact number of prisoners who heard the prefects' announcements was not disclosed to the researchers. Those who showed interest in the study were brought to the prison officer in charge, who escorted them to an office (i.e., in the Nsawam and Takoradi prisons) and a classroom (i.e., in the Kumasi prison) where the questionnaire was self-administered. Groups of five to seven people completed their questionnaires at a time. There was a maximum of seven participants in each group due to the small size of the office (in the Nsawam and Takoradi prisons) and classroom (in the Kumasi prison). Every participant was allocated an independent desk in the office or classroom. The participants were not allowed to take the questionnaires to their cells.

Although a prison officer was present while the participants completed the questionnaires, he sat at a distance so that he could not see the participants' responses. The researchers addressed the participants in groups of five to seven, explaining the aims of the study and asking the participants to sign a consent form. The authors ensured that the participants' concerns were addressed regarding items on the questionnaire that were unclear to them. The participants were also assured of the confidentiality of their responses. To allay their fears, the researchers told the participants that the study was not being conducted on behalf of any security agency, including the Ghana Prisons Service. To maintain the participants' anonymity, we assigned codes to the completed questionnaires so that responses could not be linked to individuals. The completed questionnaires were dropped in a box provided in the office. The participants did not hand over the questionnaires to the researchers or the prison officer. It took 15 minutes on average for the participants to complete the questionnaires. The study did not pose any risk to the participants.

Data Collection Measure

The first part of the questionnaire requested demographic information, such as age, highest education level attained and religious affiliation. It also elicited information regarding childhood abuse and offending history. We included items such as 'This is the first time that I have been convicted of taking someone's belongings/property with force' and 'This is the second/more time that I have been convicted of taking someone's belongings/property with force' to determine whether the inmates were robbery reoffenders. To determine whether the participants had ever experienced child abuse, we asked, 'Were you abused as a child?' Eleven items on the questionnaire measured the respondent's history of drug use. Several of those items were excluded from the analysis in this study because they were part of a broader study that also elicited information from the general public. To determine the respondents' drug use within different timeframes, we asked, 'Have you used marijuana within the past year?', 'Have you ever used any other drugs?', 'Do you currently use marijuana?' and 'Do you currently use any other drugs?'. The researchers clarified to the participants that 'ever used' and 'presently use' referred to the past year and the past 30 days, respectively. Except for the item for age, participants were asked to respond either 'Yes' or 'No' to all of the items used in the analysis. To ensure that the items elicited the required responses, we provided other names for marijuana in the items that measured marijuana use. The items were crafted based on the first author's experience in gathering information regarding drug use and recommendations from members of the ethics committee of the Noguchi Memorial Institute for Medical Research. We also followed guidance from Friestad and Kjelsberg (2009), who simply asked their participants to indicate all of the types of drugs they had ever used. They also asked prisoners to indicate their number of incarcerations (Friestad & Hansen, 2005).

Data Analysis

First, we inputted the data into IBM SPSS version 22. Then, due to the dichotomous responses of the dependent variables, we used binary logistic regression to perform our data analysis. The independent variables were continuous (i.e., age) and dichotomous (i.e., a history of child abuse and a history of offending behaviour). The objective of the study was to reveal any possible associations between age, a history of child abuse, a history of offending behaviour and a history of marijuana or other drug use, which are not measured on an interval or ratio scale. Thus, binary logistic regression was the appropriate statistical test to perform. The dichotomous variables were dummy coded before we began the analysis.

Results

Less than half of the participants had used marijuana (40.7%), and less than a third had used other drugs (27.2%) within the past year (Table 13.2). Eighty-two (32.8%) had used marijuana within the past 30 days, and 17.7% had used other drugs within the same period (Table 13.2).

The logistic regression analysis results show that two of the variables, age and child abuse, significantly contributed to whether an offender

Table 13.2 Prevalence of drug use among participants

Drug use	Yes (%)	No (%)
Ever used marijuana within the past year	101 (40.7)	147 (59.3)
Ever used any other drug within the past year	68 (27.2)	182 (72.8)
Ever used marijuana within the past 30 days	82 (32.8)	168 (67.2)
Ever used any other drug within the past 30 days	44 (17.7)	204 (82.3)

Table 13.3 Summary of logistic regression analysis for variables predicting whether a prisoner had ever used marijuana within the past year

Predictors	B	SE	Wald χ^2	p	e^B	95% CI
Age	−0.04	0.02	4.22	0.040*	0.96	[0.93, 0.99]
Ever been abused during childhood	1.02	0.31	10.74	0.001***	2.78	[1.51, 5.11]
Ever been convicted of robbery	0.39	0.32	1.49	0.222	1.48	[0.79, 2.77]
Re-offender-robbery	0.55	0.46	1.40	0.236	1.73	[0.69, 4.27]

*$p < 0.05$, ***$p < 0.001$; model- $\chi^2 = 24.22$ ($df = 4$, $p < 0.001$); Hosmer-Lemeshow goodness-of-fit test: $\chi^2 = 6.86$ ($df = 4$, $p > 0.05$); Nagelkerke's adjusted $R^2 = 0.15$

used marijuana within the past year (Table 13.3). The Hosmer–Lemeshow goodness-of-fit result is not significant ($\chi^2_{(4, n = 197)} = 6.86$, $p > 0.05$). There is no significant difference between the observed probabilities and the theoretical model probabilities. Thus, the model had a good fit. We conclude that the equation containing the variables (Table 13.3) explains 15% (Nagelkerke's adjusted $R^2 = 0.15$) of the variance in whether a prisoner used marijuana within the past year. Compared with younger prisoners, older prisoners were less likely to have used marijuana within the past year ($OR = 0.96$, $p = 0.040$). Prisoners with or without a robbery conviction were equally likely to have used marijuana within the past year ($OR = 1.48$, $p > 0.05$). Those who were robbery reoffenders and those who were not were equally likely to have used marijuana within the past year ($OR = 1.73$, $p > 0.05$). Prisoners who had been abused in childhood were about three times more likely to have used marijuana within the past year than those who had not been abused in childhood ($OR = 2.78$, $p < 0.001$).

Table 13.4 Summary of logistic regression analysis for variables predicting whether a prisoner had ever used any other drugs within the past year

Predictors	B	SE	Wald χ^2	p	e^B	95% CI
Age	−0.05	0.02	4.96	0.026*	0.95	[0.91, 0.99]
Ever been abused during childhood	0.94	0.35	7.19	0.007**	2.56	[1.28, 5.09]
Ever been convicted of robbery	0.45	0.35	1.62	0.204	1.56	[0.78, 3.11]
Re-offender-robbery	1.78	0.48	13.64	0.000***	5.94	[2.31, 15.27]

*$p < 0.05$, **$p < 0.01$, ***$p < 0.001$; model- $\chi^2 = 35.72$ ($df = 4$, $p < 0.001$); Hosmer–Lemeshow goodness-of-fit test: $\chi^2 = 17.54$ ($df = 4$, $p = 0.025$); Nagelkerke's adjusted $R^2 = 0.23$

The logistic regression analysis results indicate that three of the variables, age, child abuse and robbery reoffending, significantly contributed to whether a prisoner had used any other drugs within the past year (Table 13.4). The Hosmer–Lemeshow goodness-of-fit result is not very good ($\chi^2_{(4, n = 198)} = 17.54$, $p = 0.025$). There could be a difference between the theoretical model probabilities and the observed probabilities. Although the model is not a very good fit, it affords a good classification in 72.7% of the cases. We conclude that the equation containing the variables (Table 13.4) explains 23% (Nagelkerke's adjusted $R^2 = 0.23$) of the variation in whether a prisoner used any other drugs within the past year. Prisoners who were older were less likely to have used other drugs within the past year ($OR = 0.95$, $p = 0.026$). Prisoners with or without a robbery conviction were equally likely not to have used any other drugs within the past year ($OR = 1.56$, $p > 0.05$). Those who were robbery reoffenders were about six times more likely to have used other drugs within the past year than those who were not ($OR = 5.94$, $p < 0.001$). Prisoners who had experienced child abuse were about three times more likely to have used other drugs within the past year than those who had not been abused in childhood ($OR = 2.56$, $p = 0.007$).

The logistic regression analysis results show that all of the variables—age, child abuse, robbery conviction and robbery reoffending—significantly contributed to whether a prisoner had used marijuana within the past 30 days (Table 13.5). The Hosmer–Lemeshow goodness-of-fit result

Table 13.5 Summary of logistic regression analysis for variables predicting whether a prisoner had ever used marijuana within the past 30 days

Predictors	B	SE	Wald χ^2	p	e^B	95% CI
Age	−0.04	0.02	3.58	0.059*	0.96	[0.92, 1.00]
Ever been abused during childhood	1.41	0.36	15.89	0.000***	4.11	[2.05, 8.24]
Ever been convicted of robbery	1.01	0.35	8.27	0.004***	2.73	[1.37, 5.42]
Re-offender-robbery	1.42	0.48	8.75	0.003***	4.13	[1.61, 10.55]

*$p < 0.05$, ***$p < 0.001$; model- $\chi^2 = 46.62$ ($df = 4$, $p < 0.001$); Hosmer-Lemeshow goodness-of-fit test: $\chi^2 = 4.63$ ($df = 4$, $p > 0.05$); Nagelkerke's adjusted $R^2 = 0.29$

is not significant ($\chi^2_{(4, n = 199)} = 4.63$, $p > 0.05$). There is no significant difference between the theoretical model probabilities and the observed probabilities; thus, the model had a good fit. The equation containing the variables (Table 13.5) explains 29% (Nagelkerke's adjusted $R^2 = 0.29$) of the variation in whether a prisoner had used marijuana within the past 30 days. Those who were older were less likely to have used marijuana within the past 30 days ($OR = 0.96$, $p = 0.059$). Prisoners who had been convicted of robbery were about twice as likely to have used marijuana within the past 30 days as those without a robbery conviction ($OR = 2.73$, $p = 0.004$). Similarly, those who were robbery reoffenders were about four times as likely to have used marijuana within the past 30 days as those who were not robbery reoffenders ($OR = 4.13$, $p = 0.003$). Prisoners who were abused as children were about four times more likely to have used marijuana within the past 30 days than those who were not abused in childhood ($OR = 4.11$, $p = 0.001$).

The logistic regression analysis results show that all of the variables—age, child abuse, robbery conviction and robbery reoffending—significantly contributed to whether a prisoner had used any other drugs within the past 30 days (Table 13.6). The Hosmer–Lemeshow goodness-of-fit test result is not significant ($\chi^2_{(4, n = 198)} = 6.92$, $p > 0.05$). There is no difference between the theoretical model probabilities and the observed probabilities; thus, the model had a good fit. The equation containing the variables (Table 13.6) explains 23% (Nagelkerke adjusted $R^2 = 0.23$) of

Table 13.6 Summary of logistic regression analysis for variables predicting whether a prisoner had ever used any other drugs within the past 30 days

Predictors	B	SE	Wald χ^2	p	e^B	95% CI
Age	−0.05	0.03	4.01	0.045*	0.95	[0.90, 0.99]
Ever been abused during childhood	1.04	0.42	6.07	0.014**	2.84	[1.24, 6.51]
Ever been convicted of robbery	0.78	0.41	3.65	0.056*	2.19	[0.98, 4.89]
Re-offender-robbery	1.75	0.49	12.93	0.000***	5.73	[2.21, 14.83]

*$p < 0.05$, **$p < 0.01$, ***$p < 0.001$; model- $\chi^2 = 30.78$ ($df = 4$, $p < 0.001$); Hosmer-Lemeshow goodness-of-fit test: $\chi^2 = 6.92$ ($df = 4$, $p > 0.05$); Nagelkerke's adjusted $R^2 = 0.23$

the variation in whether a prisoner had used any other drugs within the past 30 days. Compared with younger prisoners, older prisoners were less likely to have used any other drugs within the past 30 days ($OR = 0.95$, $p = 0.045$). Prisoners who had been convicted of robbery were about twice as likely to have used other drugs within the past 30 days as those without a robbery conviction ($OR = 2.19$, $p = 0.056$). Those who were robbery reoffenders were about six times more likely to have used other drugs within the past 30 days than those who were not robbery reoffenders ($OR = 5.73$, $p < 0.001$). Prisoners who had experienced child abuse were about three times more likely to have used other drugs within the past 30 days than those who had not been abused in childhood ($OR = 2.84$, $p = 0.014$).

Discussion

Four research questions guided this study: (1) What is the association between age and the use of marijuana or other drugs among prisoners in Ghana? (2) What is the relationship between a first-time robbery conviction and the use of marijuana or any other drugs among prisoners in Ghana? (3) What is the relationship between robbery reoffending and the use of marijuana or any other drugs among prisoners in Ghana? (4) What is the association between childhood abuse and marijuana or other drug use among prisoners in Ghana? We observed that compared with younger prisoners, older prisoners were less likely to have used marijuana within the past year or the past 30 days. Prisoners who were older were less likely to have used other drugs within the past year and the past 30 days. Prisoners with or without a robbery conviction were equally likely to have used marijuana within the past year. Nonetheless, prisoners who had been convicted of robbery were more likely to have used marijuana within the past 30 days than those without a robbery conviction. Prisoners with or without a robbery conviction were equally likely not to have used any other drugs within the past year. Nevertheless, prisoners with a robbery conviction were more likely to have used other drugs within the past 30 days than those without a robbery conviction. Those who were robbery reoffenders and those who were not were equally likely to have used marijuana within the past year. However, those who were robbery reoffenders were more likely to have used marijuana within the past 30 days than those who were not robbery reoffenders. Those who were robbery reoffenders were more likely to have used other drugs within the past year than those who were not. Likewise, those who were robbery reoffenders were more likely to have used other drugs within the past 30 days than those who were not robbery reoffenders. Prisoners with a history of child abuse were more likely to have used marijuana and other drugs within the past year and the past 30 days than those who had never suffered child abuse.

Compared with younger prisoners, older prisoners were less likely to have used marijuana or any other drugs within the past year or the past 30 days. Our findings confirm the report of Davoren et al. (2015) that younger prisoners use more illicit drugs than older prisoners. Fazel et al. (2016) established that compared with younger inmates, older inmates were less likely to use drugs in prison. The use of marijuana has been documented among young prisoners (Cope, 2000), whereas Arndt et al. (2002) found that older prisoners were likely to use (predominantly) alcohol. Edgar and O'Donnell (1998) indicated that older adult prisoners use more drugs in prison than younger prisoners. The divergence of these findings may be attributed to the differences in the normalisation that young people (Parker et al., 1998) and adults (Duff et al., 2012) experience in the prison context. The dynamics of drug supply into and within prison may also explain why older prisoners are less likely to use drugs than younger prisoners. O'Hagan and Hardwick (2017) demonstrated that social relationships established within prison can facilitate drug use among prisoners. Young prisoners' organisational skills may enable the effective distribution of drugs (Cope, 2000). Compared with older prisoners, they are also more likely to have networks outside prison (Majekodunmi et al., 2017), which can facilitate the provision of drug supply in prison. On one of the researcher's visits to one of the prisons, a person was arrested for smuggling marijuana into the facility. The culprit inserted the marijuana inside *banku*, which is a local dish in Ghana, to be given to a young prisoner.

We found that prisoners with or without a robbery conviction were equally likely to have used marijuana within the past year. Nonetheless, prisoners who had been convicted of robbery were more likely to have used marijuana within the past 30 days. Prisoners who had been convicted of robbery and those who had not were equally likely not to have used any other drugs within the past year. However, prisoners with a robbery conviction were more likely to have used other drugs within the past 30 days. Prisoners have reported using illicit drugs on the day of the robbery that they committed (Brochu et al., 2001). Brochu et al. (2001) suggested that criminal behaviour was probably the result of drug addiction because people may need to engage in crime to raise funds to support their drug use. Pernanen et al. (2002) showed that prisoners in a federal prison in Canada reported that they had committed robbery to buy illicit drugs. Such offenders probably continue to use drugs in prison as long as they are available. Thus, in this study, the participants who had been convicted of robbery for the first time were more likely to have used marijuana and other drugs within the past 30 days than those without a robbery conviction. This finding corroborates Cope's (2000) study, which established that those who commit robbery also use marijuana and other drugs, such as heroin, in prison.

This study established that prisoners who were robbery reoffenders and those who were not were equally likely to have used marijuana within the past year. However, those who were robbery reoffenders were more likely to have used marijuana within the past 30 days than those who were not. Robbery reoffenders were more likely to have used other drugs within the past year than those who were not. Similarly, robbery reoffenders were more likely to have used other drugs within the past 30 days than those who were not reoffenders. This finding supports Mannerfelt and Håkansson (2018), who showed that drug abuse is associated with criminal recidivism. If a robbery was committed to raise funds to feed an addiction, and the convicted robber is not rehabilitated in prison and continues to feed his addiction in prison, he will continue to commit crime when released into society. Belenko (2006) showed that prisoners who often use drugs in prison are likely to reoffend. The cycle will continue if the prisoner is not rehabilitated. Our finding of drug use among robbery reoffenders may be because prisoners with drug use problems who are not rehabilitated in prison are likely to reoffend when released into society.

We observed that prisoners with a history of child abuse were more likely to have used marijuana and other drugs with the past year and the past 30 days than those who had not suffered abuse in childhood. These findings confirm those of Swogger et al. (2011), who showed that prisoners who have a history of childhood abuse are more likely to use drugs. This association has also been established among prisoners in Greece (Sergentanis et al., 2014). Teixeira et al. (2017) posited that this category of prisoner uses addictive drugs to help them cope with the stress associated with their traumatic childhood experiences. Our findings support the suggestion of Ibrahim et al. (2015) that inmates in some prisons in Ghana suffer mental distress. Such prisoners are more likely to resort to drugs (Bengtsson, 2012).

Limitations and Recommendation

The researchers took measures to reduce social desirability. However, the authors acknowledge that some of the items could have still evoked socially desirable responses. We also admit that although the prison officer sat at a distance, his presence could have influenced the prisoners' dispositions. Although instructive, the findings could have provided further details if the other types of drugs that prisoners used had been explicitly investigated. Future studies should examine the association between other types of offense and other illicit drugs (e.g., cocaine, heroin, methamphetamines and amphetamines). Asking prisoners to indicate whether they suffered child abuse is acceptable. Nevertheless, validated instruments to verify the extent to which prisoners suffered child abuse could be used in future studies. The lack of data on the actual number of invited prisoners made it impossible to indicate the number of prisoners who declined participation. These data are missing due to the unavailability of a register for each cell and the researchers' inability to contact and invite prisoners personally. Future qualitative studies should explore why certain types of prisoners use marijuana or other illicit drugs in prison.

Conclusion

The findings of this study lend credibility to Kolind and Duke's (2016) assertion that prisons are a high-risk environment for drug use. They support studies that have found drug use among prisoners in other African countries, such as Kenya (Kinyanjui & Atwoli, 2013) and Uganda (Uganda Prisons Service, 2009). We can conclude that drug use not only cuts across the social fibre of the general public (Adu-Gyamfi & Brenya, 2015) but is also a problem in prisons in Ghana. The prevalence could be attributed to the lack of proper screening among prisoners, which are needed to identify drug use problems for possible rehabilitation. This study showed that offenders processed through the criminal justice system could have mental illnesses (Edgely, 2009), and may continue to use drugs to cope with life in prison (Bengtsson, 2012). Unfortunately, the lack of proper screening of offenders in Ghana (Adjorlolo, 2016) makes it difficult to identify problematic drug users who commit robbery to fund their addiction and continue to use drugs in prison. Likewise, inmates with a history of child abuse, who may resort to drug use, may need therapy, but they are not currently identified. Proper screenings of offenders are needed before they are incarcerated. The criminal justice system needs to identify those who might have a mental illness because they may need to be diverted from incarceration or receive therapy in prison. By doing so, the Ghana police will fulfil their mandate to ensure that offenders are carefully screened and consequently diverted from the criminal justice system. Separate prison facilities also need to be established. They should provide some form of therapy for prisoners with robbery convictions who use drugs and prisoners with a history of child abuse.

Acknowledgments The authors express their gratitude to the Ghana Prisons Service and all the prisoners who took part in the study. Commanders of the Takoradi, Kumasi and Nsawam medium security prisons including Supt Constance Dokumah (Takoradi prisons) and Supt Robert Kavi (Nsawam prisons) are hereby acknowledged.

References

Adjorlolo, S. (2016). Diversion of individuals with mental illness in the criminal justice system in Ghana. *International Journal of Forensic Mental Health, 15*(4), 382–392. https://doi.org/10.1080/14999013.2016.1209597

Adu-Gyamfi, S., & Brenya, E. (2015). The marijuana factor in a University in Ghana: A survey. *Humanities & Social Sciences, 11*(8), 2162–2182. https://doi.org/10.17516/1997-1370-2015-8-11-2162-2182

Affinnih, Y. H. (1999a). A preliminary study of drug abuse and its mental health and health consequences among addicts in Greater Accra, Ghana. *Journal of Psychoactive Drugs, 31*(4), 395–403. https://doi.org/10.1080/0279107 2.1999.10471769

Affinnih, Y. H. (1999b). Drug use in Greater Accra, Ghana: Pilot study. *Substance Use & Misuse, 34*(2), 157–169. https://doi.org/10.3109/10826089909035641

Aning, K., & Pokoo, J. (2014). Understanding the nature and threat of drug trafficking to national and regional security. *Stability: International Journal of Security and Development, 3*(1), 8, 1–13. https://doi.org/10.5334/sta.df.

Antwi, A. (2015). *Social reintegration of offenders and recidivism in Ghana.* Unpublished doctoral thesis, University of Ghana, Accra.

Arndt, S., Turvey, C. L., & Flaum, M. (2002). Older offenders, substance abuse, and treatment. *American Journal of Geriatric Psychiatry, 10*(6), 733–739. https://doi.org/10.1097/00019442-200211000-00012

Belenko, S. (2006). Assessing released inmates for substance-abuse-related service needs. *Crime & Delinquency, 52*(1), 94–113. https://doi.org/10.1177/0011128705281755

Bengtsson, T. T. (2012). Boredom and action-experiences from youth confinement. *Journal of Contemporary Ethnography, 41*(5), 526–553. https://doi.org/10.1177/0891241612449356

Brochu, S., Cousineau, M., Gillet, M., Cournoyer, L., Pernanen, K., & Motiuk, L. (2001). Drugs, alcohol, and criminal behaviour: A profile of inmates in Canadian federal institutions. *Coming Up in Forum on Corrections Research, 13*(3), 20–24. Retrieved from http://www.ncjrs.gov/App/publications/abstract.aspx?ID=202443

Bullock, T. (2003). Changing levels of drug use before, during and after imprisonment. In M. Ramsay (Ed.), *Prisoners' drug use and treatment: Seven research studies* (pp. 23–48). Home Office Research, Development & Statistics Directorate.

Cope, N. (2000). Drug use in prison: The experience of young offenders. *Drugs: Education, Prevention and Policy, 7*(4), 355–366. https://doi.org/10.1080/dep.7.4.355.366

Davoren, M., Fitzpatrick, M., Caddow, F., Caddow, M., O'Neill, C., O'Neill, H., et al. (2015). Older men and older women remand prisoners: Mental illness, physical illness: Offending patterns and needs. *International Psychogeriatrics, 27*(5), 747–755. https://doi.org/10.1017/S1041610214002348

Duff, C., Asbridge, M., Brochu, S., Cousineau, M., Hathaway, A. D., Marsh, D., et al. (2012). A Canadian perspective on cannabis normalization among adults. *Addiction Research & Theory, 20*(4), 271–283. https://doi.org/10.310 9/16066359.2011.618957

Edgar, K., & O'Donnell, I. (1998). *Mandatory drug testing in prisons: The relationship between MDT and the level and nature of drug misuse* (Research Study No. 189). Home Office.

Edgely, M. (2009). Common law sentencing of mentally impaired offenders in Australian courts: A call for coherence and consistency. *Psychiatry, Psychology and Law, 16*(2), 240–261. https://doi.org/10.1080/13218710802242037

Erickson, P. G., & Hathaway, A. D. (2010). Normalization and harm reduction: Research avenues and policy agendas. *The International Journal on Drug Policy, 21*(2), 137–139. https://doi.org/10.1016/j.drugpo.2009.11.005

Fazel, S., Hayes, A. J., Bartellas, K., Clerici, M., & Trestman, R. (2016). Mental health of prisoners: Prevalence, adverse outcomes, and interventions. *Lancet Psychiatry, 3*(9), 871–881. https://doi.org/10.1016/S2215-0366(16)30142-0

Friestad, C., & Hansen, I. L. S. (2005). Mental health problems among prison inmates: The effect of welfare deficiencies, drug use and self-efficacy. *Journal of Scandinavian Studies in Criminology and Crime Prevention, 6*(2), 183–196. https://doi.org/10.1080/14043850510035100

Friestad, C., & Kjelsberg, E. (2009). Drug use and mental health problems among prison inmates—Results from a nation-wide prison population study. *Nordic Journal of Psychiatry, 63*(3), 237–245. https://doi.org/10.1080/08039480802571044

Galtung, J. (1961). Prison: The organisation of dilemma. In D. Cressey (Ed.), *The Prison* (pp. 107–145). Holt, Rinehart and Winston.

Ghana Prisons Service. (2019). *Inmates' statistics.* Ghana Prisons Service. Retrieved from http://www.ghanaprisons.gov.gh/statistics.html

Ibrahim, A., Esena, R. K., Aikins, M., O'Keefe, A. M., & McKay, M. M. (2015). Assessment of mental distress among prison inmates in Ghana's correctional system: A cross-sectional study using the Kessler Psychological Distress Scale. *International Journal of Mental Health Systems, 9*(17), 1–6. https://doi.org/10.1186/s13033-015-0011-0

Kendler, K. S., Bulik, C. M., Silberg, J., Hettema, J. M., Myers, J., & Prescott, C. A. (2000). Childhood sexual abuse and adult psychiatric and substance use disorders in women: An epidemiological and cotwin control analysis. *Archives of General Psychiatry, 57*(10), 953–959. https://doi.org/10.1001/archpsyc.57.10.953

Kinyanjui, D. W. C., & Atwoli, L. (2013). Substance use among inmates at the Eldoret prison in western Kenya. *BMC Psychiatry, 13*(53), 1–8. https://doi.org/10.1186/1471-244X-13-53

Klantschnig, G. (2016). The politics of drug control in Nigeria: Exclusion, repression and obstacles to policy change. *International Journal of Drug Policy, 30*, 132–139. https://doi.org/10.1016/j.drugpo.2015.10.012

Kolind, T., & Duke, K. (2016). Drugs in prisons: Exploring use, control, treatment and policy. *Drugs: Education, Prevention and Policy, 23*(2), 89–92. https://doi.org/10.3109/09687637.2016.1153604

Kumah-Abiwu, F. (2019). Changing trends in West Africa's drug policy terrain: A theoretical perspective. *Commonwealth & Comparative Politics, 57*(1), 52–70. https://doi.org/10.1080/14662043.2018.1514553

Majekodunmi, O. E., Obadeji, A., Oluwole, L. O., & Oyelami, O. (2017). Depression and associated physical co-morbidities in elderly prison inmates. *International Journal of Mental Health, 46*(4), 269–283. https://doi.org/10.1080/00207411.2017.1345040

Mannerfelt, C., & Håkansson, A. (2018). Substance use, criminal recidivism, and mortality in criminal justice clients: A comparison between men and women. *Journal of Addiction,* 1–9. https://doi.org/10.1155/2018/1689637

Mjåland, K. (2016). Exploring prison drug use in the context of prison-based drug rehabilitation. *Drugs: Education, Prevention and Policy, 23*(2), 154–162. https://doi.org/10.3109/09687637.2015.1136265

O'Hagan, A., & Hardwick, R. (2017). Behind bars: The truth about drugs in prisons. *Forensic Research & Criminology International Journal, 5*(3), 1–12. https://doi.org/10.15406/frcij.2017.05.00158

Oteng-Ababio, M., Owusu, G., Wrigley-Asante, C., & Owusu, A. (2016). Longitudinal analysis of trends and patterns of crime in Ghana (1980–2010): A new perspective. *African Geographical Review, 35*(3), 193–211. https://doi.org/10.1080/19376812.2016.1208768

Parker, H. (2005). Normalization as barometer: Recreational drug use and the consumption of leisure by young Britons. *Addiction Research and Theory, 13*, 205–215. https://doi.org/10.1080/16066350500053703

Parker, H., Aldridge, J., & Measham, F. (1998). *Illegal leisure: The normalisation of adolescent recreational drug use.* Routledge.

Pennay, A., & Moore, D. (2010). Exploring the micro-politics of normalisation: Narratives of pleasure, self-control and desire in a sample of young Australian 'party drug' users. *Addiction Research and Theory, 18*(5), 557–571. https://doi.org/10.3109/16066350903308415

Pernanen, K., Cousineau, M., Brochu, S., & Sun, F. (2002). *Proportions of crimes associated with alcohol and other drugs in Canada.* Canadian Centre on Substance Abuse.

Read, U. M., & Doku, V. C. (2012). Mental health research in Ghana: A literature review. *Ghana Medical Journal, 46*(2 Suppl), 29–38.

Ritter, C., Broers, B., & Elger, B. S. (2013). Cannabis use in a Swiss male prison: Qualitative study exploring detainees' and staffs' perspectives. *International Journal of Drug Policy, 24*, 573–578. https://doi.org/10.1016/j.drugpo.2013.05.001

Sergentanis, T. N., Sakelliadis, E. I., Vlachodimitropoulos, D., Goutas, N., Sergentanis, I. N., Spiliopoulou, C. A., et al. (2014). Does history of childhood maltreatment make a difference in prison? A hierarchical approach on early family events and personality traits. *Psychiatry Research, 220*(3), 1064–1070. https://doi.org/10.1016/j.psychres.2014.10.019

Swogger, M. T., Conner, K. R., Walsh, Z., & Maisto, S. A. (2011). Childhood abuse and harmful substance use among criminal offenders. *Addictive Behaviours, 36*(12), 1205–1212. https://doi.org/10.1016/j.addbeh.2011.07.025

Teixeira, C. A. B., Lasiuk, G., Barton, S., Fernandes, M. N. F., & Gherardi-Donato, E. C. S. (2017). An exploration of addiction in adults experiencing early-life stress: A metasynthesis. *Revista Latino-Americana de Enfermagem, 25*(e2939), 1–11. https://doi.org/10.1590/1518-8345.2026.2939.

Tompkins, C. (2015). There's that many people selling it: Exploring the nature, organization and maintenance of prison drug markets in England. *Drugs: Education, Prevention and Policy, 23*(2), 144–153. https://doi.org/10.310 9/09687637.2015.1085490

Turnbull, P., Stimson, G., & Stillwell, G. (1994). *Drugs in prison*. Avert.

Uganda Prisons Service. (2009). *A rapid situation assessment of Hiv/Sti/Tb and drug abuse among prisoners in Uganda*. Uganda Prisons Service and United Nations Office on Drugs and Crime.

UNODC. (2015). *World drug report 2015*. United Nations.

West Africa Commission on Drugs (WACD). (2014). Not just in transit: Drugs, the state and society in West Africa. Retrieved from https://www.globalcommissionondrugs.org/wacd

Wheatley, M. (2007). Drugs in prison. In *Handbook on prisons* (pp. 399–422). Willan Publishing.

World Prison Brief. (2019). *World Prison Brief data: Africa*. World Prison Brief. Retrieved from https://www.prisonstudies.org/country/ghana

Zhang, Z. (2004). *Drug and alcohol use and related matters among arrestees, 2003*. U.S. Department of Justice, National Institute of Justice.

14

Crossing the Social Boundary: Racial and Ethnic Representation of Black Female Offenders inside South African Institutions of Incarceration

Nontyatyambo Pearl Dastile

Introduction

This chapter explores the possibilities of studying black women's trajectories to crime from a sociological-cultural perspective that is sensitive to non-legal and non-structural factors that are often ignored in mainstream criminological studies. Such an approach departs from traditionally Western legalistic and positivist criminological approaches which are not well suited to engage with issues of class, gender or culture, and with societal perceptions, prejudices, and stereotypes about black women who commit crime. The women's narratives reveal that these sociocultural factors do impinge on the processes of rehabilitation of women who are incarcerated in correctional centres as offenders. Therefore, this chapter

N. P. Dastile (✉)
Department of Criminology and Security Science, University of South Africa, Pretoria, South Africa
e-mail: dastinp@unisa.ac.za

© The Author(s), under exclusive license to Springer Nature Switzerland AG 2021
H. C. O. Chan, S. Adjorlolo (eds.), *Crime, Mental Health and the Criminal Justice System in Africa*, https://doi.org/10.1007/978-3-030-71024-8_14

has chosen to study women's incarceration as socially embedded and situated phenomena and activities. The women reported on lived through a multiplicity of experiences that led them to come into conflict with the law. The focus areas aim to discuss how black women cross social boundaries, thus bringing the subject of black female offending into the mainstream of criminological research in South Africa.

A focus on the black female offender is very important in that it deals with that social constituency that is vulnerable and open to numerous stereotypes within societies that are male-dominated. In these male-dominated societies the criminal justice system is generally not fully 'ungendered'. However, due to the democratic transition that began in 1994, South African criminal justice system has been undergoing restructuring to take into account gender issues. These changes are far too few and too slow in the context of the increasing numbers of black female inmates within South African institutions of incarceration. This reality provokes new research questions:

- What circumstances produce black female offenders?
- Is the criminal justice system gendered enough to be sensitive to these female offenders?
- Are the institutions of incarceration well suited to accommodate female offenders?
- What can be done to improve the daily lives of female offenders within institutions of incarceration?

These are some of the key questions that are explored in this chapter as it grapples with the broader circumstances of the black female offender within South African institutions of incarceration.

The chapter is structured in the following way. First the historical trajectories to female offending in the African context are given. This is followed by the profile of black women incarcerated in South African correctional centres. What is discussed next is the discussion on women's racial and ethnical profile together with the employment status of women. A move towards engendering correctional centres in South Africa is given as well as a conclusion to the chapter.

Historical Trajectories to Female Offeding in the African Context

In the African context, lived realities of black women such as cultural scripts (for example forced and arranged marriages) underpin women's vulnerabilities, leading them to engage in crime (El-Ashmawi, 1981; Modie-Moroka & Sossou, 2001). El-Ashmawi (1981), who examines female criminality in three areas in Egypt (modern cities, villages among the Bedouin communities, and women who live on desert islands/oases), reveals the varied social conditions that lead to criminal involvement among women in these three locations. According to El-Ashmawi (1981), the women included in her study represent not only the living circumstances of women, but also how issues of religion, tradition, and lifestyle contribute to women's involvement in offending. Among urban dwellers, for example, women in the middle-income group commit offences such as prostitution and fraud in order to meet the exorbitant costs of living in the cities. Among women at college and university, who also reside in urban centres, the absence of a guardian and their perceived freedom from parental constraints are cited as some of the reasons for these women's involvement in crime. These offences are less common in the nomadic areas, where life is still primitive and is restricted to age-old traditions (El-Ashmawi, 1981). Among Bedouin women, the cultural practice of forced marriage has been cited as a reason for women's involvement in crime (El-Ashmawi, 1981). These are women who commit crimes such as murder in response to the violent abuse they have to endure in their marriages. Although El-Ashmawi's (1981) study is now dated, it rightly suggests the heterogeneity of African women, by pointing out how geographical location and cultural norms and values influence women's trajectories to criminality. It cautions against generalisations such as using the existing pathways suggested by male-centred or Western feminist studies, which may not correlate with African women's lived realities.

In other countries, such as Zimbabwe, Tsanga (2003) and Samakayi-Makarati (2003) have investigated the cultural, social, economic, and religious factors that contribute to women's involvement in crime. Tsanga (2003) notes that the divergent social profiles of women involved in crime point to the heterogeneous nature of the communities that the women hail from. She explains that some women who commit crime come from polygynous families, where incidents of economic hardships are reported, and women in these polygynous households are often forced to share limited resources. In some cases, women offenders reported how their mothers were left homeless after their father's separation from or abandonment of an older wife in favour of a younger wife. This in turn affects the women's access to education and may cause further exposure to domestic abuse from relatives and family members (Samakayi-Makarati, 2003). These studies speak to the prevalence of patriarchal practices in these societies, and how such practices are reinforced by cultural norms and values. But mostly, these studies depict the racial and social class disparities that intersect with African patriarchal traditional beliefs which impact mainly on black women in rural areas and in poor households.

El-Ashmawi (1981) in Egypt and Oloruntimehin (1981) in Nigeria trace back the circumstances that lead women to incarceration to the social and cultural dictates of what women should and should not do. According to El-Ashmawi (1981), societal prescriptions dictate that women should be submissive, should remain at home and therefore should be excluded from education in preparation for marriage and domestic duties. Women are marginalised and married off at a very young age, resulting in a higher propensity to domestic violence within the home. El-Ashmawi (1981) observes that women were subject to various societal definitions such as being "sober, submissive, tender and passive figures" (p. 72). Women's roles were thus limited to the home, with restricted involvement or contact with criminally inclined individuals. Patriarchal attitudes to education are evident in cases where women are not sent to school, as the fathers believe that women will end up being married off and will spend their lives cooking and raising families. In that case, educating women is regarded as a "wasted effort, and this was even more [evident] in for instance Nigerian black communities" (Oloruntimehin, 1981, p. 161). Such exclusion has resulted in women being socially marginalised. Marginalisation from the public sphere also affected women's participation in the labour force, leading to overrepresentation of women in less skilled jobs such as domestic cleaning and secretarial positions. Konate (2003) argues that, in Senegal, some women resorted to criminal behaviour to survive, as these were jobs that paid very little, compared to higher-skilled managerial positions.

In addition to women's domestic roles, El-Ashmawi (1981) observes that, in Egypt, urbanisation has resulted in increased participation by women in white-collar and male gang-related offences. Women involved in these traditionally male-oriented offences have been described as possessing male attributes because of the way in which they conduct themselves. Changes in persona, language, and dress style are examples of the lengths to which women go to carry out gang-related offences and be accepted as members of gangs (El-Ashmawi, 1981).

The Zimbabwean situation as described by Stewart (2003) details the circumstances that lead to women's incarceration in Zimbabwe as "tales of lives characterised by tragedy" (p. 1). Women from impoverished backgrounds, with little or no formal education, continue to be increasingly incarcerated for offences ranging from theft to shoplifting. This is because gender roles demand of women as mothers, grandmothers, aunts, and sisters to support the financial needs of children. However, Stewart (2003) cautions that despite the women's impoverished backgrounds, the majority should not be described as hopeless or as having no sense of agency to improve their circumstances. She states that once women are released from incarceration, they often, though with greater difficulty and social challenges, manage not to commit further offences. This can be supported by statistics which indicate that the majority of women in these prisons are first-time offenders (Stewart, 2003).

In her study on female offending in Botswana, Modie-Moroka (2003) observes that women's economic impoverishment (which results in inadequate nutrition, health-care problems, and inadequate housing), the persistence and maintenance of poverty, unemployment, and illiteracy in the household create an unfortunate status for women, leading them towards a life of crime. This is largely because the resources available to women determine whether a woman can maintain relationships materially and emotionally while staying free of crime (Modie-Moroka, 2003).

A study conducted by Artz, Hoffman-Wanderer, and Moult (2012) in South Africa reveals the familial circumstances, relationships, trauma, poverty, histories of abuse, experiences of domestic violence, and caretaking responsibilities, as well as addiction histories in women's lives prior to incarceration. Similar prior studies are those of Luyt and Du Preez (2010) and Haffejee, Vetten, and Greyling (2006), which reached similar conclusions. Haffejee et al. (2006) explored the various forms of sexual abuse that women experience—these range from sexual assault to rape, attempted rape, being forced to engage in sexual acts by two or more people, and being forced to have sex with men in exchange for money. Reporting on their experiences of violent behaviour in intimate relationships, the women in this study commented on their exposure to economic or financial abuse (defined in the study as men's failure to provide money for household and basic necessities, while money was spent on other things) (Haffejee et al., 2006). It is clear from the literature that most women had lived through emotional abuse, such as "insults, belittlement, physical abuse in the form of slapping, having objects thrown at them, and being kicked" (Haffejee et al., 2006, pp. 42–44). While this literature is helpful, it fails to connect the pre-incarceration existential realities of women to the broader contexts of colonialism, and pre-independence, apartheid, and post-apartheid history. These histories cannot be ignored, as their legacy continues to have a negative impact on the social position of women in African states, even decades after colonialism, post-independence.

Ally (2013) points out that the widespread feminisation of witchcraft signals the rhetoric of patriarchy, social class, racism, and seniority. Because there are limited narrative accounts of women's routes to allegations of suspected witchcraft; for example, among the Azande of the Congo, researchers have attributed these allegations to "social instability such as famine, rapid change, oppression and economic distress" (Onyinah, 2002, p. 109). It is mostly black and elderly women who are subject to allegations of witchcraft, as such women's positions suggest that they might harbour resentment towards and jealousy for both male privilege and women who occupy higher positions in society such as queens or wives of kings (Mgbako & Glenn, 2011). However, women who occupy higher positions are not insulated against allegations of witchcraft, particularly if and when they challenge male authority.

In systems where cultural norms permitted woman-to-woman marriages, for example, incidents of subordination by elderly women occurred

(Magubane, 2004; Weir, 2007). Woman-to-woman marriages were mostly practised by elite women, who could afford to pay *lobola*. By marrying a wife, these women managed to absolve themselves of domestic duties and, in some cases, even childbirth, as the "wife" married by the elite woman might be expected to bear children for her female "husband" in her stead (Jean, 1998). Such experiences are omitted from a literature which focuses on an analysis of white versus black people's histories. Even worse, the lived realities of sexual slavery in these woman-to-woman marriages have been silenced and erased—these women were expected to fulfil all obligatory sexual roles in order to give birth to an heir (Magubane, 2004).

For centuries, black women have faced triple victimisation, as sexual slavery was also experienced during the slave trade. Among the Khoi, there are many reports from the period of slavery of black women who were subjected to rape and forced sexual intercourse by slave owners. When women conceived from these violations, cases of infanticide occurred, where women killed their own offspring and were then punished by death (Gqola, 2007). Sometimes, these women were motivated to commit infanticide by their wish to ensure that their children would be spared a life of enslavement. It was not uncommon for these women to be diagnosed with mental illness, before being stoned to death (Gqola, 2007). Their stories were never told. Some of these forms of violation were carried over into apartheid South Africa. Hence, this history still "retains a haunting presence" (Gqola, 2007, p. 35), especially in post-apartheid South Africa, where many women report experiences of victimisation and violation prior to incarceration as part of their trajectory to offending and being incarcerated.

African leaders initially unquestioningly adopted the precepts of colonial rule, and more and more women, especially in the rural parts of South Africa, continued to be incarcerated on the basis of allegations of witchcraft and for infanticide. This resulted in burgeoning numbers of black women in institutions of incarceration. Relatively little attention has been paid to the impact of this history in today's debate, and this is visible in the dearth of literature available about these women's experiences. Very few women have written about their experiences—few women wrote about these experiences, not only because there were fewer women than men in correctional centres, but also because the majority of black women could not write (Vera, 1995; Walker, 1991).

Black Women Incarcerated in Correctional Centres

South Africa, and mostly post-apartheid South Africa, has black women's resistance to gender violence documented in prison memoirs and chronicles. Nevertheless, such resistance is demonstrated by "voices in a public and unhidden platform", such as political marches and gatherings in township areas (Vera, 1995, p. 184). This has had a cumulative effect of women being confined to the domestic arena and removed from public discourses. Attitudes and beliefs about women can be seen in statements such as "if woman is matter ... man is mind" (Vera, 1995, p. 209). The perceived irrationality of women's thinking has resulted in their relegation to that which requires less thinking and strategising. Ruth First (1965) records a phallocentric gaze on women, which women defied through writing and public political demonstrations. Thus First (1965) observes that public demonstration became acts of defiance and resistance in the lives of racialised and genderised women. Moreover, forms of resistance were not devoid of diversity of race, social class, and geographic location.

Emma Mashinini, in her memoir *Strikes Have Followed Me All My Life*, exposes the layered identities which were "social determinants" (Vera, 1995) of how Mashinini experienced apartheid rule. Mashinini writes of her life as a "daughter, mother, grandmother and black person"—roles which reveal all her gendered position, social class, and racial identity. She describes herself in this memoir as "a daughter with black origins, a mother to black children, a grandmother to her children", and tells of how her political activism implied that all these facets would lead her and her children and grandchildren to detention because of her racial and gender identity.

In the colonial and in apartheid eras, it was predominantly black African girls who were incarcerated in various institutions (cited in

Walker, 1991). The girls housed in reformatories were described as more "fierce and resistant" than delinquent boys (Chisholm, 1987; cited in Walker, 1991, p.293). The level of violence by these girls stood in contrast to the societal norms of females as passive. The official reasons given for the violent behaviour of these girls was that such girls were "feeble-minded and thus prone to irrational behaviour and that the absence of a punishment encouraged collective resistance which underpinned violence as a source for masturbation and lesbianism". Such explanations called for mental examinations by psychiatrists, psychologists, and social workers, after which some girls would be referred to mental institutions, or a "suitable punishment" for them would be recommended. Such mental evaluations alleged that poverty was linked to female criminality, and to behavioural traits and low intelligence levels. These young girls were also seen to be (overly) sexually active and it was claimed that signs of mental defects were more prominent among delinquent girls and boys. This stereotyping ties in with expectations that women should be subservient, particularly in the public sphere.

Very apparent during the apartheid era was social scientists' views on female criminality. Black girls and women were perceived to be at the opposite end of the scale from civilisation. Chisholm (1987; cited in Walker, 1991) expressed the opinion that these black girls should be seen as a source of corruption and disease—he saw female sexuality in general, and black sexuality in particular, as epitomising deviant sexuality. Thus the incarceration of black girls in reformatories was seen as symbolic of instilling social order, while white girls' criminality was attributed to an "abandonment of their allegiance to civilization". Criminality among white girls was seen as threatening white dominance, thus potentially leading to a deterioration of the white race. Hence they were detained with black girls, who were deemed out of control. The vast majority of African girls (black and coloured girls) were sentenced for crimes such as theft, stock theft and housebreaking with intent to steal, poisoning, murder, assault, arson, desertion from employment, and trespassing. White girls were most likely to be detained for offences such as theft, and offences of a sexual nature, such as prostitution and interracial sex. Thus, white girls were punished, among other things, for their deceitfulness towards the white community, while black girls were punished for a violation of class laws and property-related offences.

The limited information available on the involvement of women in crime during the apartheid era paints a picture of women involved in public order crimes. One of the reasons for the low numbers of recorded female offending or female offenders arrested for offences which were not political in nature may be a lack of statistical evidence on female criminality during this era. In this regard, Duvenage points out that even though most prisons were not exclusively for political prisoners, admission records and registers of offenders are difficult to access. The apartheid government did not distinguish between political and non-political offenders. Furthermore, the conditions under which prisons filed these documents were less than ideal, and they made retrieval of the data very difficult. Some documents were held "in rooms that allowed for moisture, in light and humid conditions and [were] extremely disorganised". Some documents were damaged, others were transferred to various prisons for storage, and some were archived.

There is little documentation on women's routes to incarceration other than for political reasons. The memoirs of activists such as Ruth First (1965) and Emma Mashinini (1991), to name but a few, unmask the implications of race, social class, and gendered subjectivities in women's lives. Vera (1995) explains that both writers wrote "from different material conditions, and from different positions within the same cultural and geographical location ... *both illuminate* the racialised background on which apartheid rests and the dehumanising political construct" [my emphasis] (p. 187). Both women were subjected to patriarchal domination, but Ruth First as a white woman still had white privilege, which conferred better treatment during arrest and confinement, whereas Mashinini was exposed to both patriarchy and racial segregation. Hence Vera (1995) argues that Cherry Clayton (1993, also cited in Vera, 1995) was right in describing women as "half-colonised" and Mashinini as "doubly-colonised" (p. 203). First (1965) admits that white privilege allowed her to live a good life in society, and even in prison, while black women were subject to forms of racial segregation such as carrying passes and being separated from their own families because of the Pass Laws. Nevertheless, both women operated in the male-dominated space of political activism and experienced "grotesque" feminine stereotyping. As Vera (1995) puts it, women did "not only encounter apartheid but also its patriarchal necessity to reproduce itself through the very women it oppresses" (p. 195). Hence, both the colonial and apartheid era are important markers which formed the "conditions of female oppression" in the South African landscape. Both eras managed to erase women's voices, thereby contributing to the rhetoric of a female body as a "flawed body ... a woman without objectivity" (Vera, 1995, p. 205).

Unfortunately most contemporary studies fail to examine how this history has culminated in the dearth of discussion of female offending in the African and South African context. Vera (1995) argues that a double colonisation of black women in the African context should be emphasised in order to examine and understand the confluence of race and class gendered subjectivities in the lives of women. Because of the limited narratives of black women's routes to incarceration, the author in her dialogues with incarcerated women, supports what Ruth First (in Vera, 1995, p. 203) observed during her incarceration, as depicted in her memoir: a black woman gradually learns to write her own story through oral recitation in order to make her voice heard. Such narratives aim to depict the peculiarities of African women's circumstances and protect them from being portrayed as passive recipients of norms and values. Describing women only in terms of their vulnerabilities fails to acknowledge the forms of resistance that women adapt to respond, for example, to patriarchal oppression.

The Profile of the Incarcerated Black Women in South Africa

This section aims to disrupt the profile of a "typical female inmate" (Bosworth, 1999, pp. 2–3; De Leon Relucio, 2008)—depictions of women as victims from an impoverished background, mostly black or people of colour, uneducated, and underemployed. Bosworth (1999, p. 2) points out with regard to these depictions that result in women's incarceration that they are *abstractions [which] are little more than descriptive categories with scant intrinsic meaning. They form an image of a normative type, removed from any content ... yet it is precisely the women's subjectivity—their motivations and sense of self—that can elaborate how they evaluate and negotiate power.*

When women speak about their trajectories and journeys from home through to crime and incarceration, it is clear that they have agency, and an ability to "make meanings" and sense of their lives and selves (Bosworth, 1999, p. 3). Hence, incarcerated women cannot be considered "universal" victims. Rather, women's agency is demonstrated by how, in spite of diverse "herstories", women negotiate victim experiences by fighting their abusers, or by resisting hunger by resorting to stealing, for example.

Women are caught up in contested identities, as most women are not only genderised, but racialised and ethnicised in the South African context. It is thus through recognising women's subjectivities, as Bosworth (1999) notes, that one can begin to examine women's pre-incarceration experiences in order to debunk the myth of a typical female offender trajectory and to reintroduce every woman as a subject who can "construct her own theoretical space that challenges some appropriation and negation that assigns her as the 'other'" (De Leon Relucio, 2008, p. 1). Dry generalisations which do not explain the genealogy of a female offender continue to dominate the literature. Often this is because women's stories are not told by women themselves, rendering invisible the suppression of the lived realities and sociocultural circumstances that expose women to multiple subjectivities and vulnerabilities in society and in the institutions that are supposed to mediate these realities. Universal categories or depictions of women are essentialised, and little attempt is made to understand each woman's individual circumstances versus everyday forms of resistance. More than 30 years ago, Adler (1981) already observed that the "hardest to tell is the story of the African experience", and this remains a reality in criminological discourses.

Perhaps the starting point should be to illuminate the voices of incarcerated women by enabling women to narrate their own stories. Such oracy is poignant, as even the judiciary has limited space for women's narratives, and in fact continues to be deeply androcentric. Cowan (2006) claims that with the rise of democracy in South Africa (and the rest of

Africa), it would seem that racial equality took precedence over gender equality. When black women face the justice system, they are, in most instances, confronted with traditionalists whose loyalty to customary law and traditional practices overshadows the ideals entrenched by the *Constitution*. Moreover, black women as judges, advocates, and prosecutors who can appreciate the historical legacies and double jeopardies faced by black women remain underrepresented in the judicial system (Cowan, 2006). Gender and cultural sensitivity in dealing with women's routes to crime and incarceration therefore remain in the periphery in the justice system. Cowan (2006) posits that the invisibility of women in the judiciary and court cluster leads to a situation where women "get lost in the crowd of men partly because more high powered positions are held by men" (p. 313). Ultimately the minuscule representation of women may influence the outcomes for women who appear before the courts as suspects.

Questions similar to those posed by Stewart (2003) in Zimbabwe need to be investigated to achieve appropriate gendering of the criminal justice system's processing of women. In this chapter, female offending is contextualised within the unique history of South Africa's system of apartheid as an unjust, exclusionary, and inhumane system which imposed on the oppressed practices of impunity and repression.

Women's Racial Identities

Michel Foucault (1977) describes the incarceration of black women as an imprisonment of the body. This is particularly significant because black women, compared to white, Indian, and coloured women, are more likely to be affected by high unemployment rates and underemployment, which are leading trajectories to crime among black women. The racial profiles of women incarcerated in correctional centres in South Africa reveal a numerical overrepresentation of black women. This racial profile resembles the national racial profile of women incarcerated in correctional centres across South Africa. International trends regarding incarcerated women also reveal the overrepresentation of black and African American women in correctional centres (Agozino, 1997; Muraskin,

2003; Richie, 1996; Spalek, 2008; Van Wormer, 2010). These studies show that the majority of women in correctional centres are black, but it is imperative to locate an analysis of black women's incarceration within the contextual realities of black women's positions in South Africa. As discussed earlier, black women have a specific historical reality that contributes to their marginalisation and racialisation in all spheres of life.

Given the situation of black women in Africa, Ogundipe-Leslie (1995) argues that, in discussing the circumstances that lead women to prison, an analysis of the marginalisation of particularly a black woman should consider seven areas, namely, "her body, her person, her immediate family, her society, her nation, her continent and her location" (p. 103). What Ogundipe-Leslie (1995) advocates is an analysis of black women's lived realities in relation to "the oppression from outside in the form of colonialism and neo-colonialism, oppression from traditional structures, her own backwardness, her man, her colour or her race, and how the woman herself has internalised these oppressions". In relation to colonialism and neocolonialism, Thiam (1995) observes the following about the positions of black women in Africa:

> [W]hile women from industrialized countries are focusing their attention on the problem of creating a typically female language, their daughters of black Africa are still at large seeking their own dignity, for the recognition of their own specificity as human beings [...] refused them by white colonialists or neocolonialists and by their own black males. (Thiam, 1995, p. 94)

Hence, it remains important that the existential realities of black women in South Africa are analysed from this viewpoint in order to highlight the legacies of colonialism, neocolonialism, and apartheid struggles, and the indelible marks they have left on women's lives. As this chapter emphasises, the social location and positioning of black women has a huge impact on women's access to basic resources, such as education, employment, and better living conditions. The majority of the black women interviewed by the researcher in a study she conducted were unemployed and/or underemployed. They had to rely on child income grants for their own survival, particularly younger black women. They had left school at an early age, which impacted negatively on their livelihoods. As Thiam (1995) argues, "the black African woman, be she town-dweller or villager, married, divorced or single, has a deplorable life" (p. 95).

Even though black women are disproportionately represented among incarcerated women in South Africa, black women's identities cannot be subsumed under one category, as they belong to different ethnic groups and even nationalities. One of the main flaws of criminal classifications is the absence of ethnic identifiers in classification schemes (Tonry, 1997). The Department of Correctional Services does indicate nationality in the statistical representation of inmates, but it fails to delineate ethnic identities among the incarcerated population. Because of this oversight, it is impossible to make any comparisons on the basis of ethnic identities to determine the groups most likely to offend.

Ethnic representations are important as they "enable one to theorize how different generations living in the diaspora can understand their ethnic and national backgrounds" (Radhakrishnan, 2003, p. 119). An examination of ethnic identities among women may shed light on the customs and cultural practices that have an impact on women's lives. Describing her ethnic identity, 45-year-old Monica Mase said:

> Monica Mase: As VhaLemba, we are not pure Venda. Originally we come from Zimbabwe, right next to the border.
> Researcher: Are you totally different from VhaVenda?
> Monica Mase: Yes totally different. The language (if we are together as VhaLemba we don't speak the same language). Even when we are together we have different religions. She [pointing to one of the inmates seated outside] is also VhaLemba. There are only three of us in this prison. No, we are Venda but not the same things. We have our own beliefs.

Monica Mase therefore points out to the importance of stratifying women on the basis of ethnic orientations, as blackness alone does not necessarily define a woman's identity.

Ethnic Representations of Women

The ethnic orientations of the sample of women included in this study was as follows: of the 28 women interviewed at the Johannesburg Female Correctional Centre, 4 indicated that they were of Zulu origin, 3 were of Tswana origin, 2 were Xhosa, 1 was Pedi, 1 was Shangaan, 1 was Swazi, and 1 was Ndebele. In the Johannesburg Female Correctional Centre, the ethnic representation was thus in line with the pluralistic ethnic representation in the Gauteng province in its entirety—Johannesburg is often described as the economic hub of South Africa which attracts people from many ethnic backgrounds.

In the Thohoyandou Centre of Excellence, which is in a Venda-dominated area, diverse ethnic orientations were also observed, as it is the only female correctional centre in the region designated to accommodate inmates from neighbouring towns and cities. From a sample of 21 women, 8 defined themselves as Venda and another 8 as Shangaan. A smaller representation of women from other ethnic groups, namely 2 VhaLemba women, 1 Tsonga woman, and 1 Ndebele woman, also formed part of the study. The East London Centre of Excellence is in a province dominated by Xhosa-speaking communities, and all but one black woman in the sample belonged to the Xhosa ethnic group. The closure of many correctional centres near women's places of birth or homes meant that women from as far away as Port Elizabeth were incarcerated in this centre. Five of the coloured (Afrikaans-speaking) women interviewed had just been transferred from a Port Elizabeth correctional centre which was upgrading its facilities. This points to the fluidity of the inmate population, which is not necessarily related to the release of inmates but to operational issues in each province. Notwithstanding the dominance of local or indigenous people who describe themselves as Xhosa (seven), there was one exception, an isiZulu-speaker (Nothemba, 54 years old), who had been transferred from a Kwa-Zulu Natal correctional centre due to a prison riot and a disturbance she was involved in.

In the East London female correctional centre, it was interesting that while the Xhosa speaking women spoke the same language, they came from different clans, which in itself presented diverse cultural backgrounds in terms of their belief systems and cultural practices. The influence of belonging to a particular clan was an important consideration when addressing women by their names or clan names. For instance, at this correctional centre, three women expressed their desire to be called by their clan names rather than their first names. These women were all in the age category of 50 years and above. Referring to women by their clan names was a sign of respect for their dignity. As Manyathi (55 years old) indicated, for some women, being invited to narrate their stories using their clan identities reassured them that they would be understood. This enabled them to tell their stories in a way they felt comfortable with, and which validated their stories. For instance, in a conversation with Manyathi (55 years old), she said:

> Call me Mamu Manyathi. You know there are so many things that happen in our lives. You know what happens here, for instance there was this old woman called Nomnqa and he used to understand me. I was very close to doing what I think I will do with you because he could listen. So now if I have to speak English, which I cannot, what can I say and how do I say it. Then I have to change everything and not say the things and out them the way I want to.

Acknowledging ethnic orientation is valuable to highlight differences among women and some ethnic groups, and also to validate the women's self-hood. It serves as a reminder that a person still belongs to a clan, even while incarcerated. When women presented themselves and voiced their preference for being called by their clan names, they engaged in a process of self-reclamation. In describing women's identities here, the aim is not to emphasise the features they share, or to dehumanise them, but rather to point out the significance of these different ethnic identities and belief systems, which may have formed a component of their trajectories to criminality. Ethnic identities further impacted on how the women responded to each other and how they may be marginalised by other women within correctional centres.

The Shona inmates, for example, are mostly from Zimbabwe, and Naledi Mbotha (26 years old) mentioned that they are always referred to as "*makwerekwere*", a derogatory term used in Zimbabwe to describe Africans from neighbouring countries. Even though this is a non–South

African marker which relates to citizenship, the term is used in this context as an ethnic reference when women speak about their ethnic orientations. For instance, South African Shona people have different belief systems from non–South African Shona people, and different ways of presenting themselves. All these differences and diversities have an impact on how women are accepted and treated by other women in correctional centres. Hence cultural sensitivity to the existence of culturally pluralistic identities is an important consideration.

These identities and the associated challenges are also inherent in society, where cultural and ethnic identities may create an impression that some ethnic groups are more prone to violence than others. Tonry (1997) argues that it is still important to examine "distinctive patterns" among certain groups in order to move beyond single-focused analysis and to develop theories that are culturally relevant for intervention and rehabilitation in correctional facilities (pp. 18–19). But most importantly, especially among black women, ethnic orientations also underscore the significance of women's age groups, which are discussed next.

Women's Employment Status and Education

One of the challenges of post-democratic South Africa is chronic unemployment and underemployment, particularly among underprivileged groups. Several reasons for this have been cited, including the "historic inequalities" which are a legacy of apartheid and related histories of colonialism. The symptoms of such inequalities in the criminal justice system are evident in "the poor being underrepresented in privileged institutions yet overrepresented in prisons". These observations are evident in the correctional settings, and in the wider community, where higher unemployment rates have resulted in

> chocolate cities and vanilla suburbs, white fear of black crime, and the urban influx of poor people and immigrants—result[ing] in further unemployment, hunger, homelessness and sickness in millions. (West, 1992, pp. 352–353)

Black women, particularly young women, remain marginalised because of a complex range of interrelated factors, such as access to education, cultural constraints, and early teenage pregnancies (as examined in the next chapters). Given this background, it is not surprising to note that in a sample of 55, the majority (34 women) reported that they had never been employed. The young women under the age of 25 cited reasons such as a lack of funding or financial assistance to pursue university or college education (Lerato, 20 years old), a lack of interest in school (Thembakazi, 22 years old, dropped out of school in Grade 4 and indicated that there were no role models to persuade her to go to school), dropping out of school, a forced marriage, and homelessness with no emotional or financial support (Noluntu, 24 years old), and teenage pregnancy, depression, and anxiety from neglect by her mother and not knowing who her own father is. Other reasons included loss of interest in pursuing college or university education, despite the ability of parents to provide financial support (Naledi, 28 years old). These narratives, which are also explored in-depth in the next chapter, point to the gendered and racial nature of unemployment and education in South Africa.

A point of interest was how women survived in their communities. Several of them, because they had children, indicated that as a form of survival they depended on their live-in partners (Matlou, 25 years old; Fumi, 30 years old; and Mudzhanani, 29 years old), parents, mostly their mothers (Lerato, 20 years; Patience, 20 years old; Noxolo, 19 years old; Peace, 19 years old; Eva, 18 years old; and Nancy, 22 years old), extended family members (Naledi, 28 years old), survival sex (Lebo, 26 years old), and grandmothers and uncles (Noluntu, 24 years old). All the reasons given are not explored in entirety, because they are so multifaceted, but it is important to note from this summary of reasons that there is not one single factor that can be isolated to explain women's unemployment status. A multitude of these factors needed to be considered to reveal the women's intersubjective experiences. Some of these examples resonate with the available literature, but in the African context there are a myriad of cultural factors in especially the black communities which can impede the employability and the education of women, even among adult women.

Five of the women who indicated that they had never been employed ranged in age from 55 to 75 years. Mantuli (57 years old), a chief in her village, indicated that she had only attended school up to Grade 2. As the next person to inherit and take over the throne from her father, this meant that Mantuli (57 years old) did receive training towards some of the responsibilities that this position entailed. She explained that her position did not require conventional education or employment, as the skills she needed were passed on orally from generation to generation.

The other four older women (Monica Mase, 45 years old; Nothemba, 54 years old; Mundzhelele, 60 years old; and Elisa, 54 years old) explained often mysterious and incurable conditions that they suffered from during their school-going years. These unexplained sicknesses were described as inherent forms of a sickness which is typical to the calling for a person to be a *sangoma*. These women came from families of *isangoma*, and if they had failed to respond to the calling, they would have faced life-threatening situations, including death.

> *Monica Mase: I never went to school. I passed Standard A and never went back to school.*
> *Researcher: What made you become a* sangoma?
> *Monica Mase: I was very ill and that is why I approached a* sangoma.
> *Researcher: Is this also in the family?*
> *Monica Mase: Yes and my family. When I started to be a* sangoma, *my parents were alive and now they passed on.*
> *Researcher: Were any of them sangomas?*
> *Monica Mase: Yes my mother did not train other people, but she just dreamed and would help people.*

As the training is not always time-specific, these women could neither leave their calling to find employment nor continue with formal education. For them, their everyday livelihood came from the income earned through consultation with clients. These women were the least educated of all the categories, but in fact, formal education for them was not a necessity, and might have been an encumbrance in their respective culture-specific roles.

The participants also included women who indicated that they had never been formally employed. Upon discussing the women's familial structures, it emerged, however, that seven of them were self-employed.

They occupied entrepreneurial positions such as director (companies), owner and principal of a day-care centre, restauranteur, shebeen owner, and taxi owner. Because of the varied positions which the women occupied, their formal educational qualifications varied. Largely, the women in directorship positions held the highest educational qualifications, while those who indicated that they were shebeen and taxi owners mostly had lower educational achievements. One of the interviewees was Ntombifikile (55 years old):

> *Ntombifikile: I did all my businesses without any education. I did it all without education. My kids never went to bed without food. Look even my son went as far as Std 6 and the two passed their matric and I sent them to school even though I had only passed a Standard 4. I don't want the school anymore.*
> *Researcher: What about something on business skills?*
> *Ntombifikile: Even that I don't want because I did my business and excelled at it without any education.*

These women are respected in the township and rural locations where they reside. Despite these positions, they are likely to be misrepresented as uneducated and uninformed, although their status within their communities does not tally with the urban conception of what employment and earning an income should be. Owning shebeens and taxis are indeed everyday forms of survival common in township and rural areas through which women earn an income and provide for their families.

Among the women who indicated that they were formally employed, ten, of whom eight were black and two coloured, indicated that they held low-paying jobs (women were employed as cashiers, cleaners, shop assistants, call girls, metal polishers in a scrapyard, and domestic helpers). The women's educational achievements were also relatively low. Matlou (25 years old), who dropped out of school due to limited finances, indicated that her lack of skills impeded her ability to apply for most jobs, and so she worked as a hairdresser, earning R50 a day in a construction company. Fumi (30 years old) worked in a scrapyard because she had run away from poverty and an abusive stepfather. Nomsa May (21 years old) dropped out of school due to an undiagnosed illness, which resulted in her grandmother's chasing her away from home and her being neglected by her mother, abused by her stepfather, and finally moving to the city and being employed as a domestic worker. Yvonne (22 years old) also dropped out of school due to a teenage pregnancy, and was employed as a cleaner. Buhle (21 years old), who left Zimbabwe when her parents could not afford to pay for her education, arrived in South Africa and worked on smallholdings as a farm labourer, and as a street vendor. The two coloured women in this age group were also underemployed. Anna (25 years old) described having left school early because of a lack of emotional support, and depression caused by neglect by her father and an absent mother due to work commitments. She sporadically got jobs, including ones as a cleaner and a waitress. Joyce (19 years old) worked as a cashier in a local shop, and also dropped out of school due to a teenage pregnancy. The low wages these women earned are related to these blue-collar jobs. Some, for instance, indicated that they could barely afford their daily living expenses and that of their children (the women's position vis-à-vis their children are discussed in the next section). Some women earned as little as R50 a day, while some (Nomsa May, 21 years old; Grace, 18 years old) indicated that they earned R700 per month as domestic helpers.

Coquery-Vidrovitch (1997) argues that among black women, unemployment, underemployment, and illiteracy levels point to a lack of emancipation and development. This situation is exacerbated by the fact that "group rights are still favoured over individual rights" (Coquery-Vidrovitch, 1997, p. 232). In the struggle for gender equality in employment and other sectors of the economy, calls for women's rights fail to account for the domestic and private spaces that thwart the development and emancipation of women. For women in urban areas, or *ekasi*, the practice of trading in front of one's home, at the taxi rank, and in neighbourhood stalls still prevails. As husbands' income reduced or when they failed to earn an income or send it home, women's work purpose changed. Therefore, city life and this informal trading were an impetus for providing "daily bread" (Coquery-Vidrovitch, 1997, p. 137). Tiny profit margins led some women to engage in shoplifting. These women remain breadwinners responsible for their children. Today, large cities survive on female labour, which leaves women tired and meagrely paid

(Coquery-Vidrovitch, 1997). Coquery-Vidrovitch (1997) therefore points out that "women need development by women and the only path is education" (p. 234). The women's lived circumstances and how they navigate such constraints to make their lives meaningful are not explored in this chapter.

An analysis of the 21 women who indicated that they were formally employed demonstrates that 11 were professionally trained in their respective careers. These women possessed the highest qualifications in the sample (higher education degrees and postgraduate diplomas). Their employment categories ranged from training coordinator to retail store manager, bookkeeper, chief social worker, reflexologist, personal assistant, group sales marketer, police officer, educator, carpenter, and creditor's clerk. Coquery-Vidrovitch (1997) describes such women as "intelligent, determined" (p. 181). The majority of these women were breadwinners, which for some became a source of vulnerability, as it exposed them to antagonistic and ambivalent attitudes from their partners and families. In terms of their racial categories, five of the women in this group were black, three were white, and two coloured. Interestingly, these women, in terms of vulnerabilities within their families, homes, and employment positions, were not immune from the broader heteronormative and gender-based violence and patriarchies that other women are confronted by in society.

These vulnerabilities may be worsened by the gendered roles and responsibilities inherent in their roles. The exposition of employment and women's educational status, which may determine their position in the economy and their status, cannot be discussed without considering the gendered responsibilities they have towards their children. Motherhood in Africa is a social construction that is a given, and it is significant for a woman's status within the family, community, and society at large.

Engendering Correctional Policies and Systems

New and alternative ways to fight gendered inequalities can be located in an intersectionality thesis, which the coloniality of gender seeks to advance. It is imperative when studying incarcerated women's lives to trace the marginalisation of women in society and to examine how gender, race, and class intermesh, resulting in women's subjection to gross inequalities and injustice. Overlooking it through such intersections results in under-theorisation of the nexus between women and crime in South Africa.

Engendered approaches to crime and justice in the South African context require a mental shift, a delinking from existing ways of approaching a study on women and a more embedded focus on examining the cultural idiosyncrasies that are located in women's experiences. For instance, black women continue to be subjected to repressive customs and cultures. These forms of oppression are exacerbated by poverty and racism embedded in society. This approach enables researchers to understand women's gendered needs and gender-specific challenges, such as the marginalisation of women and girls in education, particularly among black women, inequalities in terms of job opportunities, discriminatory legal structures, and discrepancies in the rights and privileges of women at societal level. These injustices are specific to African women, and, as Kolawole (1997) argues, cannot be "thrust under one single ideology as the solution to these hydra-headed problems [is] inclusive" (p. 34). Gendering the approaches to a study of incarcerated women requires holistic paradigms that may reveal both the visible and invisible forms of marginalisation that women endure prior to incarceration. In addition to gender, race, and class intersectionalities, engendering also implies an analysis of intermeshing identities.

Within an analysis of race there are also ethnic and generational considerations which should be studied and understood. Ensuring that gender is incorporated in the ways we study incarcerated women implies a social understanding of women's lived experiences to inform institutions such as corrections and social development. This cannot be done if the approaches remain gender-neutral, and ignore the experiences of the oppressed. As Imam suggests,

> [t]he individual threads can be traced, but to understand the design of the cloth, one must also appreciate how each thread[] relates to the others. [...] These are the threads that run through every context and situation, even when they appear on the surface to be absent, if the cloth is turned over and the weave is examined, these threads run along underneath.

An examination of the centrality of women's experiences must also include consideration of rehabilitation programmes designed to assist women upon their re-entry to society. The unique conditions of African women necessitate the development and formulation of African-centred endogenous paradigms. The basis of these paradigms should be indigenous methodological approaches, and tools which are cognisant of women's histories and experiences.

An in-depth understanding of the underlying circumstances that lead to female offending is important, as the incarceration of a woman for a crime affects not only the woman herself, but also her children (if she has any). If the pre-incarceration circumstances which may lead to offending among women are not properly examined, there is no clear basis for correctional assessment and rehabilitation programmes for such inmates. In this context, Caputo (2008) raises a valid question—she examines the livelihoods of shoplifters prior to incarceration, in an attempt to add to research on female offending and rehabilitation, and she asks: "[W]ithout science driving these practices, how can we know whether they are suitable or biased?" (Caputo, 2008, p. 3). The narratives of women's lives prior to their incarceration can thus broadly inform and enlighten us on three areas, namely a conceptualisation of female offending, a multifaceted assessment of women's risks and related needs, and the formulation of a theory or framework on which both assessment and rehabilitative programming can be based.

Conclusion

In part, this chapter disrupts existing hegemonic stories which depict incarceration in male-centred terms, which assume the sameness of women's routes to incarceration, while erasing historical injustices to and violations of women. Victim discourses about black women's trajectories to crime and incarceration abound, and such discourses have a negative impact on the development and introduction of context-specific intervention programmes in correctional facilities. The chapter exposes, for instance, the lived structural conditions of women, tracing these from the gender injustices which permeate the family, household, and immediate societies in which women live.

Scholars in African countries that have addressed the phenomenon have conducted studies in Botswana, Nigeria, Zimbabwe, and Egypt. In other countries, researchers seem to have neglected the issue, and there is no literature available on those countries' response to the problem. The limited amount of literature available from these countries exposes the diverse circumstances that lead women to incarceration, and the fact that Africa is a diverse continent whose people we cannot generalise about. Diversity manifests itself in the social and cultural landscapes of these countries, and most importantly in the histories of women's positions in each of these countries.

References

Adler, F. (1981). *The incidence of female criminality in the contemporary world.* New York University Press.

Agozino, B. (1997). *Black women and the criminal justice system: Towards the decolonization of victimization.* Ashgate.

Ally, Y. (2013). *Witchcrafts in modern South Africa: An under-represented facet of genderbased violence.* Fact Sheet. Retrieved October 29, 2013, from http://www.mrc.ac.za

Artz, L., Hoffman-Wanderer, Y., & Moult, K. (2012). *Hard time(s): Women's pathways to crime and incarceration.* Gender, Health and Research Unit, University of Cape Town.

Bosworth, M. (1999). *Engendering resistance: Agency and power in women's prisons*. Ashgate.

Caputo, G. (2008). *Out in the storm: Drug addicted women living as shoplifters and sex workers*. North Eastern University Press & University Press of New England.

Coquery-Vidrovitch, C. (1997). *African women: A modern history*. Westview Press/HarperCollins.

Cowan, B. (2006). Women's representation on the courts in the Republic of South Africa. *Race, Religion, Gender and Class, 6*, 291–318. Retrieved from https://digitalcommons.law.umaryland.edu/cgi/viewcontent.cgi?article=1017&context=wle_papers

De Leon Relucio, M. A. (2008). Centrality of experiences and Third World Women. *MP: An Online Feminist Journal*, July, 1–7.

El-Ashmawi, A. W. (1981). Female criminality in Egypt. In *The incidence of female criminality in the contemporary world* (pp. 176–187). New York City University Press.

Foucault, M. (1977). *Discipline and punish: The birth of the prison*. Pantheon Books.

Gqola, P. D. (2007). Like three tongues in one mouth: Tracing the elusive lives of slave women in (slavocratic) South Africa. In *Women in South African history* (pp. 21–41). HSRC Press.

Haffejee, S., Vetten, L., & Greyling, M. (2006). *Violence and abuse in the lives of women and girls incarcerated at three Gauteng women's prisons. CSVR Research Brief*, No. 3, Feb. Weaver Press.

Jean, C. R. (1998). Woman to woman marriage: Practices and benefits in Sub-Saharan Africa. *Journal of Comparative Family Studies, 29*(1), 97–117. https://doi.org/10.3138/jcfs.29.1.89

Kolawole, M. M. E. (1997). *Womanism and African consciousness*. Africa World Press.

Konate, D. (2003). Ultimate exclusion: Imprisoned women in Senegal. In A. Isaacman & J. Allman (Eds.), *A history of prison and confinement in Africa: Social history of Africa* (pp. 155–164). Heinemann.

Luyt, W. F. M., & Du Preez, N. (2010). A case study of female incarceration in South Africa. *Acta Criminologica: African Journal of Criminology & Victimology, 23*(3), 88–114. Retrieved from https://journals.co.za/content/crim/23/3/EJC29047

Magubane, Z. (2004). *Bringing the empire home: Race, class and gender in Britain and Colonial South Africa*. University of Chicago Press.

Mgbako, C. A., & Glenn, K. (2011). Witchcraft accusations and human rights: Case studies from Malawi. *George Washington International Law Review, 43*, 389–418. Retrieved from https://www.researchgate.net/publication/256019981_Witchcraft_Accusations_and_Human_Rights_Case_Studies_from_Malawi

Modie-Moroka, T. (2003). Vulnerability across a life course: An empirical study: Women and criminality in Botswana prisons. *Journal of Social Development in Africa, 18*(1), 145–180. https://doi.org/10.4314/jsda.v18i1.23823

Modie-Moroka, T., & Sossou, M. (2001). Women, criminality and multifocal empowerment response: Some aspects for Botswana. *Journal of Social Development in Africa, 16*(2), 6–30. https://doi.org/10.4314/jsda.v16i2.23871

Muraskin, R. (2003). *It's a crime: Women and justice*. PrenticeHall.

Ogundipe-Leslie, M. (1995). African women, culture and development. In *Theorising black feminisms: The visionary pragmatism of black women* (pp. 102–117). Routledge.

Oloruntimehin, O. (1981). A preliminary study of female criminality in Nigeria. In *The incidence of female criminality in the contemporary world* (pp. 158–177). New York City University Press.

Onyinah, O. (2002). Deliverance as a way of confronting witchcraft in modem Africa: Ghana as a case history. *Asian Journal of Pentecostal Studies, 5*(1), 107–134. Retrieved from https://www.semanticscholar.org/paper/Deliverance-as-a-way-of-confronting-witchcraft-in-%3A-Onyinah/231da93fadf718d48d0497ac2b34aa4fb7d60f58

Radhakrishnan, R. (2003). Ethnicity in an age of diaspora. In *Theorising diaspora* (pp. 120–131). Blackwell.

Richie, B. (1996). *Compelled to crime: The gender entrapment of battered, black women*. Routledge.

Samakayi-Makarati, J. N. (2003). Female prisoners in "male" prisons. In *Women in prison in Zimbabwe* (pp. 11–22). Weaver Press.

Spalek, B. (2008). *Ethnicity and crime: A reader*. Open University Press.

Stewart, J. (2003). Introduction: A tragedy of lives: Women in prison in Zimbabwe. In *A tragedy of lives. Women in prison in Zimbabwe* (pp. 1–10). Weaver Press.

Thiam, A. (1995). *Black sisters, speak out: Feminism and oppression in Black Africa*. Pluto Press.

Tonry, M. (1997). *Ethnicity, crime and immigration. Comparative and cross-national perspectives*. University of Chicago Press.

Tsanga, A. (2003). Conclusion. In *A tragedy of lives: Women in prison in Zimbabwe* (pp. 315–320). Weaver Press.

Van Wormer, K. (2010). *Working with female offenders: A gender-sensitive approach.* John Wiley and Sons.

Vera, Y. (1995). *The prison as a colonial space: Narratives of resistance.* Unpublished Doctoral Thesis, York University, Toronto.

Walker, C. (1991). *Women and resistance in South Africa.* David Phillip/Oxford University Press.

Weir, J. (2007). Chiefly women and women's leadership in pre-colonial Southern Africa. In *Women in South African History. They remove boulders and cross rivers* (pp. 3–20). Human Sciences Research Council Press.

West, C. (1992). Learning to talk race. In *I am because we are: Readings in Black philosophy* (pp. 350–355). University of Massachusetts Press.

15

Satisfied and Committed Prison Officers? A Qualitative Exploration of Job Satisfaction and Organisational Commitment among Prison Officers in Ghana

Thomas Akoensi

Introduction

Prisons represent an important institution in the criminal justice system and, as with many organisations, are confronted with the task of ensuring that staff are satisfied with their work and sufficiently committed to the ideals of the institution. While Locke (1976, p. 1304) defined job satisfaction as "a pleasurable or positive emotional state resulting from the appraisal of one's job or job experiences", Spector (1997, p. 214) defined job satisfaction as the extent to which an employee likes his or her job. Despite these differences, 'affect', that is emotion, is an underlying theme of job satisfaction, although a critical assessment of Locke's (1976) definition adds a further cognitive dimension involving an interaction between

T. Akoensi (✉)
School of Social Policy, Sociology and Social Research, University of Kent, Medway, UK
e-mail: t.akoensi@kent.ac.uk

© The Author(s), under exclusive license to Springer Nature Switzerland AG 2021
H. C. O. Chan, S. Adjorlolo (eds.), *Crime, Mental Health and the Criminal Justice System in Africa*, https://doi.org/10.1007/978-3-030-71024-8_15

cognition and affect. Job satisfaction is thus a subjective feeling resulting from the individual's assessment of whether his needs and wants are being met in the job or not. Organisational commitment, another crucial employee attitude, transcends attachment to the employees' job, work group or belief in the importance of work itself, encompassing the employees' bond to the organisation as a whole. Meyer and Allen (1991, 1997) have conceptualised organisational commitment as constituting three main components: affective commitment (based on a desire to belong to the organisation); normative commitment (based on a sense of obligation to the organisation) and calculative commitment (based on the belief that leaving the organisation will be costly to the employee in terms of sunk costs such as pension and benefits).

General academic and industry interest in job satisfaction and organisation commitment is not without reason. These vital attitudes have been linked to impact staff behaviours, and other important organisational efficiency and effectiveness indices such as productivity, turnover intent and voluntary turnover. In a meta-analysis, Dowden and Tellier (2004) found these attitudes to be robust predictors of job stress. Research from private and public-sector prisons in the UK has shown that staff attitudes influence behaviour and, consequently, the prison ethos (Crewe, 2011; Crewe, Liebling, & Hulley, 2011). Given the importance of attitudes in shaping the prison ethos and the implementation of prison policy reforms (Liebling, 2008), it is vital to explore the determinants of officer attitudes, especially job satisfaction and organisational commitment.

Despite efforts to explore the nature and determinants of prison staff job satisfaction and organisational commitment, the extant research suffers some limitations. First, research on these attitudes, although mainly Anglo-Saxon, is regarded as generalisable to other cultures and thus sparsely examined in contexts such as Ghana, yet cross-cultural research has shown that culture plays a pivotal role in the development of satisfaction and commitment (Clugston, Howell, & Dorfman, 2000; Kirkman & Shapiro, 2001). Despite attempts at addressing cross-cultural prison dynamics (e.g. Boateng & Hsieh, 2019), much exploration remains on satisfaction and commitment among prison officers. Second, research on both job satisfaction and organisational commitment has been mainly quantitative in orientation, involving the use of standardised scales whose contents are mainly imposed by the researchers rather than derived from the informants. This approach tends to mask differential effects and ignore individual differences caused by the 'interactions between the person and the environment' (Van Ginneken, 2016, p. 219). Finally, research into the antecedents of job satisfaction and organisational commitment has been compromised by the aggregation of correctional staff and treatment staff, thus limiting our understanding of the attitudes of prison or correctional officers, even though they represent a distinct and unique set of prison employees with considerable influence in shaping the prison environment for good or ill. The aim of this study is to explore empirically via the lived experiences of Ghanaian prison officers the factors that shape job satisfaction and organisational commitment.

Previous Research on Job Satisfaction and Organisational Commitment

Job satisfaction is acknowledged as one of the most important and widely researched constructs in the literature of industrial and organisational psychology and management. Low job satisfaction impacts negatively on prison staff. While Lombardo (1981) found that low job satisfaction increased absenteeism, Lambert, Edwards, Camp, and Saylor (2005) found that decreased job satisfaction resulted in increased use of sick leave. Turnover is another costly consequence of low job satisfaction, because of the expense of recruiting, selecting, training and placing of new staff (McShane, Williams, Schichor, & McClain, 1991). Notably, most prisons rely on human beings for the management of other human beings, and technology cannot replace staff in the running of prisons. Thus, the direct costs (e.g. recruitment and training) and indirect costs (e.g. loss of productivity and anxiety among existing staff as well as tension between new and existing staff) of prison staff turnover are considerable (Archambeault & Fenwick, 1988).

The effects of job satisfaction are not confined to staff but also affect prisoners' well-being and the wider prison environment. Research among prison officers supports a strong positive relationship between job satisfaction and support for offender rehabilitation (Hepburn & Knepper, 1993). Similarly, Nacci and Kane (1984, p. 49) concluded in their study of sex and sexual aggression among federal prison prisoners that "[w]hen officers indicated greater job satisfaction, prisoners were likely to say that their environment was more free from the danger of sexual assault". Aside from its relationship with a safe environment, job satisfaction among officers enhanced favourable staff–prisoner relationships and increased officers' maintenance of correctional standards and conditions (Farkas, 1999; Lambert, Barton, & Hogan, 1999; Styles, 1991). Nevertheless, Farkas (1999) found that when officers reported high job satisfaction, there was increased social distance between prisoners and officers, but officers' abuse of authority was significantly reduced. This was mainly because officers attributed their high job satisfaction to extrinsic aspects of the job such as pay and benefits. It can be safely argued from the literature that the impact of officer job satisfaction on prisoner outcomes is contingent upon the source of satisfaction, where intrinsic sources are more important for favourable prisoner outcomes.

Organisational commitment has become synonymous with affective commitment because of its strong predictive validity, positive association with job satisfaction and strong negative correlation with turnover and stress (Brunetto & Farr-Wharton, 2003; Mathieu & Zajac, 1990). Commitment comprises three major elements: loyalty (belief in the goals of the organisation), identification (pride and internalisation of organisational goals) and involvement (making personal sacrifices for the sake of the organisation) (Mowday, Porter, & Steers, 1982).

Despite theoretical problems such as the high correlation between affective and normative commitments (Meyer, Stanley, Herscovitch, & Topolnytsky, 2002), the works of Meyer and Allen (1991, 1997) have gained wide endorsement and validation. Of the three organisational commitment components, the affective and normative dimensions, which are attitudinal in nature, have received much research attention and have been found to be more strongly aligned with organisational outcomes than the behavioural dimension (Mathieu & Zajac, 1990; Randall, 1990; Somers, 1995).

Culliver, Sigler, and McNeely (1991) report a strong relationship between officer commitment and job performance. They established that officers who were rated at a minimum of job performance by their supervisors reported lower levels of organisational commitment. However, officers rated as delivering desirable and acceptable levels of job performance were found to report favourable organisational commitment. The researchers consequently established a link between organisational commitment and pro-social job efforts or behaviours such as organisational achievement, empathy and help towards prisoners, and facilitating the flow of work in the prison. They concluded that "it is probable that these correctional officers are motivated in their work behaviour by what they perceive to be the best for the organization" (Ibid: 283). Similarly, Lambert, Hogan, and Griffin (2008) reported that organisational commitment was linked to organisational citizenship behaviour (OCB).

On the antecedents of job satisfaction and commitment among prison staff, it has been found that officers cite intrinsic reasons for work in corrections, supervisory support, opportunities to make contributions to decision-making, promotional opportunities, pay and incentive programmes, procedural justice and distributive justice in enhancing both job satisfaction and commitment (Hepburn & Knepper, 1993; Lambert et al., 2008; Lambert & Paoline, 2008). Conflict between work and family roles, perceptions of the job being dangerous, job stress and role strain have also been found to reduce job satisfaction and organisational commitment (Hepburn & Knepper, 1993; Hogan, 2006; Lambert & Paoline, 2008).

Situating the Ghana Penal System

Ghana's prisons like most other African nations are a colonial legacy. Upon political independence from British colonial rule in 1957, Ghana inherited 33 prisons, a prison population of 52 per 100,000 of the population, with an overcrowding rate in excess of 48% and a paramilitary management structure. Currently, there are 43 prisons in Ghana with an average daily custody population of 15,203 (or 50 per 100,000 of the population), an overcrowding rate in excess of 52.87% above full capacity of 9945 places, and a staff population of almost 6000 (Ghana Prisons Service [GPS], 2016, 2020). The paramilitary organisational structure and most of the prisons inherited are in full use today. The Prisons Decree (1972), which specifies the safe custody and welfare of prisoners, guides prison work in Ghana and relegates offender rehabilitation and reformation as a secondary and optional goal.

The poor working conditions of prison officers—office space facilities, conditions of incarceration, overcrowding, staff shortages, working equipment, officers' accommodation as well as low pay and limited promotional and career development opportunities—engender officers' stress (Akoensi, 2014). High youth unemployment and job security, however, make state security or uniform roles like prison officers an attractive option despite poor work conditions. Rising incidents of prison officers' misconduct involving corruption, dealings in narcotics, officer brutalities of civilians and prisoners reported mainly in the print and electronic media have brought about discussions of officers' job satisfaction and organisational commitment in public and academic circles.[1] Recently, Boateng and Hsieh (2019) found in their cross-sectional survey of 169 officers located in five prison establishments that organisational justice and income of prison officers were important determinants of officers' satisfaction and organisational commitment. They found that whilst procedural justice predicted officers' commitment, both procedural and distributive justice predicted job satisfaction. Officers' low pay largely undermined both job satisfaction and organisational commitment. Although this study provides important insight, what remains is the lived experiences of prison officers and how this affects their job satisfaction and organisational commitment in officers' own voices.

---

[1] There have been reported cases of prison officers smuggling cell phones into prisons (https://www.ghanaweb.com/GhanaHomePage/NewsArchive/Officers-Smuggling-Mobile-Phones-Into--Prisons-227889), officers assaulting members of the public (https://www.bbc.co.uk/sport/football/47870661) and an officer dealing in narcotics being arrested and sentenced for his crimes (https://www.peacefmonline.com/pages/local/news/201805/351208.php).

Methodology

Bergman (2006) asserts that paramilitary organisations show high organisational commitment due to high norms of obligations, internalisations and identification. Among prison officers in Ghana, commitment is further reflected in the officers' oath of loyalty to the Ghana Prisons Service (GPS). Research has shown that employees in collectivist societies (who are characterised by their intense emotional attachments to the in-group) exhibit high social identification with their organisations (Chew & Putti, 1995; Markovits, Davis, & van Dick, 2007).

The exceptionally low turnover rate as reflected in the resignations and desertions of the GPS by officers despite reflecting limited job alternatives and avenues could also indicate strong prison officers' organisational commitment. For example, in 2009, only 19 (of 4753) and in 2010 only 16 (of 4593) officers resigned from the service (GPS Annual Reports, 2009, 2010). It was therefore necessary in the fieldwork not to refer to the term 'commitment' or attempt to define it while pursuing a line of questioning reflecting commitment.

In 20 of the 43 prison establishments in Ghana, 78 in-depth semi-structured interviews were conducted with a purposive sample of front-line officers. Interviews were conducted in offices, prison workshops, kitchens, visit areas and other locations. The interviews were tape-recorded with the expressed permission of the respondents, and with standard assurances of confidentiality. These were transcribed verbatim. In addition to the interviews, extensive observations of prison officers as they discharged their daily routines were also undertaken. The sample reflects the typical frontline staffing levels of prisons, including senior and subordinate officers, male and female officers, officers with long service and those who had served very few years at the various prison establishments (see Table 15.1). After creating an abstract of narratives, thematic analysis was then employed to identify categories and themes emerging from the data. This method facilitated an objective and inductive approach in the identification of the relevant categories and thematic patterns embedded in the materials in a systematic manner. The various categories were then grouped into four broad non-mutually exclusive themes

Table 15.1 Table indicating ranks of prison officers and the corresponding number of participants (*N* = 78)

Category	Rank	Number of respondents
Subordinate officer corps	Second Class Officer	5
	Lance Corporal	9
	Corporal	2
	Sergeant	2
	Assistant Chief Officer	5
	Chief Officer	10
	Senior Chief Officer	6
	Total	39
Superior officer corps	Assistant Superintendent of Prisons	6
	Deputy Superintendent of Prisons	7
	Superintendent	7
	Chief Superintendent of Prisons	9
	Assistant Director of Prisons	5
	Deputy Director of Prisons	5
	Total	39

reflecting negative or positive attributes towards job satisfaction and organisational commitment.

Findings

Job Satisfaction

In all, 51 prison officers spoke about their job satisfaction and its determinants. When officers were asked which aspects of their work they derived satisfaction or fulfilment from, the question surprised many of the participants as they admitted that they had never thought about positive aspects of their jobs. Nevertheless, they provided responses that were varied and interesting.

Reformation

A recurrent theme in officers' narratives was that professional elements of the role such as the counselling that assists offender reform was a key element of job satisfaction. Satisfaction was derived from teaching skills to prisoners, religious counselling, helping prisoners to find meaning in their lives, and observing changes in prisoners' attitudes and behaviours. Seventeen officers perceived their role in reform as an integral part of their work, as prisons were under-resourced and had no staff specialising in offender rehabilitation.

> The most rewarding and satisfying aspect of my job is to be able to train an inmate and realizing that he has picked up the skills. When such an inmate is discharged and he manages to come and visit, you realize that the person is doing well. Sometimes some of them are able to establish their own shop or are working with someone and leading a good life. When you realize that the person is not in a position to return to prison again, it is very satisfying. (Female, Sergeant)

For some officers, the mere fact that prisoners were going on discharge was enough to trigger satisfaction. Prison conditions were poor, and officers acknowledged it, so a discharge was an opportunity for prisoners to make progress in their lives. This was usually the case when a prisoner successfully appealed against his/her conviction and was set free:

> The happy and satisfying moments are any time I see that a prisoner had filed an appeal and later on becomes a victor. I remember one of them filed an appeal [against his conviction] and was discharged at the court. I was so excited with my colleagues. (Female, Sergeant)

Such officers derived satisfaction from helping prisoners but not from the organisational routines. This could potentially be a source of conflict between job satisfaction and organisational commitment: officers feel they are doing 'right' and their actions benefit others, but they do not see the prison service as moral and 'right', and so they lack commitment.

This could also explain why some officers stay in the job even though they lack commitment to the organisation.

Benefit-Finding or Personal Growth

Nine officers reported deriving satisfaction from the benefits inherent in prison work. Officers argued that there were many lessons to be learned from their interactions with prisoners. Their recognition of positive aspects of prison work was evidence of the fulfilment motivating them to continue in the job.

> For me, being an officer has helped me because when I was enlisted into the prison service, there were a lot of things I was doing formerly that I didn't know were unlawful. So in my interactions with the prisoners, I realized that those things I was doing that I got away with, prisoners were serving sentences for doing same. I have since abstained from such acts. [*What are some of those acts you were doing?*] Yes. I am a warrior. This cut [he shows me cut marks on his wrists and other parts of his body]. If you hold a knife in an attempt to stab me, I will hold the knife. Every punch of mine will cut you. True. Honestly, if you like ask my wife [standing from a distance of about 2 meters from interview point] and my children. They will all tell you. [...] So I stopped after becoming an officer. [...] So I have learnt a lot since becoming a prison officer. (Male, Chief Officer)

This extract indicates that the informant had learnt self-control and patience since becoming a prison officer. Officer narratives on benefit-finding contrast with the prevailing assumptions that prison work impacts only negatively on prison officers in the form of stress, burnout, a constant threat of danger, post-traumatic stress disorder, the monotony and the emotional labour involved (e.g. Crawley, 2004; Lombardo, 1981). It is striking that officers locate benefits or inherent meaning in a work environment that is often characterised as negative and hostile. Benefit-finding is an interpretive process involving the location of positive changes in the negative or traumatic environment of the prison. These benefits may not be concrete or objective but their recognition helps to modify behaviour. "[I]f men define situations as real, they are real in their consequences" (Thomas & Thomas, 1928, p. 572), and this depicts the interpretive nature and potential impact of benefit-finding on officers.

Helping Prisoners

The opportunity to help prisoners was an initial motivating factor for some applicants seeking employment with the GPS. That aside, the possibility of helping prisoners was a source of job satisfaction for some informants. These officers derived fulfilment in offering material and emotional support to prisoners:

> When I see prisoners happy, I feel satisfied and motivated. I like listening to their problems and helping them solve it. When it is solved, I'm happy. There is no day I come to work without a prisoner approaching me with a problem. That is what keeps me coming. (Male, Assistant Superintendent)

Offering help to prisoners was not confined to junior officers who had more daily interactions with prisoners. High-ranking officers including prison governors also offered direct assistance to prisoners:

> I get satisfaction when I'm able to help solve the myriad of problems facing prisoners. [...] Sometimes, I use my personal cell phone to invite police officers and relatives of prisoners to help solve prisoners' problems. For example, I just got answers as to why an inmate on remand's warrant has expired but still in prison. (Male, Assistant Director)

This finding replicates Liebling, Price, and Shefer (2011), who found that helping prisoners was an important antecedent of job satisfaction among prison staff in England. The desire to help prisoners was important for officers as it indicated their readiness to make the prison community a better place despite the inadequate material conditions.

A Good Day

Prison officers felt satisfied if at the end of the day there were no major disturbances and prisoners were happy. Officers referred to this success as having a 'good day':

> At the end of the day if everything has been done well, there is no problem especially with our main mandate of safe custody. So at the end of the day if everyone is safe, no prisoner has escaped, nothing has happened to any officer, then you feel satisfied that at least you have performed your duties well. (Female, Deputy Director)
>
> The most rewarding and satisfying aspect of the job is when you come to work and at the end of the shift, you were able to discharge your duties peacefully and successfully. If prisoners have had their food and there were no complaints and they are happy, the day becomes a successful and peaceful one. You feel really satisfied. (Female, Second Class Officer)

Ghanaian officers' descriptions of a 'good day' echo those of officers in England and Wales (Liebling et al., 2011).

Recognition and Praise for Work

Two officers said that praise from their supervisors gave them satisfaction. Praise and recognition were quite rare and so praise for a job well done went a long way towards making the job fulfilling. It also communicated to these officers that their work was important and sustained officers' enthusiasm for their work:

> When my boss appreciates everything that I do, I really like it; I feel satisfied and motivated to do more and to work harder. […] Anytime I make a mistake, he calls me into the office and informs me. He adds that next time, do it this way. So it gives me much satisfaction. (Female, Second Class Officer)

Pay and Benefits

The aforementioned themes may be termed intrinsic job factors, since they are linked directly to officers' role. Prison officers also mentioned extrinsic factors. Salary and benefits such as free housing were extrinsic factors for some officers. Yet the relevance of salary and benefits is not so much related to fiscal value or to the amount of compensation *per se* but to the extent to which officers believed salaries and benefits were commensurate with their merit. Four male officers emphasised satisfaction from their pay and benefits, not from their work:

> The satisfaction comes from the salary because we all work for [money]. That is the first thing everybody has in mind when going to work. So when I get my salary, I'm happy and nothing else. (Male, Sergeant)

Job Dissatisfaction

Pay and benefits are uncertain sources of job satisfaction, as officers who cited that they were dissatisfied with their work were also quick to refer to their meagre salaries, and to job stress and poor working conditions. Five officers, all male, professed job dissatisfaction:

> I do not find anything rewarding or satisfying about this job as a prison officer. This is because of the low remuneration including the salaries and also because there is tension in this job. (Male, Sergeant)
>
> I will say that the reward of the prison officer is in heaven. Because when it comes to our salaries, nil! The motivation and satisfaction is not there. Look at the conditions under which we are working. Very poor. Even the feeding rate for the inmates is meagre and at times, we the officers have to sacrifice and then support the prisoners. So when we talk about job satisfaction, the salary is meagre and there is nothing to write home about. (Male, Chief Superintendent)

These extracts point to the importance of adequate remuneration in addressing issues of officers' job dissatisfaction as implicated in the work of Boateng and Hsieh (2019).

Organisational Commitment

Fifty-four officers responded directly to questions and prompts about organisational commitment. Their narratives demonstrated a mixed relationship with the GPS: while 26 prison officers professed high organisational commitment, 28 officers indicated poor organisational commitment. Themes underlying high and low organisational commitment are presented.

High Organisational Commitment

Prison officers professing high organisational commitment described their experiences, which featured all organisational commitment components found in the literature, namely affective, continuance and normative. Regarding affective commitment, officers mainly instanced benefit-finding or personal growth as their main motivation. Thirteen officers expressed the belief that, given the level of wisdom, vigilance and the various forms of education that working in prison had taught them, they were proud of the prison service.

> I have told you previously that I have learned a lot which has shaped and moulded my life in such a way that certain misbehaviours I engaged in, had I not joined the service I would have still be[en] engaging in them. So joining the service alone had made me change. (Male, Assistant Superintendent)

Prison work and the experiences garnered shaped officers' character overtime. One officer's account of benefit-finding was particularly revealing:

> I was married before I joined the service and then, on 30th June 1980, I went to work. I was for afternoon shift. I went home after work but my wife was not home. I went to check with a friend if my wife was at theirs but she wasn't there. After I returned home, I came to meet my wife with another man. Because of this work, I have met some people who have been condemned to death, and those who were killed right in front of me through executions. It made me think. It reminded me and because of that, I kept my cool and left the scene. I went and reported the matter to the

police. The police inspector was particularly full of praises for my efforts. And this always teaches me a lesson. You see, if not because of this work, I don't know what would have happened. I met my wife with another man on my matrimonial bed. It was June 30th 1980. I will never forget and will never forget. (Male, Chief Officer).

This officer's exercise of self-control was remarkable and, hence, the immediate praise from police officers. The virtue of self-control developed from his interactions with prisoners in general and those who have found themselves in similar situations in particular helped him considerably to steer off violence that could have landed him in prison. Due to the predominant adherence to patriarchal values in Ghana, strong cultural abhorrence is attached to female infidelity and to the extent that adultery was committed in the officer's matrimonial bed engendered deep sentiments and moral outrage. Frequently, even cases of intense suspicion of female spouse or intimate partner involved in a sexual affair with another man end up with the man committing lethal violence or homicide of both the female victim and male assailant (Adinkrah, 2014).

Continuance/Calculative Commitment

Eight officers expressed continuance commitment. They said that benefits in terms of pay, educational opportunities and prestige would be lost should they decide not to return to the service if they had the opportunity again in life. These opinions reflect a cost–benefit analysis on their part, or what Becker (1960) refers to as 'side-bets'. Becker (1960) suggested that where benefits far outweighed the costs of leaving the organisation, employees were likely to remain committed. These employees were committed to the GPS because of the perceived costs of leaving it:

My life depends on the prison service; it is a good occupation. I earn a salary, which has made my family and I prosperous. I have enrolled my kids in secondary schools. (Male, Assistant Chief Officer)

I haven't regretted joining it [Prison Service]. I came here with a Master's degree and through the help of the service, I now [have higher qualifications]. [...] I like the job because it has made me who I am now. I am enjoying every bit of the facilities that the service has given me. I am enjoying a three-bedroom house; I don't pay rent, water, electricity and telephone bills. So even though I was a teacher and left that profession to join the service, I didn't go back to teaching. Why am I still here? It is because I like the job and the benefits. (Male, Superintendent)

These findings speak to the work of Boateng and Hsieh (2019) about the role of low pay in shaping officers' commitment.

Normative Commitment

Five officers said that their commitment to the GPS rests solely on their wish to help prisoners. They were therefore expressing their normative commitment to remain in the GPS for its own sake:

I always want to see the prisoners. [...] Some of them see me and share their stories and make up stories to share with me. They make me laugh all the time and sometimes, I even forget I have problems. Their happiness makes the shift and the work easy and smooth. [...] I like to see the prisoners and to be there for them. (Female, Lance Corporal)

These prisoners are needy and people must take care of them. You go to hospital and there are people to take care of patients. Though they might not be happy working there, yet they do. So people must sacrifice for others and I will come back to this work. (Male, Assistant Director/OIC)

As these extracts show, officers' commitment was not based on any rewards or benefit-finding, but on the moral obligation of helping prisoners who are required by law only to be detained. To remain an employee of the GPS then was to continue to help prisoners.

Low Organisational Commitment

Low commitment was enmeshed in a variety of factors relating to the lack of affective, continuance and normative commitment to the prison service. Often poor experiences at the hands of the GPS were the main reason for poor commitment to an organisation whose norms and values they could not internalise. Since officers' accounts of low commitment involved all three aspects of commitment, themes emerging from their narratives are described under the appropriate stressors.

Organisational Injustice

The lack of organisational justice was a recurrent reason given by some officers for their lack of commitment to the GPS. Specifically, they mentioned deficient interpersonal treatment at the hands of the service, as well as arbitrary allocation of incentives and punishments.

> The discipline and punishment is too much and people tend to infringe on your rights a lot. (Male, Assistant Director)
>
> Not that I have regretted joining the service, but with the bad experiences in the service I won't. [Can you share some of these experiences?] I have seen colleagues who have been dismissed from the service for very trivial violations simply because they don't have a say in the affairs of GPS. One afternoon, a colleague was dismissed and at the same time, his family was asked to vacate the accommodation. The service vehicle was at their house to convey them. Where were they going without an alternative place of abode? […] Another officer was also dismissed for a very minor incident too after spending 22 good years in the service. So this job is not worth dying for. (Male, Chief Officer)

These extracts indicate that unfair treatment (procedural injustice) and harsh punishments for minor violations of the prison rules (distributive injustice) were important in shaping organisational commitment. This aligns with findings from Boateng and Hsieh (2019) about the importance of organisational justice in shaping officers' commitment.

Pay and Benefits

Pay and conditions of service were the next most frequently cited themes. Officers argued that the poor state of their residential accommodation, their meagre salaries, harsh environmental working conditions and the lack of career development opportunities were responsible for their poor dedication to the GPS.

> I don't think there is any prison officer who goes home happy. It's all got to do with remuneration and motivation. I have been in this service for 37 years. [...] Is it not pathetic, sad, melancholic that to date, I can't even boast of a fowl coop? Every Prison officer relies on the end of service benefit, which is nothing to write home about. That means, as I am here, I have nothing at the bank. I have three children. One just completed the university, the other polytechnic and the last is in secondary school. With this burden, how can I put up a house? I am a debtor. [Officer beats his chest] There is no officer in this facility that is not a debtor. We are all debtors. I surely won't return to this service. (Male, Superintendent)

Concerns about benefits extended to limited career development opportunities:

> I have missed a lot of opportunities. There are limited opportunities to study both locally and internationally in the service. If I get a second chance in life, I would like to join another organization and not the prison service. (Male, Assistant Director)

For other officers, their motive in joining the service was a decisive factor in their low organisational commitment. They argued that enlisting in the GPS was a last resort. Thus, they were not motivated to internalise GPS' values in the first place, let alone build on them:

> [Officer sucks teeth] Nothing inspired me to join the service in the first place. I only joined because I just needed a job and that was the only opportunity that came my way. (Female, Corporal)

Lack of Job Autonomy or Powerlessness

The lack of job autonomy was the third most frequently cited reason for low organisational commitment. Officers cited the lack of discretion at work and their lack of voice in decision-making:

> Progressing in the service is a problem. You can't have your way to do things the way you would want to. You always have to work by the rules. Even though it may not be the best, you are compelled to work by the book. [...] I would like to be in an organization where I can use my discretion to do things that will benefit the work and the organization rather than coming back to the prison service. Here, you can even go to meetings, and they will admonish you to feel free to talk; woe betide you if you say something that is in bad taste to the superiors. They will not punish you directly but you will suffer for speaking at that [meeting] that you were asked to speak. So, I will not return to such an organization. (Female, Sergeant)

Job Characteristics (Perceived Job Dangerousness, Work–Family Conflict and Public Image of Prison Service)

Four officers described job and organisational characteristics as mainly impacting on their affective commitment. Two officers cited the danger and threat of assault inherent in their work. As one male officer said, "Why should I return to this job and continue to risk my life in the course of duty? I won't".

Another officer cited his inability to make time for his family as the source of his low commitment:

> You cannot express your feelings in this job. You cannot also socialize with your family. As I'm sitting here, I have lost my mother-in-law and I won't be allowed to go and pay my respects because I have already enjoyed my annual leave. I can't also attend my village festival, which I enjoy so much. [...] My extended family relationship has deteriorated due to this job. My father called me from Accra to relate some sad issues with me about my

behaviour: he says whenever there were funerals I did not attend. He was angry. [...] (Male, Assistant Chief Officer)

Another officer cited the poor public image of the prison service as contributing to his poor commitment:

It appears that no matter how much effort the prison officer puts in his job, he is not given the recognition. Compared to other security agencies, we are not regarded. It appears that the public hatred for the prisoner has been transferred to us officers. Because of this, members of society don't want to feed prisoners three times a day, clothe them properly, provide them with proper bedding, house them in well ventilated structures, etcetera. This hatred for prisoners has greatly affected the image of the prison officer. Since society thinks prisoners are nothing, how can they attach any importance to the prison officer? This is why I won't return to this job. (Male, Deputy Superintendent)

Conclusion

Discussions of job satisfaction and organisational commitment have hitherto been based almost exclusively on quantitative empirical evidence from studies in Europe and North America, with sparse research from sub-Saharan Africa. The present study therefore sought to examine job satisfaction and organisational commitment and what shaped them among prison officers, in the predominantly collectivist culture of Ghana. The findings indicate that while officers were generally satisfied with their jobs, their relationship to the organisation via organisational commitment was mixed. Nevertheless, satisfaction and commitment cannot be regarded as a fixed or static state. While satisfaction implies a transient emotion based on retroactive information (i.e. how they have been treated, the personal rewards achieved), commitment is the concept of an individual's current and future involvement with the organisation. Satisfaction can change from day to day, but commitment is a long-term and stable trait.

Despite officers' expressions of job satisfaction, officers' level of commitment (expressed through pride, involvement and internalisation of norms and values of the prison service) was heterogeneous. Similar proportions of officers professed favourable and negative organisational commitment. Whilst intrinsic rewards, including benefit-finding and helping prisoners in accord with their values, was associated with high commitment, extrinsic rewards, including pay and benefits career development opportunities, were important drivers of poor organisational commitment. Regarding the components of organisational commitment, it was established that all three components identified by Meyer and Allen (1991, 1997) are important in this African penal context. While affective commitment was vital in enhancing organisational commitment, normative and calculative/continuance commitment were important components associated with poor commitment.

Negative organisational commitment was predicated on several factors, which had a telling effect mainly via behavioural considerations. Although quantitative studies endorse affective commitment as an important determinant of organisational commitment, normative commitment and calculative commitment are equally important in determining commitment. Following suggestions by Reiner (2000) and Kleinig (1996) about commitment among police officers in the West, it is plausible that officers join the GPS with pre-existing ideals. Their commitment either increases or decreases, depending on their job experiences and the internal climate or organisational dynamics. The paramilitary organisational structure connotes military discipline, as well as the fear and respect for the hierarchy and the ideals of prison work instilled into new recruits and officer cadets. Officers' accounts further depict an interplay of interactions among affective, normative and calculative/continuance considerations in determining organisational commitment.

This study is not without limitations. Similar to qualitative studies employing purposeful samples, it is important that these findings are interpreted with caution. The nature of the sampling indicates that the findings cannot be generalised beyond the sample for this study. This limitation notwithstanding, some findings about job satisfaction and organisational commitment among prison officers in Ghana are noteworthy. First, intrinsic elements of prison work were important in shaping both officer satisfaction and commitment. Most importantly, benefit-finding (or personal growth) was remarkable in this respect, and so was helping prisoners. Social altruism is an important aspect of the Ghanaian cultural fabric. It is traditionally believed that providing and sharing material and non-material items with the less fortunate in society accrues spiritual blessings and life satisfaction for the benefactors, irrespective of their religious orientation. Social altruism does not only promote societal inclusiveness and integration but also preserves the spiritual continuity of communities and their ancestors. Secondly, job stressors, including pay and benefits in particular, were important determinants of both job dissatisfaction and low commitment. Motivation for enlisting in the GPS also appeared to be a crucial factor as it determined states of satisfaction and commitment at the outset, which might then increase or decrease, depending on job conditions. Satisfaction and commitment are contingent states and uncompleted performances that change and are influenced by a variety of factors and probably play off each other in given situations, depending on individual and institutional characteristics.

Overall, there appears to be congruence between cultural values and social practices on the one hand, and job satisfaction and organisational commitment on the other. This might account for the positive levels of intrinsic satisfaction and work commitment found among Ghanaian prison officers. Thus, in helping to improve satisfaction and commitment, opportunities for officers to exhibit qualities that would encourage a stronger emotional and moral attachment to their jobs would be more important than improving pay and conditions. Officers' personal values would therefore be congruent with those of the GPS, resulting in increased productivity expressed in increased satisfaction and commitment. The Ghanaian prison officer culture is shaped such that while officers derive satisfaction from and are committed to their work with prisoners in line with local culture and values, officers lack commitment to the prison service.

Benefit-finding shows the extent to which prisons can positively impact their inhabitants, especially officers, in the development of virtues. Benefit-finding had meaning for officers, and impacted officers' overall quality of life and well-being positively. Benefit-finding is applicable in other contexts but this has not been found and given the research attention and profile it deserves. The benefit-finding cases identified here are transferable to the West, but they may not have been found if this study had commenced in the West and if a quantitative research approach had been adopted. Thus, the incorporation of cultural and societal influences via interviews enhanced the value of this study and brought to light themes that have previously not been found in the literature (e.g. benefit-finding). The findings from this research illustrate the importance of context-specific and participant-led research for understanding not just issues of job satisfaction and organisational commitment, but also informing future research (both qualitative and quantitative) among prison officers in Ghana particularly and in countries with similar prison characteristics globally.

Future studies on job satisfaction and organisational commitment among prison officers will benefit from including specialist staff in their samples. For example, we have very limited knowledge about how prison officers who primarily work in sentry positions feel about their jobs. Owing to the very demanding nature of their job requiring constant attention, concentration and the use of an assault rifle, and their location, sitting high above prison fence walls, assessing them for interviews can be quite daunting. Future researchers might also consider concentrating on frontline senior prison officers in governor grades in order to illuminate our understanding of their feelings towards their demanding jobs of making decisions that affect not just prisoners, but prison officers as well.

References

Adinkrah, M. (2014). Homicide-suicide in Ghana: Perpetrators, victims, and incidence characteristics. *International Journal of Offender Therapy and Comparative Criminology, 58*(3), 364–387. https://doi.org/10.117 7/0306624X12470530

Akoensi, T. D. (2014). *A tougher beat? The work, stress and well-being of prison officers in Ghana*. University of Cambridge.

Archambeault, W., & Fenwick, C. (1988). A comparative analysis of culture, safety, and organizational management factors in Japanese and U.S. prisons. *The Prison Journal, 68*, 3–23. https://doi.org/10.1177/003288558806800103

Becker, H. (1960). Notes on the concept of commitment. *American Journal of Sociology, 66*, 32–40. Retrieved from https://www.jstor.org/stable/2773219?seq=1

Bergman, M. (2006). The relationship between affective and normative commitment: Review and research agenda. *Journal of Organizational Behavior, 27*, 645–663. https://doi.org/10.1002/job.372

Boateng, F. D., & Hsieh, M. L. (2019). Explaining job satisfaction and commitment among prison officers: The role of organizational justice. *Prison Journal, 99*(2), 172–193. https://doi.org/10.1177/0032885519825491

Brunetto, Y., & Farr-wharton, R. (2003). The commitment and satisfaction of lower-ranked police officers: Lessons for management. *Policing: An International Journal of Police Strategies & Management, 26*(1), 43–63. Retrieved from https://www.emerald.com/insight/content/doi/10.1108/13639510310460297/full/html

Chew, I., & Putti, J. (1995). Relationship on work-related values of Singaporean and Japan. *Human Relations, 48*, 1149–1170. https://doi.org/10.1177/001872679504801003

Clugston, M., Howell, J. P., & Dorfman, P. W. (2000). Does cultural socialization predict multiple bases and foci of commitment? *Journal of Management, 26*, 5–30. https://doi.org/10.1177/014920630002600106

Crawley, E. (2004). *Doing prison work: The public and private lives of prison officers*. Willan Publishing.

Crewe, B. (2011). Soft power in prison: Implications for staff-prisoner relationships and legitimacy. *European Journal of Criminology, 8*(6), 455–468. https://doi.org/10.1177/1477370811413805

Crewe, B., Liebling, A., & Hulley, S. (2011). Staff culture, use of authority and prisoner quality of life in public and private sector prisons. *Australian & New Zealand Journal of Criminology, 44*, 94–115. https://doi.org/10.1177/0004865810392681

Culliver, C., Sigler, R., & McNeely, B. (1991). Examining prosocial organizational behaviour among correctional officers. *International Journal of Comparative and Applied Criminal Justice, 15*, 277–284. https://doi.org/10.1080/01924036.1991.9688973

Dowden, C., & Tellier, C. (2004). Predicting work-related stress in correctional officers: A meta-analysis. *Journal of Criminal Justice, 32*(1), 31–47. https://doi.org/10.1016/j.jcrimjus.2003.10.003

Farkas, M. (1999). Correctional officer attitudes toward inmates and working with inmates in a "get tough" era. *Journal of Criminal Justice, 27*(6), 495–506. https://doi.org/10.1016/s0047-2352(99)00020-3

Ghana Prisons Service. ([2010] 2016). *Annual Report: Ghana Prisons Service*. Accra.

Ghana Prisons Service. (2020). *Inmate statistics*. Retrieved from http://www.ghanaprisons.gov.gh/statistics.html

Hepburn, J., & Knepper, P. (1993). Correctional officers as human service workers: The effect on job satisfaction. *Justice Quarterly, 10*, 315–338. https://doi.org/10.1080/07418829300091841

Hogan, N. L. (2006). The impact of occupational stressors on correctional staff organizational commitment: A preliminary study. *Journal of Contemporary Criminal Justice, 22*, 44–62. https://doi.org/10.1177/1043986205285084

Kirkman, B., & Shapiro, D. (2001). The impact of cultural values on job satisfaction and organizational commitment in self-managing work teams: The mediating role of employee resistance. *Academy of Management Journal, 44*, 557–569. https://doi.org/10.5465/3069370

Kleinig, J. (1996). *Ethics of policing*. Cambridge University Press.

Lambert, E. G., Barton, S. M., & Hogan, N. L. (1999). The missing link between job satisfaction and correctional staff behavior: The issue of organizational commitment. *American Journal of Criminal Justice, 24*, 95–116. https://doi.org/10.1007/bf02887620

Lambert, E., Edwards, C., Camp, S., & Saylor, W. (2005). Here today, gone tomorrow, back again the next day: Antecedents of correctional absenteeism. *Journal of Criminal Justice, 33*(2), 165–175. https://doi.org/10.1016/j.jcrimjus.2004.12.008

Lambert, E. G., Hogan, N. L., & Griffin, M. L. (2008). Being the good soldier: Organizational citizenship behaviour and commitment among correctional staff. *Criminal Justice and Behavior, 35*, 56–68. https://doi.org/10.1177/0093854807308853

Lambert, E. G., & Paoline, E. A. (2008). The influence of individual, job, and organizational characteristics on correctional staff job stress, job satisfaction, and organizational commitment. *Criminal Justice Review, 33*, 541–564. https://doi.org/10.1177/0734016808320694

Liebling, A. (2008). Why prison staff culture matters. In *The culture of prison violence* (pp. 105–122). Pearson Education Inc.

Liebling, A., Price, D., & Shefer, G. (2011). *The prison officer* (2nd ed.). Willan Publishing.

Locke, E. (1976). The nature and causes of job satisfaction. In *Handbook of industrial and organizational psychology* (pp. 1297–1343). Rand McNally.

Lombardo, L. (1981). *Guards imprisoned: Correctional officers at work*. Elsevier.

Markovits, Y., Davis, A., & van Dick, R. (2007). Organizational commitment profiles and job satisfaction among Greek private and public sector employees. *International Journal of Cross Cultural Management, 7*, 77–99. https://doi.org/10.1177/1470595807075180

Mathieu, J. E., & Zajac, D. M. (1990). A review and meta-analysis of the antecedents, correlates, and consequences of organizational commitment. *Psychological Bulletin, 108*, 171–194. https://doi.org/10.1037/0033-2909.108.2.171

McShane, M., Williams, F., Schichor, D., & McClain, K. (1991). Early exits: Examining employee turnover. *Corrections Today, 53*, 220–225.

Meyer, J., & Allen, N. (1991). A three-component conceptualization of organizational commitment. *Human Resource Management Review, 1*, 61–89. https://doi.org/10.1016/1053-4822(91)90011-z

Meyer, J., & Allen, N. (1997). *Commitment in the workplace: Theory, research, and application*. Sage.

Meyer, J. P., Stanley, D. J., Herscovitch, L., & Topolnytsky, L. (2002). Affective, continuance, and normative commitment to the organization: A meta-analysis of antecedents, correlates, and consequences. *Journal of Vocational Behavior, 61*, 20–52. https://doi.org/10.1006/jvbe.2001.1842

Mowday, R., Porter, L., & Steers, R. (1982). *Employee-organization linkages: They psychology of commitment, absenteeism and turnover*. Academic Press.

Nacci, P., & Kane, T. (1984). Sex and sexual aggression in federal prisons: Inmate involvement and employee impact. *Federal Probation, 48*, 46–53. Retrieved from https://psycnet.apa.org/record/1987-32498-001

Randall, D. (1990). The consequences of organizational commitment: Methodological investigation. *Journal of Organizational Behavior, 11*, 361–378. https://doi.org/10.1002/job.4030110504

Reiner, R. (2000). *The politics of the police*. Oxford University Press.

Republic of Ghana. (1972). *The prisons service decree (NCRD 46)*. National Redemption Council.

Somers, M. J. (1995). Organizational commitment, turnover and absenteeism: An examination of direct and interaction effects. *Journal of Organizational Behavior, 16,* 49–59. https://doi.org/10.1002/job.4030160107

Spector, P. (1997). *Job satisfaction.* Sage.

Styles, S. (1991). Conditions of confinement suits. *Federal Prisons Journal, 2,* 41–47. Retrieved from https://heinonline.org/HOL/LandingPage?handle=hein.journals/fedprsj2&div=29&id=&page=

Thomas, W., & Thomas, D. S. (1928). *The child in America: Behavior problems and programs.* Alfred A. Knopf.

Van Ginneken, E. (2016). Making sense of imprisonment: Narratives of post-traumatic growth among female prisoners. *International Journal of Offender Therapy and Comparative Criminology, 60*(2), 208–227. https://doi.org/10.1177/0306624X14548531

16

Perceptions of the Police and Courts in Ghana

Akosua A. Adu-Poku

Introduction

Scholars and policymakers have long contemplated how citizens' views and attitudes on the formal justice system affect the image and legitimacy of the police and courts. Citizens' perspectives are fundamental to the overall functioning of the justice system. When citizens have a poor image of the justice system, they do not respect its authority. Citizens' perceptions, support and confidence are important in measuring and improving the performance of legal institutions. When trust in the justice system is low, so are compliance with civil suits, dispute resolution and jury and witness participation. These dynamics can undermine the process, and people may pursue justice through political connections and bribery or circumvent the system altogether (Benesh, 2006; Reisig & Parks, 2000).

A. A. Adu-Poku (✉)
Department of Sociology, University of Ghana, Accra, Ghana
e-mail: sadu-poku@st.ug.edu.gh

© The Author(s), under exclusive license to Springer Nature Switzerland AG 2021
H. C. O. Chan, S. Adjorlolo (eds.), *Crime, Mental Health and the Criminal Justice System in Africa*, https://doi.org/10.1007/978-3-030-71024-8_16

365

Justice systems worldwide have been challenged by scandals involving violence, bribery and corruption, which negatively affect citizens' attitudes, trust, support and confidence in the law (Brown & Benedict, 2002; Tankebe, 2008b; Wilson, 2012). Individuals who have negative perceptions of the police are less likely to report crimes, rely on the police for assistance or provide vital information to law enforcement officers (Cao & Zhao, 2005; Ren, Cao, Lovrich, & Gaffney, 2005; Tyler, 1990). Personal experiences continue to rank high among citizens' determinants of perceptions, attitudes and evaluations of their justice systems (Cheurprakobkit, 2000; Orr & West, 2007; Skogan, 2009; Weitzer & Tuch, 2005). This chapter elucidates the perceptions of the police and courts of people who have used the legal system in Ghana.

The Justice System in Ghana: A Historical Overview

Numerous efforts have been made to reform the formal legal system in Ghana to increase people's access to justice. Precolonial, colonial and postcolonial developments and reforms have taken place in the police and the judiciary process. Citizens' perceptions, attitudes and utilisation of the continually reformed system have been shaped by historical, structural and cultural nuances. This section provides a historical overview of the formal justice system in Ghana and the reforms that have been made to instill trust and access to justice.

Policing in Precolonial, Colonial and Postcolonial Ghana

Prior to colonisation, the police service looked quite different than it does today in many African societies. But to say 'that policing as currently known to us did not exist prior to the colonial period in most African societies is hardly an original observation' (Tankebe, 2008a, p. 68). Policing in the Gold Coast was organised by traditional authorities. Chiefs and kings deployed messengers who carried out police and judicial functions in their respective communities. For instance, there were highly developed and bureaucratised states such as the Ashanti Empire that had special units which could be deployed on urgent security assignments. While these special units may be less sophisticated in organisation, some were sufficiently well organised and vested with authority to patrol and enforce bye-laws of the traditional polity. Some of these units were even 'salaried' for performing policing functions. An example is the road warders called 'Akwansrafo' of the Ashanti state that patrolled trade routes and controlled the movement of travellers as well as collected taxes on behalf of their chiefs (Wilks, 1966 cited in Tankebe, 2008a).

Formal policing in Ghana dates to 1831, when Governor George McClean stationed a small number of officers at the courts of prominent chiefs across the Gold Coast. These police officers were meant to 'keep him informed on everything that was going on' (Ward, 1948, p. 184 cited in Tankebe, 2008a). Policing in the colonial Gold Coast had two goals. The first was to enforce and maintain security for trade in European goods and aid the expansion into the hinterland to exploit agricultural and mineral resources. The second was to protect the ruling and propertied classes. The police in colonial Ghana did not enjoy public trust. Citizens were concerned about the institution's moral standing as colonial policing regulated conduct that ran contrary to colonial rules and regulations. In 1851, the government withdrew the West India Regiment and replaced it with a locally raised police force due to financial constraints. This force was disbanded due to its lack of discipline and mutinous behaviour. Then, arms-bearing soldiers were deployed to patrol the major cities and towns, which resulted in riots between the troops and the locals. A new paramilitary police followed to perform general police duties. The initial police officers, who were ill-equipped and poorly paid, were later replaced by a better-educated force (Gillespie, 1955 cited in Tankebe, 2008a).

In 1868, the police's poor performance was attributed to the force's recruitment from the native population and a belief that a stranger would be more trustworthy. This sentiment resulted in the recruitment of Hausa people from Nigeria to replace the local officers. The new external police force widened the gap between the police and the local residents, as the colonial police came to be perceived as 'an intrusive alien force'. Successive governors saw the police as 'worse than inefficient' and 'so thoroughly unfit for their work that it is not surprising that they are decried and distrusted' (Deflem, 1994, p. 52; Gillespie, 1955, pp. 27–30 cited in Tankebe, 2008a). The police had a negative image, which persisted even after the decolonisation of British rule.

In 1957, when Ghana gained independence, the police continued enforcing the rules and regulations that had been set by colonial administrators. However, new frameworks for establishing police effectiveness and legitimacy were developed. Before independence, many police officers had little or no education, which affected the quality of the service they could provide. Most of the police officers in the Gold Coast (57.5%) were illiterate. According to Twum (2011), there was an effort to encourage graduates to enter the police service after independence. Educational programmes were introduced to inform the public about police–citizen relations. Public relations campaigns involved 'meet the people' musical programmes that aimed to improve the public's image of the Ghanaian police. Another important reform was the police five-year development plan that brought to fruition modern equipment and logistical advances. Coupled with the expansion of personnel in all units, these reforms have improved the police service (Twum, 2011).

The 1992 Constitution of the Republic of Ghana permits the police to perform its traditional role of maintaining law and order, which was established with the Police Service Act of 1970 (Act 35). An ongoing structural development that has helped improve the Ghana police service has been the establishment of other institutions, such as the Commission on Human Rights and Administrative Justice. This commission is mandated to investigate complaints of violation of fundamental rights, abuse of power and unfair treatment of citizens by public officers. The Select Committee on Defence and Interior was introduced to ensure the democratic accountability of the police. This institution is charged with the provision of security oversight responsibilities. These constitutional and institutional arrangements are meant to establish the police's legitimacy (Tankebe, 2013). However, negative perceptions of policing in Ghana remain. Anecdotal and empirical evidence suggests that most Ghanaian residents perceive the police negatively. The police continue to be associated with bribery and corruption, and public outrage over the Ghana police seems to have increased. Tankebe (2008b) argued: 'If it was thought that with political independence in 1957, this "alien institution" would undergo a fundamental restructuring—organisationally and ideologically—such aspirations were dashed' (p. 190). The colonial militaristic approach to policing, with its quintessential lack of accountability and respect for the fundamental rights of citizens, remains intact. Police misconduct appears to have worsened since the colonial period. Historical antagonism between the police and citizens, reports of basic human rights violations and increasing crime levels corroborate residents' negative outlooks on the police.

Judiciary in Precolonial Ghana

The establishment of the modern formal judiciary in Ghana can be traced to the colonial Gold Coast era. Prior to colonisation under British rule, there were no formal probation services, court systems or modern prisons. The maintenance of law and dispute resolutions was pursued through the chief or the lineage head depending on the nature and seriousness of the crime or dispute. Among the Akans, for instance, crimes and disputes within the lineage referred to as 'efisem' were usually settled by the 'abusuapayin' or lineage head. Crimes considered serious such as murder, adultery, treason, sexual intercourse with a menstruating woman and suicide called 'oman akyiwadie' were believed to be against the collective conscience of the community and was resolved by the 'omanhene' or chief (Nukunya, 2003).

The Ghana Judicial Service (2013) traces the historical development of the formal justice system from the colonial Gold Coast period to the present. Prior to colonisation, the British government's trading forts and settlements on the Gold Coast were vested in the Company of Merchants, which was a successor to the Royal African Company of England. British possessions on the Gold Coast were under the control of the governor of Sierra Leone. The West Africa Act of 1821 dissolved the Company of Merchants, its forts and other possessions vested in the British Crown. In 1843, the British Settlements Act established the Order in Council and permitted the establishment of laws, institutions and ordinances for peace and order. By September 1844, the Order in Council required judicial authorities in the Gold Coast to observe the local customs as compatible with the principles of the law of England.

On 6 March 1844, the Bond of 1844 was signed with the local Fanti chiefs at Cape Coast. The document outlined basic human rights and criminalised several customary practices, such as human sacrifices and panyarring, that the British considered barbaric. Serious crimes were to be tried at the Queen's Court by the Queen's judicial officers together with the local chiefs. Less serious crimes were to be tried in the customary courts. At the trials of serious criminal cases, local chiefs sat alongside the judicial personnel to ensure that the verdicts and practices in the new British legal system coincided with customary practices.

By 1853, the national Supreme Court of Her Majesty Forts and Settlement on the Gold Coast was established by Supreme Court Ordinance. It was presided over by a chief justice who was given the civil and criminal jurisdiction equivalent to the Courts of the Queen's Bench, Common Pleas and Exchequer at Westminster. This ordinance was shortly replaced by the Court of Civil and Criminal Justice, which merged the Gold Coast, Sierra Leone, Lagos and Gambia under The Governor of Four West Africa Settlements. In 1866, the Supreme Court was abolished and replaced by the Court of Civil and Criminal Justice. In July 1874, the Royal Charter, issued under the British Settlements Act, revoked the Commission of 19 February 1866 so far as it applied to the Gold Coast and Lagos and constituted these territories as a separate colony under the title of the Gold Coast Colony. The Royal Charter was repeated with little variation in March 1877 when the seat of government was moved from Cape Coast to Accra.

In 1876, the Supreme Court Ordinance was re-established. The court was divided into a two-tier system consisting of the higher court (Supreme Court) and lower courts (District Commissioners). The Supreme Court Ordinance provided room for the application of customary laws alongside the formal legal system. The traditional justice system was given the right to operate as long as the traditional laws and uses did not violate the law of the constitution, and serious criminal cases were sent to the formal system to be resolved. According to Ghana Judicial Service (2013), 1925 saw significant constitutional advances in the legislation. The Gold Coast

Colony (Legislative Council) Order in Council gave the colony elected representation for the first time. The new legislative council included the governor plus 15 official and 14 unofficial members. The Ordinance of 1876 was extended to the entire Gold Coast. Magistrate courts replaced district commissioners' courts, and district magistrates and district commissioners ceased to form part of the Supreme Court. In 1944, the Native Courts (Colony) Ordinance marked a revolutionary change in Ghana's judicial history. For the first time, the governor was given the power to set up entirely new courts and appoint members instead of the old customary law tribunals. Native authorities were given the power to exercise functions usually under the jurisdiction of local government, and default powers were given to the provincial commissioner. The pluralistic legal system continues to exist with few changes in postcolonial Ghana.

The Ghana Judicial Service (2013) observed that the Ghanaian Constitution of 1957 gave legislative power to the Ghanaian government. With the establishment of the constitution, the prime minister had the authority to appoint the chief justice and other justices of the superior courts. Executive and legislative powers were given to the Ghanaian parliament and prime minister, respectively. However, ultimate legislative and executive powers were still held by the Queen of Britain until 1960, when her authority was displaced by the establishment of the First Constitution of the Republic of Ghana. This legal framework was used until 1966, when Dr Nkrumah was overthrown by the National Liberation Council, which resulted in several structural changes in the judiciary. According to Smith (2008), the Supreme Court was abolished by the Courts Decree of 1966, which vested power in a two-tier court system comprised of the Superior Court of Judicature and the inferior courts. No changes were made until 1979, when the Armed Forces Revolutionary Council (AFRC) established the AFRC Special Tribunals. The purpose of these tribunals was to remove corrupt officials from Ghana. However, they fuelled suspicions, as judicial power was exercised without due process or respect for the rule of law (Smith, 2008). In 1981, the National, Regional, District and Community Public Tribunals were established.

A major turning point of the judiciary system occurred in 1992 with the Constitution of the Republic of Ghana. This constitution incorporated several innovations, including fundamental human rights and freedoms and the creation of the Commission of Human Rights and Administrative Justice. It also established the structure and hierarchy that continue to operate today. At the apex of the judiciary is the chief justice. The head of the judiciary is responsible for the administration and supervision of justice throughout the country. This constitution also provides for a judicial council, which is responsible for the administration of justice. Chaired by the chief justice, the council works independently to uphold the accurate interpretation of the constitution. As prescribed by the Constitution of Ghana, the council can propose government judicial reforms to improve the administration of justice and efficiency in the judiciary. The Judicial Council also plays an advisory role and holds judges accountable. Today, the Ghanaian judiciary has two strata of courts, the Superior Courts and the Lower Courts. The Superior Courts of Judicature consist of the Supreme Court, the Appeals Court, the High Court and regional tribunals. Beneath the Superior Courts are the Lower Courts, consisting of circuit courts and district courts. Specialised courts manage particular issues of justice and include family tribunals, juvenile courts, motor courts and chieftaincy tribunals.

Despite years of reform, the Ghanaian public continues to have little confidence in the courts. The administration of justice has been associated with bribery, corruption and dishonesty. The loss of trust and confidence in the legal system has been exacerbated by the system's inability to adjudicate cases efficiently. The need for reforms to earn citizens' confidence has become clear. Various steps have been taken by the judiciary to improve the administrative system nationwide. The government has established fast-track courts, specialised commercial courts, the Public Complaints and Court Inspection Unit, court-connected alternative dispute resolution, an automated supreme court library, the Private Process Service Schemes, the Home Finance Bank Post in the Supreme Court building and Child Panels (Smith, 2008). The fast track courts are equipped with modern technology, such as computers, voice recording systems and stenographs, and are meant to clear the overwhelming backlog of cases in the judiciary. The specialised commercial courts are mandated to deal exclusively with commercial matters. The general public is sceptical of litigation as an efficient method of resolving business disputes. The alternative dispute resolution system is meant to prevent cases that can be solved amicably from going through the full court proceedings. For the purposes of legal research, a commercial law library was also established for professionals, students and the public to access.

In acknowledgement of perceived judiciary corruption, the government introduced the Public Complaints and Court Inspectorate Unit to serve as an anti-corruption tool and give citizens an opportunity to air any grievances or complaints with the judicial service and staff. The court-connected alternative dispute resolution system is meant to settle disputes outside of the formal adjudication process. Many people prefer solving their disagreements outside of court, and traditional methods of resolution were not regarded with as much scepticism by the public. The Legal Aid Scheme guarantees that all members of society, especially the poor, who cannot afford legal services have access to legal representation. The overall aim of the development of these tools has been to improve the working of the courts and increase the public's trust and confidence.

Citizens' Assessment of the Justice System

The literature on the public's perceptions of the justice system has highlighted the diversity of people's sources of information. Several studies have hypothesised that a demographic model would include citizens' views of the police and courts based on age, sex, race, education, income and other characteristics (Brown & Benedict, 2002; Jesilow & Meyer, 2001; Sun & Wu, 2006; Weitzer & Tuch, 1999). Other scholars have posited a 'symbolic attitude' model in which the public assesses government agencies from abstract orientations. In this model, the general views of politics and government agencies are the basis of the public's assessment of the justice system (Brody & Sniderman, 1977; Lau, Brown, & Sears, 1978). Closely related to the symbolic attitude model is the 'experiential' model in which the public's assessment of the police and courts is based on individuals' direct encounters with personnel.

According to the experiential model, which underpins this study, the public views and rates the justice system based on direct encounters with legal institutions. The performance of the police and courts is the basis of citizens' perceptions and assessments. Several studies measuring justice system encounters have shown that positive or satisfactory experiences yield positive attitudes and confidence, whereas unsatisfactory experiences are associated with negative perceptions and mistrust (Cheurprakobkit, 2000; Jesilow, Meyer, & Namazzi, 1995; Schafer, Hueber, & Bynum, 2003; Smith, Graham, & Adams, 1991; Tyler, 2001; Weitzer & Tuch, 2005). Winfree and Griffiths (1971) measured the differences in police performance and found that positive or negative contact with the police explained 20% of citizens' ratings of the police; only 2% were explained by social background or demographics. However, the literature is inconsistent regarding which type of encounter (positive or negative) has a stronger bearing on citizens' satisfaction (Cheurprakobkit, 2000; Dean, 1980; Jacob, 1971).

Some researchers (Decker, 1981; Reisig & Correia, 1997) have extended the debate to argue that the nature of the contact influences citizens' dichotomisation of police encounters as either negative or positive. Decker (1981) suggested that attitudes towards the police depend on whether the individual contact was initiated by a citizen or the police. He calls police-initiated encounters 'proactive'; they are not voluntary, and they spark negative attitudes. He calls citizen-initiated encounters 'reactive'; they yield more positive attitudes. Decker (1981) maintained that the supportive roles played by the police in citizen-initiated contacts generate positive attitudes.

The role of vicarious experiences on perceptions, attitudes and evaluations of the police and courts has also been highlighted in the justice system literature. Indirect experiences, such as those reported by families, friends, neighbours and the media, can influence the public's assessments of the formal justice system (Moy, Pfau, & Kahlor, 1999; Weitzer & Tuch, 2005). Few studies have qualitatively explored experiences with the justice system from citizens' perspectives. Investigating individuals' experiences and interpretations can help us better understand the justice system.

Perceptions and Attitudes Towards the Justice System: The Ghanaian Context

Ghana's constitution asserts that '[j]ustice emanates from the people', implying a close nexus between justice and the people. Since its inception, the Ghanaian justice system has been continually reinvented. The changes have largely been in response to the public's lack of confidence in the institution, which continues to be associated with bribery, corruption, dishonesty and inefficiency (Boateng, 2012; Smith, 2008; Tankebe, 2010). The public holds negative perceptions of the Ghanaian police force, which is also associated with bribery and corruption. There have been reports of violations of basic human rights, such as police beating suspects, making arrests without warrants and detaining suspects beyond the constitutionally permitted limits (Tankebe, 2008b). The courts are always congested, and cases often take years to go to trial partly because of the absence of sufficient judicial staff. This problem has proved more daunting in rural communities. In 2005, it was estimated that approximately 65% of the country's district rural courts were vacant, as many citizens could not afford to use the law (Smith, 2008). The poor and vulnerable could not afford to seek justice from the courts due to the challenges of travelling to towns far away and the costs of court fees. Reforms to improve access to justice and the public's outlook on the system became necessary. Various steps have been taken by the judiciary to improve the administrative system nationwide. However, significant challenges remain. As with many institutional reforms, efforts have come from a top-down technocratic initiative and concentrated on structural changes. Although vital to expanding access to justice, structural changes lose sight of the social and cultural specificity of the particular contexts in which justice operates. The policies relating to the reforms have been developed in the absence of the participants who are most affected by them. This unilateral approach has ignored the reality of residents' local conditions and offered few gains. Appiah (2013, p. 3) argued:

> The last two and half decades have witnessed a justice system that reflects and responds to an economy badly in need of foreign exchange and foreign investors. We have established Fast Track High Courts, Commercial Courts

and Land Courts to meet the needs of mostly foreign investors as they sue Ghanaians to claim debts for sometimes overpriced services that are poorly rendered. The filing fees for initiating a case in the Fast Track High Court (not counting legal fees) is well beyond the pocket of ordinary Ghanaians. We have also seen the establishment of Commercial Crime and Property Crime Units within the Ghana Police Service and the use of the criminal process to recover private debts for businesses. The demand for formal justice services in Ghana involves mostly the business or propertied classes as litigants.

Following these agenda-based reforms, the police and courts in Ghana have been reported to be corrupt, and the Ghanaian populace continues to have little confidence in the justice system. The Ghanaian justice system ranks high among the institutions in the country perceived to be corrupt. The Global Corruption Barometer revealed that among the various institutions in Ghana, the police force is perceived to be the most corrupt, and the judiciary is ranked third (Ghana Web, 9 July 2013). The Global Corruption Barometer also found that almost half (47%) of citizens surveyed across Africa believed police services were the most corrupt officials in their countries (Pring & Vrushi, 2019).

Negative attitudes towards the Ghanaian justice system are corroborated by citizens' engagement in 'Instant Justice'. In 2014, three young women were asked by the security personnel stationed at a local shopping mall to crawl to the main entrance of the mall on suspicion of shoplifting underwear (citifmonline.com, 25 February 2014). Similarly, three people were arrested by police officers in Tamale, the capital city of the Northern Region of Ghana, for their alleged involvement in the destruction of property at a local radio station (Radio Justice) that left four cars and motorbikes burnt beyond repair (adomonline.com, 11 March 2014). In May 2017, an officer of the Ghana Armed Forces, Maxwell Adam Mahama, was lynched when he was deployed to help curb illegal mining activities in Denkyira Obuasi in the Central Region of Ghana. There are several possible reasons for the public's involvement in instant justice despite governmental and non-governmental agencies' insistence that citizens resist such acts. First, the justice system has not met the citizens' needs. Second, there are problems in the justice system that need to be resolved. Lastly, citizens may prefer alternative avenues for justice. Understanding the public's perceptions, attitudes and utilisation of the police and courts in Ghana is important. First, public perceptions generate legitimacy and confidence in the justice system. When the public trusts the justice system, the legitimacy of legal institutions and personnel are not undermined. Second, most crimes enter the justice system through citizens' reports. If the public does not trust the justice system, individuals will be less likely to report crimes. Third, prosecution is only successful as long as citizens are willing to act as jurors or witnesses, comply with the legal institutions' decisions and participate in cases. Understanding citizens' perceptions will also allow policymakers to make informed decisions over reforms in the Ghanaian context. This research contributes to knowledge of the determinants of attitudes towards the justice system by highlighting the qualitative nature of citizens' perceptions, attitudes and utilisation of the justice system.

The Study

The findings reported in this chapter come from a qualitative study of citizens who have used the police and courts in Taifa, a peri-urban suburb of Accra, the capital of Ghana. The observations discussed earlier motivated this research. Critical speculations, the challenges of accessing justice and the dearth of qualitative studies on this topic justified the need for this study. The aims were to explore citizens' perceptions and confidence in the police and courts based on their experiences and to identify the determinants of their attitudes and future utilisation of the justice system. The study was exploratory in nature and involved analysing face-to-face interviews with citizens who had voluntarily sent their cases to the police or the court. There are other important aspects of the justice system, but the police and the courts are the most visible components. The majority of citizens have contact with these institutions, and they are structured to instil trust in the populace to fulfil their mission. As most justice interactions occur at the police or court level, investigating this level could yield more practical strategies for improving citizens' perceptions. Understanding the public's encounters with the justice system looms large for shaping policies and practices to reduce negative perceptions and increase public support.

Methodology: Sampling and Recruitment

The sampling for this study was purposive. Individuals were recruited based on whether they had used the police or court. They were identified for an interview through visits to households, the police station and the courthouse. At the police station and courthouse, visitors' contact numbers were collected, and the researcher visited their homes to conduct the interviews. The interviews were not conducted at the police station or courthouse because the researcher wanted to have sufficient time to explore the topic and did not want officials to influence the participants' responses. Other participants were recruited through participants, friends or relatives who had used the police or court. Thus, the snowball sampling technique was also used to identify possible participants. Snowball sampling is a sampling technique in which initial participants identify other participants who are eligible for the study (Yin, 2011). The sample size for the study was not defined at the start of data collection. Instead, data saturation was used to determine when sufficient data had been gathered (Yin, 2011). To ensure data saturation, the researcher engaged in a preliminary analysis during the data collection period. The overall criteria for sample consideration included citizens who were 18 years or older, had used the police or courts within the past five years and indicated a willingness to participate in an interview. The age limit was to ensure that participants were old enough to make reasonable, informed decisions regarding justice and discuss their views based on their experiences. The limit was also chosen because in Ghana, the 1992 constitution recognises persons who are 18 years and above as adults. The focus on justice system users was based on the participants' ability to offer first-hand information on the workings of the police and the courts. The researcher interviewed 17 participants who had experience with the police and/or the courts. Among them, 5 were recruited by house visits, 2 were recruited by participants who had used the law, 3 were invited by relatives and friends, 3 were recruited at the police station and 4 were recruited at the courthouse.

Demographics

Out of the 17 participants, 2 were between 18 and 30 years old, 4 were between 31 and 40 years old, 6 were between 41 and 50 years old, 4 were between 51 and 60 years old and 1 was 61 years old. The sample included 13 males and 4 females. All of the participants had received formal education. Of the participants 4 had completed junior high school, 4 had completed secondary high school and 9 had completed tertiary education. Among the participants 4 were civil servants, 4 were public servants, 3 were private formal workers, 5 were private informal workers and the remaining participant was unemployed. In this sample 5 were unmarried, 10 were married, 1 was divorced and 1 was widowed.

Data Collection

The researcher conducted in-depth interviews and observations. Face-to-face interviews were used to solicit information from the participants. The researcher sought to give the participants enough time and scope to express their opinions. The format allowed the researcher to exhaust all possible categories of data necessary for the study. The interview was open and flexible, allowing prompts, probes and digressions from the core focus of the work (Yin, 2011). The interview schedule had a cover letter explaining the purpose and ethical issues involved in the study. The interviews were conducted in both English and Twi (the local language) and were later transcribed for analysis. They were audio-recorded so that the researcher could capture and analyse all relevant information.

In the field, the researcher paid close attention, watched and listened carefully. Field researchers believe that the core of social life is communicated through mundane, trivial and everyday minutia, and they strive to discover intriguing details through listening and watching (Creswell, 2007). The researcher made observations at the police station and during court to understand the process and procedures involved in the justice system. Particular attention was paid to the interactions between the participants, who were victims, suspects, police officers or court officials. Witnessing the different roles allowed the researcher to gain deeper insights into the research problem. Notes were taken through direct and indirect observations using the observational protocol by Creswell (2007, p. 135). The researcher strictly adhered to ethical considerations, including informed consent, voluntary participation, privacy and confidentiality, throughout the entire research process. Particular attention was given to the researcher–participant relationship while in the field. The participants' informed consent was sought before data were collected, and participation was voluntary. Participants were assured of confidentiality and anonymity.

Data Analysis

In line with Yin's (2011) analytical framework of qualitative studies, the interview data analysis moved through five stages: compiling, disassembling, reassembling, concluding and interpreting. The interview audio-recordings were transcribed, and the transcriptions and field notes were compiled, dissembled, reassembled, concluded and interpreted. The key themes emanating from the analysis formed the basis of the following findings.

Findings

To Use or Not to Use: Deciding to Go to the Police or Court

Before analysing people's perceptions of the police and the courts in the Ghanaian context and the problems they may encounter, it seems fitting to chart how cases enter the formal justice system. Cases do not automatically come to the attention of the police and the courts in Ghana. When confronted with a justiciable problem, people typically define or interpret the problem as private/minor or public/severe before a concrete decision is made. When a problem is conceptualised as private, especially between close relatives, informal mechanisms are utilised. As Black (1973) argued, the social relationships enveloping a crime or dispute to a large extent predict the utilisation of the law. Persons in intimate relationships may use extra-legal avenues for criminal violation or conflict resolution and turn to formal avenues when the former does not work. The sustained utilisation of informal avenues rests on their effectiveness to resolve problems. Informal mechanisms need to be not only available but also effective to prevent the mobilisation of the formal justice system. Even when a case is between people in an intimate social relationship, the formal justice system is invoked if the extra-legal avenues are unavailable or have failed to resolve the issue. When the participants conceptualised issues as trivial or minor, they either chose to forget about the problem or decided not to report the incident to the formal justice system.

Public or severe problems are sent to the police or the courts. The participants perceived public cases as those that are serious and could only be addressed by the government, such as robbery, fraud, rape, defilement or murder. However, even the entry of these incidents into the formal justice system is not automatic. For cases that have been interpreted as public, serious or severe, many participants said they had tried informal avenues, such as calling the family members of both parties to meet, summoning the other party to a chief's palace and calling on elders, pastors or mallams to resolve the problem. These strategies are crucial when the offender and the victim are closely related. When informal avenues have been exhausted or proved ineffective, citizens send the case to the formal justice system. These interpretations and decisions over resolution mechanisms are not reached in isolation. Individuals generally seek advice from significant others, such as relatives, friends and other close relations, on how to handle the problem. Many participants noted that they consulted different people before finally deciding to go to the police or court for redress. This finding reflects the importance of context in attitudes towards the justice system; in a country in transition, formal and informal mechanisms of seeking justice coincide. Ghanaians are still socialised to contact relevant social actors such as chiefs, community elders, pastors and relatives to resolve misunderstandings. The meanings conferred on the offense or dispute determine the response to the problem. A crime or dispute may not matter in and of itself; it may be the context that matters. The context frames and determines the meanings and reactions to an incident. When a crime or dispute is conceptualised as meriting a formal solution, individuals invoke the formal justice system. For people to use the formal justice system, they must first label the case as one that merits formal attention. The invocation of formal or informal justice avenues rests on social reactions, situations and formations.

Experiences and Perceptions of the Police and Courts in Ghana

It is not uncommon to hear Ghanaians express negative sentiments towards the police and the courts. Some of these feelings emanate from vicarious experiences. The participants who voluntarily invoked the functions of the police and the court perceived their encounters negatively. Some participants recounted abuse of power by the police. They felt that the police do not respect citizens. The police's lack of respect reflected in their inappropriate use of harsh language, intimidation and condescension. A 52-year-old female business woman explained:

> The police are very annoying. Because the police think they have the power to enforce the law, they abuse it. The police were very arrogant and disrespectful yet not effective at all. I don't know what was wrong with the policemen; they were arrogant and unconcerned, as if they were not paid for their work.

Citizens who had experience with the police held unfavourable perceptions, evaluated them negatively and doubted whether they served the interest of the public. With the courts, many participants noted unsatisfactory experiences because the outcome of the case did not meet their expectations. A 33-year-old male teacher said:

> My experience with the court wasn't good. I wouldn't say that I was satisfied with the court's decision because they didn't reach a conclusion I expected. I felt that the officials could have done better. I felt that the court

could have done better. I felt so disappointed because the money was gone, and I couldn't catch the man. Although I didn't know how the law really operates, what I felt was that the court could have gone a step further by confiscating his property or something, but they didn't. At the end of the day, my money was gone, and I couldn't get the man. I felt that I did not get any justice.

Based on their unsatisfactory encounters, many participants held negative views of the courts. This connection between sentiment and experience is in line with previous studies that have shown the importance of experiences in perceptions of the justice system (Benesh & Howell, 2001; Wenzel, Bowler, & Lanoue, 2003). With reduced trust in the police and the courts, many participants expressed an unwillingness to use the formal justice system in the future. However, some expected to invoke the law in the future.

Experience, Knowledge and Future Utilisation

Previous studies (Benesh, 2006; Gibson et al., 1998) have found that when people use the justice system, they acquire knowledge of the institution and then express confidence in it. Many citizens who have invoked the police and courts in Ghana have acquired knowledge of how the justice system works despite their negative experiences. All of the participants alluded to having acquired experiential knowledge of the justice system, but their knowledge acquisition shaped how they expected to use the system in the future. For one group of participants, knowing how the justice system worked demotivated them from future usage. Their experiences eroded the positive stereotypes that they had held prior to their utilisation due to the deficiencies uncovered during their experiences. They were less confident in the justice system as a resolution mechanism, and they expressed an unwillingness to use the formal justice system in the future.

Other participants' experiential knowledge of the processes and procedures of the police and the courts served as a positive catalyst for future utilisation. Their contact with the justice system made them feel more familiar. These participants had come to know and understand how the justice system works and felt prepared to use it to resolve future problems. Some participants said that citizens they now understand the rules of the game and are willing to play it again. These participants claimed to have a better grasp of the process, procedures and information they need. They have learnt the importance of evidence through personal encounters with the formal justice system, and they now know what they could have done to make their case stronger. Although the knowledge they acquired in the process created awareness and made them confident in using the law in the future, there were other factors beyond knowledge. Mediating factors, such as socialisation, inner convictions and personal worldview, also affected future pursuance. Thus, while knowledge may influence people's willingness towards future utilisation, the decision to go to the justice system may also be influenced by the social context.

What Accounts for Citizens' Perceptions?

Several factors shaped the participants' perceptions of the justice system in Ghana, including the high cost involved in seeking resolution, the length of time needed, unexpected outcomes, ambiguity and the rigidity of court processes and procedures.

Cost

One critical question in the literature on law and society has been 'who bears the cost?', and this question influences the public's assessment of legal institutions. The issue of cost is critical, as it can serve as a potential barrier to the utilisation of the justice system. To meet ordinary citizens' needs, the justice system must be affordable enough to enable everybody, irrespective of income, to have access. For citizens who invoke formal mechanisms, justice can prove too expensive. As the police and courts have limited resources with which to operate, victims bear most of the costs involved. Some participants reported using money to support the police's efforts at an arrest. Some participants provided their own vehicles for the police to make an arrest. Another cost associated with the utilisation of the justice system is that of legal representation. For ordinary citizens, the fees charged by lawyers are very expensive. At the police station, the researcher observed a police officer in conversation with a citizen who had reported her case. He said: 'Ah, so, you don't have money, and you said you want to litigate. Or you think we are joking here?' Seeking justice requires monetary investment in the justice system, and this investment is beyond the reach of ordinary citizens.

Bribery and Corruption

State control agencies are responsible for ensuring order. Legal institutions must be credible, competent and efficient. Bribery and corruption undermine the legitimacy and effective performance of the justice system. The participants explained that these issues were a significant and costly problem. Many of the participants had to bribe the police to perform their duties. Some participants attributed their unfavourable outcomes to their inability or unwillingness to 'grease the palms' of the police and judges. Although the participants reported paying bribes, the officials did not always ask for them. Instead, the participants interpreted the officials' slowness and seeming inattention to their cases as a signal that 'something should be done' or that 'they need to be motivated' to do their work.

It is possible that reported delays were genuine rather than a ruse to elicit money from the participants. The researcher's interactions with the chief inspector of police in Taifa revealed that there were practical challenges, including infrastructure and human resources, as in the courts. During observations at the courthouse, the researcher saw that the courts were overloaded with cases, and many were handled or adjourned quickly throughout the day. The inadequate infrastructure and limited human resources of the justice system undermine the effectiveness of the functioning of the judiciary. Moreover, citizens may not always understand bureaucratic processes and procedures. They may misinterpret delays as a request for a bribe. By accepting money from citizens under such circumstances, police officers create or reinforce perceptions that access to the formal justice system is costly.

Time

The participants discussed the length of time it took for a case to be resolved as constituting another issue with the formal justice system. Their sentiments aligned with the adage 'justice delayed is justice denied'. Many participants went to the police and the courts expecting a swift response. Contrary to their expectations, they encountered a long process. They found the length of time required to be unreasonable and frustrating. The wheels of justice were moving too slowly (Benesh & Howell, 2001, p. 202), and it generated much anger in the participants and dissipated their interest in pursuing their cases. Some stopped going to the police or courts. Others tried to gain an 'upper hand' in navigating the system, using various strategies to expedite their cases. They sought the intervention of either the personnel in the police or courthouse or an influential person in their social networks to advance their cases. Their influential networks included politicians, police authorities and judges. Other participants turned to religious interventions, including consulting pastors and mallams, praying and fasting.

Expected Outcomes

People send their cases to the formal justice system with some expectations. Whether the outcomes meet their expectations is critical to people's overall assessment of the justice system. Although issues such as fairness and courteous treatment were important to the participants' evaluation of the formal justice system, the most profound dissatisfaction stemmed from case outcomes that did not meet their expectations. Some participants felt stuck, as their cases did not progress, leading them to abandon them. Many participants who had completed a police or court case had sought justice for retribution. They had expected the police or the courts to help them reclaim what they had lost, which did not happen. Moreover, implementing the police or court decisions became impractical, and the participants were unable to do anything about the outcomes. They felt disappointed and helpless, as the outcomes made no sense to them, which left them with a negative perception of the entire justice system.

Effects of Social Relationships on Assessments of the Justice System

The prior social relationships between the victim and offender also shaped the participants' assessments of the justice system. The closeness of the relationship shaped how participants interpreted legal decisions. Sometimes the participants felt that the type of justice delivered by the formal system was inappropriate because of the intimate nature of the relationships between parties. The imprisonment of the perpetrator in particular yielded dissatisfaction, as it hampered or destroyed prior social connections. In these instances, reconciliation appeared to be the best remedy. Some participants reported experiencing a breakdown in the relationship with the perpetrator's family. In other cases, the perpetrator's imprisonment left victims afraid of retaliation from the perpetrator's family members. This result was even more dissatisfying if the victims did not regain what they had lost, and the perpetrator was imprisoned. The imprisonment of the perpetrator was not beneficial to the participants. In the end, many participants who sought redress from the formal justice institution felt they had lost the time used in pursuing the case, the resources invested in the process and their social relationships.

Rigidity of Processes and Procedures

The participants' involvement in the case and the flexibility of the process were important in determining their evaluations of the police and the courts. For some citizens, the problem with the justice system was the rigidity of the processes and procedures. Many participants were unfamiliar with police and court processes and found them complicated. They felt that they were not allowed to express their opinions when they wanted to. In the court process, participants had to wait until their turn for cross-examination. In one of the court sessions I witnessed, a defendant raised his hand, asking the judge why they had not asked him to tell his side of the story. The defendant looked disappointed when the judge told him that he would be asked after all of the witnesses for the complainant were cross-examined. My interview with this participant revealed that he was expecting the judge to allow him to respond instantly to the issues his opponent raised. He said that he had been to court for the fourth time and still had not had the opportunity to tell his side of the story, which was unfair. The rigid procedures and processes also left the participants feeling excluded. The feeling of non-involvement was more pronounced in criminal cases between the state and the suspect.

Many of the participants who had gone to the police or to court with criminal cases were disappointed when they realised their cases were between the state and the suspect. The victims had hoped to actively engage in the process. They felt that their role in the process did not matter. These people felt not only dissatisfied but also disconnected. The participants misunderstood the processes and the outcomes and could not identify with the formal justice system. The dissatisfaction with criminal cases in particular was compounded by the realisation that the victims would not be paid. Some participants were not happy with the courts' verdicts, and they felt that the entire process was a waste of time and money.

Who Gets Justice?

At the core of the participants' narratives of their experiences and assessments of the formal justice system is the issue of who gets justice. Many of the participants felt that the formal justice system works for particular groups of people. Many contended that the system favours only the 'big men' in the country. They doubted whether the police and the courts served the interests of ordinary citizens. This assertion supports Genn's (1999) observation that most people think that the justice system works better for the rich than for the poor. The inability of the participants in this study to obtain satisfactory results may have been due to their low socio-economic backgrounds, which could have prevented them from engaging the services of qualified, motivated attorneys. Most of the participants interpreted their frustrations in accessing justice as stemming from their low status, as little progress had been made by contacting the influential people in their lives. They felt that their influential networks were important, as they shaped the process and outcomes of their cases. The participants from low socio-economic backgrounds did not experience the police or courts in terms of access and progression; they depended on a network of relations. A person with a low socio-economic status with an influential network may experience the formal justice system more positively than one with no influence in the Ghanaian setting. We cannot lump together all citizens with low socio-economic status and claim that they will have negative experiences with the formal justice system. Future studies should explore the extent to which networks of relations moderate or mediate the relationship between socio-economic status and experience with the justice system.

Conclusion

The aim of this chapter was to document the perceptions, attitudes and experiences of people who have encountered the police and the courts in Taifa, a peri-urban in Accra, Ghana. This chapter highlighted the major themes from the narratives of citizens who have sent their cases to the police or courts for redress. Citizens use the police and courts in complex, multidimensional ways, and their experiences shape their interpretations of the problems with the justice system. The participants' contact with the formal justice system was overwhelmingly negative. The participants recounted unsatisfactory experiences and had hard feelings about the fairness of the justice system. Several factors accounted for their unfavourable outlook. Their dissatisfaction stemmed from the high cost of justice, the slow pace of the system, unexpected or unimplemented outcomes, rigid processes and procedures, and their own limited involvement in the system. Unfavourable police or court outcomes that did not meet the participants' expectations were the greatest source of frustration among participants. Concern over the outcome of a case needs to be understood in context. Ghana is a country in transition and as in many other postcolonial states, traditionalism and modernity are at play in daily interactions (Nukunya, 2003). Most Ghanaians have been socialised to believe that traditional informal justice systems are restitutive in nature. Most of the participants went to the formal justice system thinking that they would regain what they had lost, but they did not.

The participants' perceptions, attitudes and utilisation of the formal justice system depended on the individuals' contexts and interpretations. Other factors, such as one's history, socialisation or worldview and governmental structures, also played a role. In a country where many institutions operate with scarce resources, the delivery of justice is inefficient and evokes negative perceptions. Many citizens prefer extra-legal mechanisms. The preference for informal mechanisms finds expression in its availability and effectiveness. The use of informal systems is prevalent, as it is not only logical but also necessary for people to use informal avenues to address justiciable problems that are not resolved by the formal justice system. The practical and symbolic significance of social relations joins residents together for economic, religious and political reasons. Disregard for these pertinent issues in the formal justice system renders it ineffective in the eyes of many citizens. Interventions in the justice system should incorporate the realities of people's local conditions. Such efforts should be guided by people's specific needs and preferences in terms of having their justice needs met in their communities. In the absence of this level of specificity, efforts at treating crime or resolving disputes will probably fail to improve access to justice. A justice system that meets citizens' needs requires policies and reforms that are all-inclusive and creative. It must take into consideration locals' needs, preferences, experiences and conditions.

Limitations of the Study

This study was limited due to the role of memory in potentially altering participants' accounts of their experiences. The researcher asked the participants to recall experiences as far back as five years ago. This method raises questions about recall accuracy and the reconstruction of experiences. Future studies that rely on more recent experiences, such as within the last 6–12 months, might help address this limitation. The study focused on citizens' perceptions and experiences of their interactions with the police and courts. The researcher did not interview the police or court officials involved in interactions. Thus, this chapter presents a one-sided account. Studies that capture police officers' and citizens' views about the same interaction can advance our understanding of both parties. Even when both viewpoints are captured, there is still the possibility of inaccuracy arising from exaggeration or memory failure. To overcome this challenge, some researchers have used independent observers or data from police body cameras (Nawaz & Tankebe, 2018; Worden & McLean, 2017). The Ghana police have recently obtained body cameras (Daily Graphic Online, 2019), creating the possibility for similar analysis in Ghana. Notwithstanding these limitations, this study has filled an academic lacuna and extended prior research by offering insights into several previously ignored elements of Ghana's justice system.

References

Appiah, K. (2013). *Report on access to justice: Scoping study of the justice.* Formal and Informal Sector in Ghana: Ministry of Foreign Affairs.

Benesh, S. C. (2006). Understanding public confidence in American courts. *Journal of Politics, 68,* 697–707. https://doi.org/10.1111/j.1468-2508.2006.00455.x

Benesh, C., & Howell, S. E. (2001). Confidence in the courts: A comparison of users and non-users. *Behavioral Sciences & the Law, 19,* 199–214. https://doi.org/10.1002/bsl.437

Black, D. J. (1973). The mobilization of law. *Journal of Legal Studies, 2*(1), 125–149. Retrieved from https://www.jstor.org/stable/724029?seq=1

Boateng, F. D. (2012). Public trust in the police: Identifying factors that shape trust in the Ghanaian police. (Doctoral dissertation, Washington State University).

Brody, R., & Sniderman, P. (1977). From life space to polling place: The relevance of personal concerns for voting behaviour. *British Journal of Political Science, 7,* 337–360. https://doi.org/10.1017/s0007123400001022

Brown, B., & Benedict, W. R. (2002). Perceptions of the police: Past findings, methodological issues, conceptual issues and policy implications. *Policing: An International Journal of Police Strategies and Management, 25*(3), 543–580. https://doi.org/10.1108/13639510210437032

Cao, L., & Zhao, S. J. (2005). Confidence in the police in Latin America. *Journal of Criminal Justice, 33*(5), 403–412. https://doi.org/10.1016/j.jcrimjus.2005.06.009

Cheurprakobkit, S. (2000). Police-citizen contact and police performance: Attitudinal differences between Hispanics and non-Hispanics. *Journal of Criminal Justice, 28*(4), 325–336. https://doi.org/10.1016/s0047-2352(00)00042-8

Creswell, J. W. (2007). *Qualitative inquiry and research design: Choosing among five approaches* (2nd ed.). Sage.

Dean, D. (1980). Citizen ratings of the police: The difference contact makes. *Law and Policy Quarterly, 2,* 445–471. https://doi.org/10.1111/j.1467-9930.1980.tb00225.x

Decker, S. H. (1981). Citizen attitudes toward the police: A review of past findings and suggestions for future policy. *Journal of Police Science and Administration, 9,* 80–87. Retrieved from https://www.ncjrs.gov/App/Publications/abstract.aspx?ID=77072

Genn, H. (1999). *Paths to justice: What people do and think about going to law.* Hart Publishing.

Ghana Judiciary. (2013). *Historical development of the courts after independence.* The Judicial Service of Ghana. Retrieved April 4, 2014, from http://www.judicial.gov.gh/index.php/history/after-independence

Ghana Web. (2013). *Police service most corrupt institution in Ghana.* GhanaWeb. Retrieved June 27, 2012, from http://www.ghanaweb.com/GhanaHomePage/NewsArchive/artikel.php?ID=279056

Gibson, J., Gregory, L., Caldeira, A., & Baird, V.A. (1998). On the llegitimacy of national high courts. *American Political Science Review, 92*(2), 343–358.

Graphic Online. (2019). *Ghana Police take delivery of 250 body cameras.* Graphic. Retrieved September 4, 2020, from https://www.graphic.com.gh/news/general-news/ghana-news-police-take-delivery-of-250-body-cameras.html#:~:text=The%20Ghana%20Police%20Service%20has,enhance%20police%20transparency%20and%20accountability

Jacob, H. (1971). Black and white perceptions of justice in the city. *Law and Society Review, 5,* 69–89. https://doi.org/10.2307/3052913

Jesilow, P., & Meyer, J. A. (2001). The effect of police misconduct on public attitudes: A quasi-experiment. *Journal of Crime and Justice, 24*, 109–121. https://doi.org/10.1080/0735648x.2001.9721619

Jesilow, P., Meyer, J., & Namazzi, N. (1995). Public attitudes towards police. *American Journal of Police, 14*(2), 67–88. https://doi.org/10.1108/07358549510102767

Lau, R., Brown, T., & Sears, D. (1978). Self-interest and civilians attitudes towards the Vietnam War. *Public Opinion Quarterly, 42*, 464–483. https://doi.org/10.1086/268474

Moy, P., Pfau, M., & Kahlor, L. (1999). Media uses and public confidence in democratic institutions. *Journal of Broadcasting and Electronic Media, 43*(2), 137–158. https://doi.org/10.1080/08838159909364481

Nawaz, A., & Tankebe, J. (2018). Tracking procedural justice in stop and search encounters: Coding evidence from body-worn video cameras. *Cambridge Journal of Evidence-based Policing, 2*(3–4), 139–163. https://doi.org/10.1007/s41887-018-0029-z

Nukunya, G. K. (2003). *Tradition and change in Ghana: An introduction to sociology*. Ghana Universities Press.

Orr, M., & West, D. M. (2007). Citizens' evaluations of local police: Personal experience or symbolic attitudes. *Administration and Society, 8*(6), 649–668. https://doi.org/10.1177/0095399706293989

Pring, C., & Vrushi, J. (2019). Global Corruption Barometer: Africa 2019. *Transparency International*.

Reisig, M. D., & Correia, M. E. (1997). Public evaluations of police performance: An analysis across three levels of policing. *Policing: An International Journal of Police Strategies and Management, 20*, 311–325. https://doi.org/10.1108/13639519710169153

Reisig, M. D., & Parks, R. B. (2000). Experience, quality of life and neighbourhood context: A hierarchical analysis of satisfaction with police. *Police Quarterly, 17*(3), 607–629. https://doi.org/10.1080/07418820000094681

Ren, L., Cao, L., Lovrich, N., & Gaffney, M. (2005). Linking confidence in the police with the performance of the police: Community policing can make a difference. *Journal of Criminal Justice, 33*(1), 55–66. https://doi.org/10.1016/j.jcrimjus.2004.10.003

Schafer, J. A., Hueber, B. M., & Bynum, T. S. (2003). Citizen perception of police service: Race, neighbourhood context and community policing. *Police Quarterly, 6*, 440–468. https://doi.org/10.1177/1098611102250459

Skogan, W. G. (2009). Concern about crime and confidence in the police: Reassurance or accountability? *Police Quarterly, 12*(3), 301–311. https://doi. org/10.1177/1098611109339893

Smith, D. A., Graham, N., & Adams, B. (1991). Minorities and the police: Attitudinal and behavioral questions. In *Race and criminal justice* (pp. 22–35). Albany, NY: Harrow and Heston Publishers.

Smith, S. T. (2008). *Judicial reform and its impact on the administration of justice: A monograph.* Published by The Judicial Service of Ghana in collaboration with CUSO and the National Judicial Institute.

Sun, I. Y., & Wu, Y. (2006). Citizens perceptions of the courts: The impact of race, gender, and recent experience. *Journal of Criminal Justice, 34*, 457–467. https://doi.org/10.1016/j.jcrimjus.2006.09.001

Tankebe, J. (2008a). Colonialism, legitimation, and policing in Ghana. *International Journal of Law, Crime and Justice, 36*(1), 67–84.

Tankebe, J. (2008b). Police effectiveness and police trustworthiness in Ghana: An empirical appraisal. *Criminology & Criminal Justice, 8*, 185–202. https:// doi.org/10.1177/1748895808088994.

Tankebe, J. (2010). Public confidence in the police: Testing the effects of public experiences of police corruption in Ghana. *The British Journal of Criminology, 50*(2), 296–319. https://doi.org/10.1093/bjc/azq001

Tankebe, J. (2013). In search of moral recognition? Policing and eudaemonic legitimacy in Ghana. *Law and Social Inquiry, 38*(3), 576–597. https://doi. org/10.1111/lsi.12025

Twum, H. (2011). *Indispensable police.* Media Fanbern: Ofankor-Accra.

Tyler, T. R. (1990). *Why people obey the law.* Yale University Press.

Tyler, T. R. (2001). Public trust and confidence in legal authorities: What do majority and minority members want from the law and legal institutions? *Behavioral Sciences & the Law, 19*(2), 215–235. https://doi.org/10.1002/bsl.438

Weitzer, R., & Tuch, S. A. (1999). Race, class and perceptions of discrimination by the police. *Crime and Delinquency, 45*(4), 494–507. https://doi. org/10.1177/0011128799045004006

Weitzer, R., & Tuch, S. A. (2005). Determinants of public satisfaction with the police. *Police Quarterly, 8*(3), 279–297. https://doi. org/10.1177/1098611104271106

Wenzel, J. P., Bowler, S., & Lanoue, D. J. (2003). The sources of public confidence in the state courts: Experience and institutions. *American Political Research, 3*(2), 191–211. https://doi.org/10.1177/1532673X02250295

Wilson, C. (2012). *The public and the justice system: Attitudes, drivers and behaviour a literature review.* Scottish Government Social Research.

Winfree, T., & Griffiths, C. (1971). Adolescent attitudes toward the police. In T. Ferdinand (ed.), *Juvenile delinquency: Little brother grows up.* Beverly Hills, CA: Sage.

Worden, R. E., & McLean, S. J. (2017). *Mirage of police reform: Procedural justice and police legitimacy.* University of California Press.

Yin, R. K. (2011). *Qualitative research from start to finish.* The Guilford Press.

17

Conclusion

Samuel Adjorlolo and Heng Choon (Oliver) Chan

The Emergence of an African Criminology

There is now a burgeoning literature from the African continent exploring crime, mental health and criminal justice. This is a promising development, albeit a belated one given the longstanding observation that crime and criminal activities are high on the African continent owing to such factors as poverty, the gradual breakdown of the extended family system and of social cohesion, and limited opportunities for the attainment of fundamental human needs, including such basic physiological

S. Adjorlolo (✉)
Department of Mental Health Nursing, School of Nursing and Midwifery, University of Ghana, Accra, Ghana
e-mail: sadjorlolo@ug.edu.gh

H. C. O. Chan
Teaching Laboratory for Forensics and Criminology, Department of Social and Behavioural Sciences, City University of Hong Kong,
Hong Kong, Special Administrative Region of China
e-mail: ohcchan@hku.hk

© The Author(s), under exclusive license to Springer Nature Switzerland AG 2021   **397**
H. C. O. Chan, S. Adjorlolo (eds.), *Crime, Mental Health and the Criminal Justice System in Africa*, https://doi.org/10.1007/978-3-030-71024-8_17

needs as food. Likewise, studies have shown that the burden of mental health problems is very large in Africa and in other low- and middle-income countries due to a preponderance of risk factors and limited resources and facilities to improve mental health among the population (Whiteford et al., 2013). The chapters in this book were written by African-based researchers and practitioners to provide a timely overview of crime, mental health and criminal justice in Africa. Importantly, the chapters in this book will help set the stage for future discourse on topical issues on crime and mental health in Africa.

Crime and Deviance in Africa

One of the major developmental challenges confronting countries in Africa is crime control and prevention (Tankebe, 2009). Given the social and economic consequences of criminal activities, such as endangering public safety and security and reducing investor confidence in the economy, governments in Africa have instituted several measures to address these phenomena, including retooling law enforcement agencies, thereby contributing to high rates of arrest and prosecution. Notwithstanding the short-term impact of these measures, the general observation that crime is still on the increase on the continent largely supports the view that arrest and imprisonment do not necessarily lead to reduction in crime. Instead, understanding the dynamics and mechanisms of offending, including the risk and protective factors and the modus operandi, is key to designing sensitive and tailored intervention programmes. Given the foregoing, empirically informed discourses centred on the emergence and sustenance of, and desistance from, criminal activities are a significant prospect for countries in Africa.

Consequently, the common themes across some of the chapters in this book relate to why crime and deviant behaviour occurs in Africa and the strategies to prevent and control crime. For instance, Aborisade (Chap. 2) and Andoh-Arthur and Quarshie (Chap. 8) adopt multidisciplinary approaches rooted in history, culture, criminology, mental health and other factors to explain the increasing rates of suicide in Nigeria and the antecedents of suicide laws in Ghana. Van Graan (Chap. 3) similarly provides insights into the factors contributing to the reported increase of violent crime in South Africa through a novel exploration of criminological theories and the narratives of violent offenders. The work of Eseadi and colleagues (Chap. 4) on contemporary online dating scams in Nigeria also picks up these themes. Central to the discussion are the modus operandi of the scammers, the factors underpinning the menace and the mental health challenges reported by victims of online dating scams. The chapter offers Afrocentric measures to curb online dating scams, including regulating access to and use of the internet. Oludare and colleagues (Chap. 5) analyse kidnapping, a troubling crime in Nigeria, using existing criminological theoretical frameworks pertaining to rational choice and strain.

Notwithstanding these important contributions, more studies exploring the risk and protective factors of crime/deviant behaviour, and measures to prevent the same, are warranted. Is criminal behaviour produced by psychosocial factors, biological factors or both? These intriguing questions have directed scholarly endeavours for a very long time, but discussions on the aetiology of criminal and deviant behaviour in Africa continue to centre on disordered social processes and institutions. The resurgence of the biosocial criminology movement has brought significant changes to and also broadened the understanding of criminal behaviour, not only from social or psychological perspectives, but also from a biological perspective. Biosocial researchers proceed on the assumption that there are biological predispositions to criminal behaviour and juvenile delinquency or offending (Beaver, 2008, 2011; Beaver et al., 2009; Beaver, DeLisi, Vaughn, & Wright, 2010; Boutwell et al., 2014; Connolly & Beaver, 2014). The interest is to unearth the biological underpinnings of criminogenesis, either independently or in collaboration with professionals from other disciplines with similar interests. The focus is to understand the vulnerability and predisposition to criminal behaviour from biological as well as social perspectives. The emerging trend, and almost ubiquitous conclusion, is that juvenile delinquency and antisocial behaviour can be explained by a wide array of factors ingrained in biological and social processes (Connolly & Beaver, 2014; Eme, 2009; Fabian, 2010; Nordstrom et al., 2011). Thus, the developmental trajectories of juvenile antisocial behaviour are inherent in the interaction between or the cumulative effects of two or more biological and/or social risk factors.

With this in mind, it is highly recommended that future studies examine the role of biological and social processes in criminality and deviant behaviour in Africa. This will help to situate the African literature on crime and deviance within the international literature to allow for cross-cultural discussions, while providing empirical evidence to inform crime control, prevention and management.

Crime and Mental Health in Africa

While the nexus between mental health and criminal tendencies has been discussed extensively, attention has recently shifted to the overrepresentation of persons with mental illness in the criminal justice system (Fazel & Seewald, 2012). In South Africa, 23% of 193 (Naidoo & Mkize, 2012) and 44% of 236 (Prinsloo, 2013) prisoners had been diagnosed with psychotic disorders. In Zambia, 63% of 206 inmates were found to have a severe mental illness (Nseluke & Siziya, 2011), and in Ghana, nearly 70% of 100 inmates met the criteria for moderate and severe depression (Ibrahim, Esena, Aikins, O'Keefe, & McKay, 2015). These individuals are mostly poorly represented in court by unmotivated attorneys and as a result are processed via the criminal justice system without consideration of their mental states (Adjorlolo, 2016). Once incarcerated, prison conditions further worsen their mental health status, including those without overt signs of mental disorders. These conditions include unhygienic environments, inadequate sleeping provisions, poor ventilation, poor food quality, poor recreational activities and an increase in victimisation and abuse partly due to overcrowded prisons (Adjorlolo, 2016).

Without addressing their mental health needs, these individuals are prone to harming themselves, other inmates and the general public after release from custody. An increase in reoffending will translate into higher criminal justice costs, thereby depriving the state of some of its limited resources for developing other sectors of the economy. Consequently, culturally appropriate and sustainable interventions to respond to the mental health needs of individuals in the criminal justice system in Africa are extremely important. Eseadi and Nwagbo (Chap. 10) provide highly interesting perspectives on this subject based on developments in Nigeria, where it is apparent that there are no innovative and culturally responsive interventions aimed at promoting the mental well-being of prisoners. Instead, the authors revealed several structural (e.g., lack of dedicated prison mental health services) and policy issues encumbering efforts to respond adequately to the mental health needs of the prisoner population in Nigeria. According to Swanepoel (Chap. 7), effective and feasible mental health legislation that advocates for and streamlines the organisation and delivery of mental health services to various categories of the population is one of the surest ways to meet the mental health needs of prisoners. Nevertheless, there is a clear need for additional studies on mental health and criminal justice in Africa.

Criminal Justice Systems in Africa

Just like jurisdictions in other regions, the structure and functional organisation of the criminal justice system, comprising the police, judiciary and prisons/correctional system, in African countries is extremely important for crime control, prevention and management. Indeed, as former colonies of high-income countries, including Britain and France, the criminal justice systems of most African countries have mirrored those of their former colonial masters (Adjorlolo, Abdul-Nasiru, Chan, & Bambi, 2018). Nonetheless, criminal justice systems across the continent have experienced changes that reflect contemporary African societies and their development. These changes, and the entire structure and operation of the criminal justice system in African countries, should be documented as a basis for further discussions on strengthening and supporting crime control and prevention.

In this regard, some of the chapters in this book discuss the operations of criminal justice practitioners in Africa, including the police and judiciary. Labuschagne (Chap. 6), for example, provides a rare and interesting insight into how serial murders are investigated by the police in South Africa. The discussion is carried out through case studies that enable readers to appreciate the context of each case and how the various investigations unfolded. Kwakye-Nuako (Chap. 9) report on police prosecutors' encounters and interactions with victims of child sexual abuse and their caregivers. Central points of the discussion relate to the inadequate training of police officers to handle child sexual abuse cases, and the perception of police officers as intimidating or friendly. On a related note, Adu-Poku (Chap. 16) reports that citizens' negative encounters with the police and court system in Ghana have largely contributed to a situation in which citizens appear to resolve criminal issues and disputes using informal means, such as invoking the jurisdiction of local chiefs. The police and court systems are regarded as the last resort, usually called upon only when the crime is perceived to be serious, as in the case of murder, or where the informal justice system has proven to be ineffective. The characteristics of prison populations have also received some attention. For example, Dastile (Chap. 14) expands the discourse on racial and ethnic representation in prisons. Consistent with the literature from high-income countries, such as the United States, Dastile shows that black female offenders are overrepresented in South African prisons, compared with their white counterparts. A similar observation is made for black male offenders, relative to white male offenders. Dastile argues for gender-sensitive prison systems to accommodate unique gender differences in offending patterns and responses to rehabilitation and corrections. There remains a need for more studies on the operations of criminal justice systems in Africa.

Crime, Mental Health and Criminal Justice Research Agenda

As noted previously, there is a dearth of literature on crime, mental health and criminal justice systems in Africa. The high burden of diseases and other structural issues have contributed to the limited attention paid to criminal justice by local researchers and international partners. This trend is changing, however. The collection of studies in this book is largely representative of the nature and focus of the literature on the aforementioned subject matter in Africa. The perspectives offered by some chapters also concur with trends in the literature from other regions. Prominent among these are violent crime, suicidal tendencies, stress among police officers, the commitment and satisfaction of corrections workers, drug use in prisons and representation of minority groups in prisons. Nevertheless, the chapters in this book situate the discussions within nuanced renderings of uniquely African cultures. The Afrocentric discussions and views will be of benefit to the research community by supporting comparative discussions across contexts and collaborative efforts dedicated to research and practice.

From these beginnings, it is imperative that conscious and systematic efforts are undertaken to establish a robust research agenda on crime, mental health and criminal justice systems in Africa. Research partnerships that draw on multidisciplinary approaches across different geographical contexts will provide a platform for illuminating differences and similarities in criminal justice systems across jurisdictions. This is important given that African countries are essentially homogenous with respect to the risk and protective factors of crime, and the organisation and delivery of criminal justice.

Our understanding of the intersection between crime, mental health and criminal justice systems in Africa is hampered severely by a lack of empirical studies. Among the topical issues deserving empirical attention include the practice and science of offender rehabilitation and treatment in correctional or prison systems; courts and criminal adjudication; the sociocultural and geopolitical underpinning of various crimes, such as gangs, terrorism and recidivism; the judicial decision-making process, including the role of jurors, assessors and eyewitness and expert testimony in justice delivery; risk assessment and criminal offending; the application of criminological theories to the crime situation in Africa; the architecture and functions of the criminal justice system; and transnational crimes, such as human trafficking and the drug trade, and approaches to crime prevention. Research from Africa has much to offer policymakers and practitioners on the continent and in the broader international community on crime prevention and management strategies. This collection of studies and commentaries on crime, mental health and criminal justice is pertinent to understanding the current areas of focus and thereby to inform future research plans and activities.

References

Adjorlolo, S. (2016). Diversion of individuals with mental illness in the criminal justice system in Ghana. *International Journal of Forensic Mental Health,* *15*(4), 382–392.

Adjorlolo, S., Abdul-Nasiru, I., Chan, H. C. O., & Bambi, L. E. (2018). Mental health professionals' attitudes toward offenders with mental illness (insanity acquittees) in Ghana. *International Journal of Offender Therapy and Comparative Criminology,* *62*(3), 629–654.

Beaver, K. M. (2008). Nonshared environmental influences on adolescent delinquent involvement and adult criminal behavior. *Criminology,* *46*(2), 341–369.

Beaver, K. M. (2011). Environmental moderators of genetic influences on adolescent delinquent involvement and victimization. *Journal of Adolescent Research,* *26*(1), 84–114.

Beaver, K. M., DeLisi, M., Vaughn, M. G., & Wright, J. P. (2010). The intersection of genes and neuropsychological deficits in the prediction of adolescent delinquency and low self-control. *International Journal of Offender Therapy and Comparative Criminology,* *54*(1), 22–42.

Beaver, K. M., Eagle Schutt, J., Boutwell, B. B., Ratchford, M., Roberts, K., & Barnes, J. C. (2009). Genetic and environmental influences on levels of self-control and delinquent peer affiliation: Results from a longitudinal sample of adolescent twins. *Criminal Justice and Behavior,* *36*(1), 41–60.

Boutwell, B. B., Menard, S., Barnes, J. C., Beaver, K. M., Armstrong, T. A., & Boisvert, D. (2014). The role of gene–gene interaction in the prediction of criminal behavior. *Comprehensive Psychiatry,* *55*(3), 483–488.

Connolly, E. J., & Beaver, K. M. (2014). Examining the genetic and environmental influences on self-control and delinquency: Results from a genetically informative analysis of sibling pairs. *Journal of Interpersonal Violence,* *29*(4), 707–735.

Eme, R. (2009). Male life-course persistent antisocial behavior: A review of neurodevelopmental factors. *Aggression and Violent Behavior,* *14*(5), 348–358.

Fabian, J. M. (2010). Neuropsychological and neurological correlates in violent and homicidal offenders: A legal and neuroscience perspective. *Aggression and Violent Behavior,* *15*(3), 209–223.

Fazel, S., & Seewald, K. (2012). Severe mental illness in 33 588 prisoners worldwide: Systematic review and meta-regression analysis. *The British Journal of Psychiatry,* *200*(5), 364–373.

Ibrahim, A., Esena, R. K., Aikins, M., O'Keefe, A. M., & McKay, M. M. (2015). Assessment of mental distress among prison inmates in Ghana's correctional system: A cross-sectional study using the Kessler Psychological Distress Scale. *International Journal of Mental Health Systems, 9*(1), 17.

Naidoo, S., & Mkize, D. (2012). Prevalence of mental disorders in a prison population in Durban, South Africa. *African Journal of Psychiatry, 15*(1), 30–35.

Nordstrom, B. R., Gao, Y., Glenn, A. L., Peskin, M., Rudo-Hutt, A. S., Schug, R. A., et al. (2011). Chapter 10—Neurocriminology. In D. L. B. Robert Huber & B. Patricia (Eds.), *Advances in genetics* (Vol. 75, pp. 255–283). Academic Press.

Nseluke, M. T., & Siziya, S. (2011). Prevalence and socio-demographic correlates for mental illness among inmates at lusaka central prison, Zambia. *Medical Journal of Zambia, 38*(2), 3–7.

Prinsloo, J. (2013). Offenders with mental disorders in a South African prison population: Profiling the behavioural characteristics on mental illness. *Journal of Psychology in Africa, 23*(1), 133–138.

Tankebe, J. (2009). Self-help, policing, and procedural justice: Ghanaian vigilantism and the rule of law. *Law & Society Review, 43*(2), 245–270.

Whiteford, H. A., Degenhardt, L., Rehm, J., Baxter, A. J., Ferrari, A. J., Erskine, H. E., et al. (2013). Global burden of disease attributable to mental and substance use disorders: Findings from the Global Burden of Disease Study 2010. *The Lancet, 382*(9904), 1575–1586.

Correction to: An Exploratory Study on Kidnapping as an Emerging Crime in Nigeria

Alaba M. Oludare, Ifeoma E. Okoye, and Lucy K. Tsado

Correction to:

Chapter 5 in: H. C. O. Chan, S. Adjorlolo (eds.),
Crime, Mental Health and the Criminal Justice System in Africa,
https://doi.org/10.1007/978-3-030-71024-8_5

The original chapter was inadvertently published with incorrect affiliation of one of the authors 'Ifeoma E. Okoye'. The affiliation has been corrected in the chapter as below:

I. E. Okoye
Department of Criminal Justice, West Virginia State University, Institute, WV, USA

Changed to:

I. E. Okoye
Department of Criminal Justice, Virginia State University, VA, USA

The updated version of this chapter can be found at
https://doi.org/10.1007/978-94-007-5869-8_5

Index[1]

---

[1] Note: Page numbers followed by 'n' refer to notes.